Mental Health Outcome Measures

First edition published by Springer Verlag (Berlin, Heidelberg), 1996

RCPsych Publications is an imprint of the Royal College of Psychiatrists,
17 Belgrave Square, London SW1X 8PG
http://www.rcpsych.ac.uk

British Library Cataloguing-in-Publication Data.
A catalogue record for this book is available from the British Library.
ISBN 978-1-904671-92-3

Distributed in North America by Publishers Storage and Shipping Company.

Printed by Bell & Bain Limited, Glasgow, UK.

Contents

Tables, boxes and figures

Tables

Boxes

Figures

Contributors

Thomas Becker Department of Psychiatry, University Medical Center Groningen, University of Groningen, The Netherlands

Rohan Borschmann clinical psychologist and research worker at the Institute of Psychiatry, King's College London, UK

Elaine Brohan Health Service and Population Research Department, Institute of Psychiatry, King's College London, UK

Traolach (Terry) S. Brugha Professor of Psychiatry, and Deputy Head, Department of Health Sciences, University of Leicester; Honorary Consultant Adult General Psychiatrist, Leicestershire Partnership NHS Trust, Leicester, UK

David J. Castle holds the Chair of Psychiatry at St Vincent's Hospital and The University of Melbourne, Australia.

Sarah Clement Health Service and Population Research Department, Institute of Psychiatry, King's College London, UK

Emese Csipke Research Associate at the Institute of Psychiatry, King's College London, UK

Farifteh F. Duffy Director of Quality of Care Research at the American Psychiatric Institute for Research and Education, Arlington, Virginia, USA.

Graham Dunn Professor of Biomedical Statistics, Health Methodology Research Group, School of Community Based Medicine, University of Manchester, UK

David Goldberg Professor Emeritus, Institute of Psychiatry, King's College, London, UK

Juan Luis González-Caballero Professor of Statistics and Operational Research, University of Cadiz, Spain.

Aleksandar Janca Winthrop Professor and Head of School of Psychiatry and Clinical Neurosciences, University of Western Australia, Perth, Australia.

Rachel Jenkins Director, WHO Collaborating Centre and Head, Section of Mental Health Policy, Institute of Psychiatry, King's College London, and Visiting Professor, London School of Hygiene, UK

Foreword

In my years as a junior doctor in a general medical ward, I was often impressed by the gap between what the patient had originally complained of and the leads followed by the medical team in pursuing an unexpected abnormality in a routine investigation, which in fact had little relevance to the patient's actual concerns. Later, while training in psychiatry, I was interested to observe how clinical psychiatry followed a similar pattern: procedures were carried out which made sense to the clinical team but had little relevance to the patient.

This new edition of Thornicroft and Tansella's review of outcome measures marks an important step in the development of mental health services, in that major emphasis is now given to aspects of outcome that are valued by the service users themselves. In Chapter 1, Kabir and Wykes review this important field, and point out that users are more interested in recovery and happiness than in remission of presenting symptoms. Even measures of 'satisfaction with services' that are not devised in collaboration with users come in for a critical examination.

However, another new area of interest, identified by the editors in the Introduction, is indeed the currently fashionable concept of 'recovery', which gets an extended treatment in Chapter 4. As a retired psychiatrist, I found the new enthusiasm for full recovery rather strange, as it appears to imply that such an aim is something new and (worse still) always achievable. However, it emerges from Chapter 4 that there are in fact a range of meanings ascribed to the concept of 'recovery', ranging from the fairly modest aim of living as well as possible to the more utopian one of having a fulfilling, meaningful life and a positive sense of identity founded on hopefulness and self-determination.

Failure to achieve 'full recovery' may not be due either to incompetence on the part of the clinician or to lack of motivation on the part of the patient; it is often due to the severity of the underlying disorder. It seems to me important that, rather than inwardly apologising to themselves for incomplete recovery, clinicians should adapt their energies to enabling users to achieve more personal autonomy. But for the most disabled patients with long-term severe mental disorders, enabling them to make personal choices about what they eat and giving them a more active involvement in the choices they can make in their personal lives are worthy objectives. An example of this is given in Fig. 4.1 (p. 71), where a user sets her own goals for an improvement in her autonomy.

This new edition is indispensable to researchers in health services research, as it is strikingly comprehensive, with every aspect of outcome covered, and includes all the most recent developments in the field. New measures are constantly being developed, and old measures are often re-evaluated, so that even those chapters that are similar to those in previous editions have new and important information. An example of this appears in Chapter 2, on statistical methods for measuring outcomes. Novices to the field are stepping over a statistical minefield when they rely on single, small evaluations – Dunn emphasises the importance of multicentre trials in order to achieve adequate power.

The book does what needs to be done – it brings the whole field up to date, and in doing so expands our horizons.

David Goldberg
Professor Emeritus
Institute of Psychiatry, King's College London

Foreword

Many different themes dominate the current literature on mental health services. Services should facilitate meaningful outcomes. The mission should be recovery. Interventions should be evidence based. Care should be client centred or self-directed. The mental health system should diminish stigma and foster social inclusion. Information technology should enhance efficiency. And many more! Each of these represents an endangered species. Why endangered? Simply put, philosophical movements easily become transient fads when they are not grounded in measures, numbers and data. Ideas, goals, guidelines, missions, benchmarks and plans require measurement to attain any hope of enduring reality. If nothing is measured, nothing changes. Instead, the next year brings a new commitment to yet another banner idea.

Mental health has long suffered from lack of measurement – a tradition extending back to the days when lack of measurement was valorised by clinicians who argued that the entire enterprise was too personal, ethereal or mystical to measure. Mental healthcare has, though, emerged from the dark ages. Although we still lack clear biological and physiological standards, measurement must be at the core of what we do. And measurement is no simple matter.

As the authors of the following chapters argue, measurement in mental health is serious and arduous work. We need measures that are reliable and valid, that address meaningful processes and outcomes, that uphold and reinforce our values, and that enhance rather than impede the enterprise of behavioural health. Developing, refining, testing, comparing and instantiating such measures are essential tasks if the field is to move forwards, rather than recycle old ideas in new terminology.

I commend the editors for their persistent efforts to encourage high-quality research. The chapters herein describe progress on many important fronts.

Robert E. Drake MD PhD
Andrew Thomson Professor of Psychiatry
Dartmouth Medical School, Lebanon, New Hampshire, USA

Preface: an evolving perspective of mental health outcome measures

Since the appearance of the two previous editions of *Mental Health Outcome Measures* (first published by Springer Verlag in 1996, with a second edition published by the Royal College of Psychiatrists in 2001), there have been several intriguing developments in the field. First, an even wider range of important outcome domains are now measurable using well standardised instruments than were measurable before. Second, a greater emphasis upon positive outcomes has evolved (for example referring to the concept of recovery) among researchers, service users and clinicians. Third, the voice of the service user/consumer is now centre stage to a much greater extent than in earlier years. This third edition refers to these three core themes throughout its pages. Nevertheless, the fundamentals remain unchanged, namely:

- the scales used must have known and strong psychometric properties (Chapter 2)
- evidence (both qualitative and quantitative) needs to be ascertained from the most rigorously scientifically designed studies (Chapter 3), taking into account the complexity of the intervention (Campbell *et al*, 2000, 2007; Tansella *et al*, 2006)
- in many outcome studies, symptom and social domains (such as quality of life and employment) need to be assessed concurrently (Chapters 5, 8, 9, 11, 13, 14 and 16)
- scales need to be applicable and relevant to a wide of settings to allow valid international comparisons (Chapter 17)
- an inclusive approach to the whole range of mental disorders is required, so that people are included whose conditions have sometimes been excluded from care, such as personality disorders (Chapter 15).

At the same time, a clear trend is now identifiable not so much to look at mental disorders in terms of their producing chronicity, impairment and severe disability but instead to emphasise the hope of recovery (Chapter 4). Central to this view is the participation of service users in research (Chamberlin, 2005) and a more nuanced approach to potential collaboration between people disclosing experience of mental illness, and others, in the development and use of outcome measures (Sweeney *et al*, 2009). In other words, people with direct experience of mental illnesses (both service users and family members) are gradually coming to be seen less as the 'subjects' or 'objects' of research, and more as those in fact with the greatest depth of knowledge and experience of the conditions. They are therefore in the strongest position to give valid ratings of which treatments and services confer benefit (Chapters 1, 6 and 7). This change of perspective is of fundamental importance (Rose *et al*, 2006).

In a global context, this edition documents the continued and rapid production of new scales and the translation of psychometrically well established scales into new languages (Sartorius & Kuyken, 1994; Thornicroft *et al*, 2003). Even so, the number of effectiveness studies does not distribute equitably across international settings; in particular, few, as yet, have been carried out in low-income countries (Saxena *et al*, 2004; Patel *et al*, 2007; de Jesus *et al*, 2009).

There is another sense in which outcomes are important, namely how far the results of research are used to shape and improve routine clinical practice. This applied end of the research spectrum has been referred to as 'implementation science', and is itself at present underdeveloped, under-researched and underfunded (Tansella & Thornicroft, 2009). For example, although many hundreds of papers refer to the creation of clinical guidelines, few studies have explored under what conditions clinicians actually put such guidelines into practice (Madon *et al*, 2007; Proctor *et al*, 2009).

The operational linkages between policy and practice are therefore now being scrutinised as never before, both to identify interventions which are effective and cost-effective, and to judge how to realise behavioural changes on the part of practitioners that lead to better outcomes for people with mental health problems (Chapters 10 and 18).

When the first edition of this book was published in 1996, we wrote that 'research instruments are the basic tools of health service evaluation'. We would now add that the skilful use of these tools requires, as for artists or craftsmen, a clear eye for design, a steady and relentless focus upon the needs of the consumer, and the skill to realise the creative intent – in this case better mental health (Thornicroft & Tansella, 2009).

References

Campbell, M., Fitzpatrick, R., Haines, A., *et al* (2000) Framework for design and evaluation of complex interventions to improve health. *BMJ*, **321**, 694–696.

Campbell, N. C., Murray, E., Darbyshire, J., *et al* (2007) Designing and evaluating complex interventions to improve health care. *BMJ*, **334**, 455–459.

Chamberlin, J. (2005) User/consumer involvement in mental health service delivery. *Epidemiologia e Psichiatria Sociale*, **14**, 10–14.

de Jesus, M. J., Razzouk, D., Thara, R., *et al* (2009) Packages of care for schizophrenia in low- and middle-income countries. *PLoS Medicine*, **6**, e1000165.

Madon, T., Hofman, K. J., Kupfer, L., *et al* (2007) Public health. Implementation science. *Science*, **318**, 1728–1729.

Patel, V., Araya, R., Chatterjee, S., *et al* (2007) Treatment and prevention of mental disorders in low-income and middle-income countries. *Lancet*, **370**, 991–1005.

Proctor, E. K., Landsverk, J., Aarons, G., *et al* (2009) Implementation research in mental health services: an emerging science with conceptual, methodological, and training challenges. *Administration and Policy in Mental Health and Mental Health Services Research*, **36**, 24–34.

Rose, D., Thornicroft, G. & Slade, M. (2006) Who decides what evidence is? Developing a multiple perspectives paradigm in mental health. *Acta Psychiatrica Scandinavica*, suppl. 429, 109–114.

Sartorius, N. & Kuyken, J. (1994) Translation of health status instruments. In *Quality of Life Assessment in Health Care Settings* (eds J. Orley, & J. Kuyken), vol. 1, pp. 3–18. Springer-Verlag.

Saxena, S., Sharan, P. & Saraceno, B. (2004) Research for change: the role of scientific journals publishing mental health research. *World Psychiatry*, **3**, 66–72.

Sweeney, A., Beresford, P., Faulkner, A., *et al* (eds) (2009) *This Is Survivor Research*. PCCS Books.

Tansella, M. & Thornicroft, G. (2009) Implementation science: understanding the translation of evidence into practice. *British Journal of Psychiatry*, **195**, 283–285.

Tansella, M., Thornicroft, G., Barbui, C., *et al* (2006) Seven criteria for improving effectiveness trials in psychiatry. *Psychological Medicine*, **36**, 711–720.

Thornicroft, G. & Tansella, M. (2009) *Better Mental Health Care*. Cambridge University Press.

Thornicroft, G., Becker, T., Knapp, M., *et al* (2003) *International Outcome Measures in Mental Health. Quality of Life, Needs, Service Satisfaction, Costs and Impact on Carers*. Royal College of Psychiatrists.

Michele Tansella and Graham Thornicroft

Part I
Methodological issues

CHAPTER 1

Measures of outcomes that are valued by service users

Thomas Kabir and Til Wykes

This book has many chapters on outcome assessments, from the global functioning scales to more specific and detailed measures for use in service evaluation as well as in measuring treatment outcome. So we suspect that the reader will be asking a number of questions before dipping into this first chapter, specifically on measures of outcome that are valued by service users. These we are sure will include:

- Will this chapter examine new measures of outcome that are not covered by other chapters?
- Will any new measures look radically different from those already described in other chapters?
- Why is there a chapter on outcomes that are valued by service users?

The answers to the first two questions are: yes, but not many; and probably not. But it is the answer to the last question which is key. A chapter has been specifically allocated to this topic because such measures are important in evaluations of mental healthcare. Many professionals will consider that this is just a focus on what is politically correct and that service users' experiences are not generally that helpful or, more often, that their clinical carers usually know best. We have some sympathy with the view that when healthcare resources are scarce there is a need to measure outcomes that reflect the performance of services and that this is sometimes at variance with service users' views. Service users may not be interested in symptom remission, patient throughput or even the assessment of their global functioning. They may be more interested in their definition of recovery or simply their happiness and sometimes these aspirations may lie outside the remit of mental health service provision.

But even with this understanding of different perspectives, we believe that the pendulum has swung too far and for too long in the direction of outcomes which may not be relevant to service users, may not be appropriately measured even if they are relevant, or may just be the opposite of what service users would expect of a mental health service. In this chapter we try to rebalance the field by introducing or describing outcome measures that are accepted by service users, and show how methods involving service users can be used to develop new, relevant and acceptable measures of outcome that reflect the purpose of services. It is also important that we have measures of what service users expect from services, as their models of appropriate care will undoubtedly affect the take-up of services, especially novel ones. Assessments compared from different perspectives can also provide new insights into how services might improve as well as how new treatments or types of care can be organised. This chapter may overlap with some others in this volume in its description of measures but, crucially, it highlights the need for good measures of satisfaction, service outcome and quality of life that reflect the mental health service user's experience.

What constitutes a user-valued measure?

The answer to this question is simple. A user-valued measure is one that is recognised as such by a majority of service users. A user-valued measure is one which reflects the values and experiences of a majority of service users. To use an analogy, to be a user-valued outcome measure, it would have to pass a 'Turing Test'. A majority of service users would have to be able to say from looking at the measure that it did indeed make sense and evaluate human factors that were important to them. In other words, the majority of service users that the measure applies to have to believe that the scale has been constructed *by people* who have an understanding of their situation.

But this is not the only criterion that we are going to use to judge a measure as worthy of being called a user-valued measure. Clearly, the instrument also needs to be useful in understanding services and therefore we want to know whether it can be used in different settings, with different groups of service users and in different types of mental health organisation. We would like to see evidence not only that the measure is being used in the academic literature but also that it is being used in mental health service assessment. In other words, our aspiration is to see user-valued measures used in routine practice.

Fitzpatrick *et al* (1998) propose eight essential properties of a patient-based outcome measure. These are shown in Table 1.1. One kind of measure which is clearly user valued is the method designed by Diana Rose and called user-focused monitoring (UFM) (Rose *et al*, 1998). This is a general method of involving service users in producing a schedule of assessment that is grounded in their views within a particular service setting. The questions therefore vary between services rather than being generally appropriate. So although this method is one of the best for producing a measure with user value, it does not fulfil the criteria we have set out, as each UFM measure will be service specific and therefore it would not be 'appropriate' (see Table 1.1) for the measure to be generalised.

This book concentrates on outcome measures and these are normally used in evaluations of treatments or services. We therefore need to be certain

Table 1.1 Essential properties of an outcome measure

Property	
Appropriateness	Is the content of the instrument appropriate to the question that the clinical trial is intended to address?
Reliability	Does the instrument produce results that are reproducible and internally consistent?
Validity	Does the instrument measure what it claims to measure?
Responsiveness	Does the instrument detect changes over time that matter to patients?
Precision	How precise are the scores of the instrument?
Interpretability	How interpretable are the scores of the instrument?
Acceptability	Is the instrument acceptable to the patients?
Feasibility	Is the instrument easy to administer and process?

Adapted from Fitzpatrick *et al* (1998) and Gilbody *et al* (2003).

that the information is accurate; that is, if we repeated the evaluation we would gain similar results. These psychometric qualities of any instrument therefore also need to be available for a measure to begin to be used in routine practice. The usual list includes: validity, reliability and, crucially, sensitivity to change over time. The reason for the importance of psychometric data is highlighted in a report of the outcome measures used in 300 trials randomly selected from the Cochrane database of trials in schizophrenia (Marshall *et al*, 2000). The review showed that outcome measures that were developed for a specific study and did not have adequately published reliability and validity data were more likely to conclude that the new treatment was superior to a control treatment. When pharmacological and non-pharmacological studies were independently assessed, the non-pharmacological treatments fared the worst, with nearly twice the chance of a report of clinical significance if an unpublished rather than a published scale had been used. Overall, the authors concluded that in more than one-third of all studies in this area the claims for clinical significance could not have been made if published scales had been used. Although this was a report of studies of schizophrenia, we assume that similar results would have been found for other disorders. The fact that the problems seemed to be amplified in the non-pharmacological area is of great importance to service users, who tend to prefer these sorts of treatments to medication alone. For service users, the diversion of resources into therapies which would not have been found to be useful if rigorously assessed scales had been used is a further reason to ensure that all studies use such scales.

It might be expected that this chapter would describe a set of outcomes with a specific user value attached to them. However, this is not possible, as there have been few investigations of what types of outcome measure are acceptable and have value. The approach that we have taken is to investigate those measures to which service users have contributed in any way, as these are likely to have value; we also point out ones that users may value but

5

where they have not been involved in their development. One clear research agenda would be to investigate the value expert service users (i.e. those with experience of the disorder or service) would consider as an outcome worth measuring.

It should be noted, however, that a measure need not be constructed exclusively by people with experience of using mental health services for it to be a user-valued outcome measure. It is not good scientific practice for the validity of any measure to be dependent on the background of those who constructed it. It is only necessary that the majority of service users are able to say that the outcome measure does indeed measure factors that are important to them.

In what types of study would user-valued measures be relevant?

It is not controversial to suggest that service users' views are important in assessing the value of services. Hence, most user-valued measures of outcome have come from the field of service satisfaction. But we believe that user-valued measures could be used to understand treatment outcome, including side-effects in randomised controlled trials.

Which treatments are included in guidance for healthcare in the UK is determined by the National Institute for Health and Clinical Excellence (NICE), which makes its judgements on the basis of the evidence from high-quality controlled trials. These are nearly always studies where the primary outcome is symptoms and the secondary outcomes are those of interest to the clinicians. Often the only information in the evidence base about whether service users value the treatment is their decision to opt out of the study, that is the drop-out rate. Given that most decisions about treatments are based on the balance of outcomes, surely it would be helpful to allow service users to state their choice? For instance, although efficacy is based on symptom reduction, the severity of side-effects may make it unlikely that the treatment will be prolonged. An outcome measure which shows this balance might provide clearer information to the healthcare professionals and service providers about the likely effectiveness of treatments.

There is a further reason for introducing user-valued measures, and that is the acceptance of the term 'recovery' rather than 'cure' in the mental health literature (Davidson *et al*, 2005). The acceptance of new terms will change the measurement field to include issues of balance in the service user's life between a number of competing choices; one specific measure is unlikely to reflect this complex world view. For example, consider someone who is on antipsychotic medication which has reduced their clinical symptoms to the point where they might clinically be considered to have recovered but this person has experienced significant medication-related side-effects, including weight gain, which has led to a negative self-image and social withdrawal, and drowsiness, which has impaired their ability to carry out his usual occupation. It is unlikely that a single outcome measure would capture all the information that is pertinent to this service user's situation.

The production of user-valued measures

The majority of outcome measures are produced through a process of item generation, item testing, scale feasibility testing and further work on the psychometrics. What need to be added to this list are those extra items that service users would most notice about a scale, regardless of the content. Some of these have been described by Fitzpatrick *et al* (1998). Of prime importance is the acceptability of the scale to service users, which includes the length of time needed to complete it and whether there is a chance for them to add their own context to their answers. Scales that are administered within an interview do give some time for service users to reflect on their answers (although this does depend on the skills of the interviewer). Scales with fixed items that are completed by self-report are unlikely to reflect the key issues for an individual. It is vital in this latter case to ensure that the items chosen and the categories for the answers allow service users to give an accurate rendition of their perspective. For this, they need to be involved in the production of the scale items and category assembly. Below we provide a brief description of the continuum of involvement in the outcome measures we have reviewed. This is based on a continuum adopted by a UK Department of Health funded patient involvement group called INVOLVE (www.invo.org.uk). However, we recognise that this system is too simple to distinguish some subtleties in service user involvement. In our opinion the best possible measures would be those:

- where service users had been closely involved in the development as full partners
- which have been rigorously tested for their psychometric properties (especially sensitivity to change)
- which have been tested in a variety of service settings in a variety of countries.

The few such measures on the market are described below. First, though, we describe the methods used to develop user-valued measures, as this will allow researchers to carry out similar exercises where there are gaps in the field.

Derived without user involvement

Even if a measure is derived without their involvement, the end result may still be valued by service users. It does seem unlikely that this could happen but there are some measures that have been produced with no consultation with service users which are valued. These include quality-of-life measures and some service-satisfaction measures. These scales were produced through the traditional route, by clinicians working with academics. The feasibility of the scales was tested with service users but they were not involved in item generation. An example of such a scale is the Working Alliance Inventory (WAI; Hovrath & Greenberg, 1989). The scale can be said to be user-valued partly because of its subsequent usage and because 'some of the definitions used include the client's experience of the relationship with the therapist as being helpful in achieving goals' (Tracey et al, 1989). There are two versions of this scale, one for the patient and one for the counsellor. The 36 items contained in both versions of the scale were generated by consulting seven experts in the field of working alliance and 21 randomly selected psychologists. The WAI was piloted using 29 graduate students in a 'counselling psychology program engaged in a peer counselling task' (Hovrath & Greenberg, 1989). This outcome measure was specifically chosen as an outcome in one study of motivational interviewing (Hayward et al, 2009).

Consultation

Consultation can take various forms, from representation on steering groups to surveys of service users. This can further be refined by looking at the level of representation, through service users' voluntary organisations or through representation of service user experts. Consultation does not imply that the research team (where the power lies) will accept the advice given. Outcome measures derived in this way may or may not be valued by service users – usually this has not been tested – but do show some involvement and so are more likely to be valued by service users than those measures developed with no user involvement.

Representatives of services users were involved in the development of the Carers' and Users' Expectation of Service – User Version (CUES–U; Lelliott et al, 2001; Blenkiron et al, 2003). This scale was the result of a collaboration between two Royal Colleges, the University of East Anglia, and an organisation representing service users and carers (then called National Schizophrenia Fellowship, now called Rethink). Domains that were important to service users were identified in two ways. The first was by carrying out a comprehensive literature search, including a search of the 'grey literature' and unpublished material. The second was by carrying out focus group interviews with service users. The development of the scale was also informed by the establishment of an advisory group of service users. Once the large number of domains that were important to service users was identified, then the domains were 'grouped into the smallest number of items without losing definition or meaning' (Lelliott et al, 2001). The scale was field tested using nearly 450 service users from across the UK.

The final scale is self-rated and consists of 17 items, split into three sections. The items concern: where you live; money; help with finances;

how you spend your day; family and friends; social life; information and advice; access to mental health services; choice of mental health services; relationships with mental health workers; consultation and control; advocacy; stigma and discrimination; medication; access to physical health services; relationships with physical health workers; and other issues (anything else that the service user would like to raise which has not been covered by the other 16 items). The paper reporting the development of the scale notes that service users 'appear to place less emphasis on symptom reduction than they do on improvements in other area of their lives' (Lelliott *et al*, 2001). A slightly different level of consultation took place to produce the Camberwell Assessment of Need (CAN) (Phelan *et al*, 1995, see http://www.iop.kcl.ac.uk/virtual/?path=/hsr/prism/can/).

A slightly different level of consultation took place to produce the Camberwell Assessment of Need (CAN)9 (see http://www.iop.kcl.ac.uk/virtual/?path=/hsr/prism/can/). This measure reflects the needs (both met and unmet) of people in touch with high-support services. Although the development of the items was based on consultation between clinicians and researchers, the development team also included a survey of service users about the importance of the items that were proposed to make up the scale. All the proposed items were judged to be at least moderately important but there was no opportunity for service users to contribute new items or to suggest ways in which the scale should be promoted, including the anchoring of the scale. However, at least we can be clear that this measure does include moderately important items and so has some value to service users.

Service users were also involved in a consultative way in the development Patient Reported Outcome Measures (PROMS; see http://phi.uhce.ox.ac.uk/home.php). Continuity-of-care measures where service users were certainly consulted include the CONNECT (Ware et al, 2003) and ACSS–MH (Durbin *et al*, 2004) measures.

Contribution

This term is used to denote that service users have been consulted and that their views have been taken into account. This differs from consultation, where views may be sought but need not have had any effect on the research. This terminology is taken from Sweeney & Morgan (2009), who specifically point out that 'contribution' is where some commitment to service user involvement has been agreed (unlike in consultation) but that the role is limited. For instance, it may mean only that a service user has been employed as a researcher on a project which has already been designed.

The CUES–U measure is likely to be one in which service users and carers were both consulted and made a contribution. The measure itself was in part constructed using focus groups of service users. The scale also contains a number of items, such as 'stigma and discrimination' and 'medication', which are commonly reported by service users as being important to them.

It can therefore be said that, to a reasonable degree, the CUES–U measure does indeed take into account the views of service users and carers.

A similar process was undertaken in the development of the Accommodation and Enabling Scale for Eating Disorders (AESED; Sepulveda *et al*, 2009). Two expert carers were involved in screening items for use in this questionnaire.

Partnership

Again, there is a continuum of involvement in measures that have been developed in partnership with service users. In some partnerships the academic researcher takes the lead but in others service users lead the research and develop the measures through new methodologies or participatory research.

The first measures we highlight here are those where service users took part as either paid or voluntary researchers. One example of this sort of development is a measure of the outcome of cognitive–behavioural therapy for people with psychosis (CBTp), called Choice of Outcome in CBT for psychoses, or CHOICE (Greenwood *et al*, 2010). The study team included a paid service user researcher, who was involved in the design of the study. The first step in the measure development was that topics for exploration were identified by CBTp experts and these were then discussed in service user focus groups, which were jointly led and analysed by a service user and a clinical researcher. Focus group participants then took part in a 'Delphi exercise' to work towards a consensus on the items that needed to be included. This produced a total of 26 items. An acceptability study with 15 further service users provided information on whether the questionnaire was understandable; these users also commented on different possible formats. The measure was then given to 152 further service users before and after they had received CBTp as part of a standard clinic. Reliability, validity and sensitivity were measured. The final measure covers both recovery-oriented items, such as general distress and quality of life, as well as CBTp-specific ones, such as psychosis-specific distress. There are data relating to its psychometric properties and therefore this is a measure which holds great promise for what is now a burgeoning area, not only in research studies but also in the provision of CBTp in routine care.

Another method of including service users has been developed from a health economics method called conjoint analysis, which allows service users specifically to influence the weighting of items in a scale. One measure that utilises this approach is the Older Person's Utility Scale for Social Care (OPUS; Netten *et al*, 2002). This scale measures key outcomes for social care. The research team included service users at different stages. At the first stage, 'experts' in social care, from social care policy-makers to care managers, were consulted about the topics that might be included. At the second stage, 356 older people were consulted about their preferences in relation to 27 different scenarios covering five different domains; these had been piloted in consultation with older people. In this part of the project, older people were given two descriptions which differed on two key domains, for example where personal safety was maximised in one but social participation reduced, compared with another where personal safety was reduced but social participation was increased. Each of the scenarios reflected different levels of unmet need in each of the five domains. This part of the development also included 58 people who indicated additional preferences on the basis of how much money they would pay for their choice. The results of these preference decisions were analysed using conjoint analysis, which produced weights for the different domains. There was a clear ranking by both the older people and those who were using services of the domains from least to most important: personal safety, food, and control over daily life, social participation and personal care. This method, by giving weights to the items, allows a score to be produced which can reflect, adequately, the importance of each item rather than each item contributing the same amount to the total score. Further testing showed that the scale was both reliable and valid.

Service user researchers have also led teams in the development of measures. One of these is a new participatory model based on UFM methodology and constructed by the Service User Research Enterprise (SURE) at the Institute of Psychiatry, King's College London. In this method, the service user leads the research project. The process falls into five stages:

- production of a topic guide
- pilot and then full focus groups to generate specific domains
- expert panels to comment on the item form and completeness
- feasibility study to test comprehensibility and acceptability of the measure
- formal psychometric testing including reliability, validity and sensitivity to change.

Two measures of value to service users have been developed using this method. The first is a measure of continuity of care which is thought to be important by service planners and policy-makers (CONTINU–UM; Rose *et al*, 2009). This is a measure of the perceptions of continuity of service users (which differ from service providers' and policy-makers' perceptions of continuity). The second measure developed using this method records service users' perceptions of the in-patient environment and is called VOICE. Both measures have been or will be used as a main outcome in studies investigating service and treatment changes.

The Empowerment Scale is another example of an outcome measure which has been designed using a participation action research method. The scale was developed by a defined partnership between researchers and a consumer research advisory board comprising service users and one of the researchers (Rogers *et al*, 1997).

Gaps in the market

Few service user outcome measures have been reported in the literature. It is unsurprising, then, that there are many 'gaps in the market'. Some areas where no or few service user outcome measures have been developed are:

- outcome measures specific to forensic settings
- outcome measures specifically for children and adolescents
- disorder-specific outcome measures, including:
  - anxiety, depression, obsessive–compulsive disorder, bipolar disorder, eating disorders
  - psychosis
  - personality disorders
- medication side-effects
- outcome measures adapted for specific groups (e.g. different ethnic groups).

In addition, to the best of our knowledge, none of the service user outcome measures reviewed in this chapter has been validated for any language other than English. There are some outcome measures produced by service users that are specific to particular local mental health services in specific countries but there are few that have been developed for routine use for particular kinds of service, other than in-patient settings. An exception is the Child and Adolescent Mental Health Services Satisfaction Scale (CAMHSSS; Ayton *et al*, 2007).

In relation to the lack of disorder-specific outcome measures, it can be argued that disorders such as depression are clinically defined, for example in the *Diagnostic and Statistical Manual* (DSM), and so subsequently the notion of 'outcome' is also clinically defined to a significant degree. But this approach is likely to be narrow from the perspective of service users. Even if the symptoms and severity of depression have not changed, it is still possible that the service user may have adapted to the circumstances and recovered a level of functioning that he or she had not had previously. This is likely to be an outcome which is valued by the service user but might be missed using one of the traditional outcome measures currently in use.

There has also been a lack of attention to certain groups such as Black and minority ethnic groups. It is not at all clear that service users will agree on what outcomes they value. Given the current interest in the effects of psychiatric services and psychiatric treatments on different cultural groups, an exploration of the differences between participating groups is essential and would add a different dimension to a user-valued measure.

Although the CUES–U scale does include medication as an item, medication (and its side-effects) is a domain that is not generally found in outcome scales that are in common use. These types of scale are essential in deriving the value of medication (or other therapies). Service users may value different aspects of treatment; for example, a medication which frequently produces some side-effects may be more acceptable than a medication that produces infrequent but more serious side-effects. This type of knowledge might enable drug development to proceed in a more productive manner, with new drugs not being discarded so early in development.

Conclusion

Despite our searches it has been difficult to discover many measures for which we are reasonably certain there is evidence that users value the outcomes they record. But our searches did throw up a number of methods for deriving such measures. Individual scale items, with preference weightings from conjoint analysis, can be derived using the participatory method developed by the team at SURE. We consider this type of method perhaps the zenith of what is available.

However, user-valued outcome measures can also be constructed with service users being used as active and equal collaborators in the process. This can be carried out in a number of different ways, for example by employing researchers who also have experience of using mental health services or by collaboration with a service user organisation, as was done in the production of the CUES–U scale. User-valued outcomes may also be derived simply by researchers being willing to engage fully with and take into account the views of a relatively large number of service users, as was the case for the Empowerment Scale (Rogers *et al*, 1997).

Most of the scales covered in this chapter are new and so it is unclear at present how widely they will be used. In the UK, the National Institute for Health Research's Mental Health Research Network (http://www.mhrn.info) has commissioned a library of outcome measures that are valued by service users. We hope that this resource will be used by clinical researchers.

In conclusion, there are a growing number of validated user-valued outcome scales that have been reported in the literature. Very simply, by definition, these measure the things are likely to be important to service users. This is possibly one of the strongest reasons why researchers should use such scales and construct new scales where there are none.

References

Ayton, A. K., Mooney, M. P., Sillifant, K., *et al* (2007) The development of the child and adolescent versions of the Verona Service Satisfaction Scale (CAMHSSS). *Social Psychiatry and Psychiatric Epidemiology*, **42**, 892–901.

Blenkiron, P., Mo, K. H., Cuzen, J., *et al* (2003) Involving service users in their mental care: the CUES project. *Psychiatric Bulletin*, **27**, 334–338.

Davidson, L., Harding, C. & Spaniol, L. (2005) *Recovery from Severe Mental Illnesses: Research Evidence and Implications for Practice*. Boston University Centre for Psychiatric Rehabilitation.

Durbin, J., Goering, P., Streiner, D. L., *et al* (2004) Continuity of care: validation of a new self-report measure for individuals using mental health services. *Journal of Behavioral Health Services and Research*, **31**, 279–296.

Fitzpatrick, R., Davey, C., Buxton, M. J., *et al* (1998) Evaluating patient-based outcome measures for use in clinical trials. *Health Technology Assessment*, **2**, i–74.

Gilbody, S. O., House, A. & Sheldon, T. (2003) *Outcomes Measurement in Psychiatry: A Critical Review of Outcomes Measurement in Psychiatric Research and Practice*. NHS Centre for Reviews and Dissemination, University of York

Greenwood, K. E., Sweeney, A., Williams, S., *et al* (2010) CHoice of Outcome INCbt for psychosEs (CHOICE): the development of a new service-user led outcome measure of CBT for psychosis. *Schizophrenia Bulletin*, **36**, 126–135.

Hayward, P., David, A., Green, N., *et al* (2009) Promoting therapeutic alliance in clozapine users: an exploratory randomized controlled trial. *Clinical Schizophrenia and Related Psychoses*, **3**, 127–132.

Hovrath, A. & Greenberg, L. (1989) Development and validation of the Working Alliance Inventory. *Journal of Counselling Psychology*, **36**, 223–233.

Lelliott, P., Beevor, A., Hogman, G., *et al* (2001) Carers' and users' expectations of services – User version (CUES–U): a new instrument to measure the experience of users of mental health services. *British Journal of Psychiatry*, **179**, 67–72.

Marshall, M., Lockwood, A., Bradley, C., *et al* (2000) Unpublished rating scales: a major source of bias in randomised controlled trials of treatments for schizophrenia. *British Journal of Psychiatry*, **176**, 249–252.

Netten, A., Ryan, M., Smith, P., *et al* (2002) *The Development of a Measure of Social Care Outcome for Older People*. Personal Social Services Research Unit (PSSRU).

Phelan, M., Slade, M., Thornicroft, G., *et al* (1995) The Camberwell Assessment of Need: the validity and reliability of an instrument to assess the needs of people with severe mental illness. *British Journal of Psychiatry*, **167**, 589–595.

Rogers, E. S., Chamberlin, J., Ellison, M. L., *et al* (1997) A consumer-constructed scale to measure empowerment among users of mental health services. *Psychiatric Services*, **48**, 1042–1047.

Rose, D., Lindley, P., Ford, R., *et al* (1998) *In Our Experience: User-Focused Monitoring of Mental Health Services in Kensington & Chelsea and Westminster Health Authority*. Sainsbury Centre for Mental Health.

Rose, D., Sweeney, A., Leese, M., *et al* (2009) Developing a user-generated measure of continuity of care: brief report. *Acta Psychiatrica Scandinavica*, **119**, 320–324.

Sepulveda, A. R., Kyriacou, O. & Treasure, J. (2009) Development and validation of the Accommodation and Enabling Scale for Eating Disorders (AESED) for caregivers in eating disorders. *BMC Health Services Research*, **9**, 171–184.

Sweeney, A. & Morgan, L. (2009) Levels and stages. In *Handbook of Service User Involvement in Mental Health Research* (eds J. Wallcraft, B. Schrank & M. Amering), pp. 25–35. Wiley/World Psychiatric Association.

Tracey, T. & Kokotovic, A. (1989) Factor structure of the Working Alliance Inventory. Psychological Assesment. *Journal of Consulting and Clinical Psychology*, **1**, 207–210.

Ware, N. C., Dickey, B., Tugenberg, T., *et al* (2003) CONNECT: a measure of continuity of care in mental health services. *Mental Health Services Research*, **5**, 209–221.

CHAPTER 2

Statistical methods for measuring outcomes

Graham Dunn

This book concerns promotion of the routine use of outcome measures in clinical practice; the purpose of this chapter, however, is to warn care providers to think very carefully before routinely (naively?) using such measures. Just what are the benefits of their use? What are the outcome measures intended to demonstrate? In order to try to convince the reader that there might be real difficulties in the interpretation of the results, the main body of the chapter concentrates on the difficulties in the interpretation of data from structured research projects specifically designed to evaluate an innovation in mental healthcare provision. The difficulties of interpreting haphazardly collected data as part of routine clinical or administrative practice will be far greater. One of the main purposes of an evaluative exercise is comparison: which approach to service provision is the better? If care providers really want to be involved in mental health service evaluation then their time would be much better spent in taking part in a large multicentre trial.

Outcome measures in routine clinical practice

The title of this chapter might have been better formulated as 'Statistical problems in the interpretation of outcomes'. The main aim of the chapter is to point out the great difficulties in the analysis and interpretation of routinely collected but unstructured clinical outcome data. But it will make this point by discussing the design and analysis of research programmes, on the assumption that if the reader is convinced of the difficulties of doing worthwhile research then he or she might realise how difficult it can be to make sense of data collected as part of routine clinical practice. The collection of outcome data has a cost, however well hidden that cost might be. In the context of a research study, there are staff specifically employed to collect the data. It is a very time-consuming and expensive activity. Given the cost of collecting, recording and analysing data, one must ask whether the benefits of the exercise are worthwhile. Just what are the intended benefits? What are the data meant to show, and to whom? Clearly, with the development of ever larger and more sophisticated databases (the explosion of so-called eScience) there will be ever more data available for people to analyse and from which to draw questionable conclusions. With these developments in bio-health informatics it is even more important to caution against the misinterpretation of the resulting data.

It is not the intention of the present author to try to prevent the introduction of outcome measures into routine clinical practice (and the development of the associated databases), but to stop clinicians and other care providers from enthusiastically rushing to collect data without giving very careful thought to the costs and the potential benefits of the exercise. Much routinely collected data will be unanalysable because they are unstructured, full of holes (missing values) and laden with subjective biases. The last are likely to arise because the outcomes are likely to be measured by the clinicians themselves rather than by neutral observers. For the same reason, much of the information collected by medical audit is of little value.

The author's conclusion is that anyone really wishing to evaluate the clinical services he or she is instrumental in providing should get involved in some sort of formal and appropriately planned evaluation exercise, that is, some sort of controlled healthcare trial. The rest of this chapter is concerned with statistical approaches to the design and analysis of such a trial, partly to underline the enormous difficulties in drawing inferences from outcome data, and partly to convince the reader of the benefits of multicentred evaluations involving cluster randomisation. We start by explaining what is meant by a healthcare trial.

What is a healthcare trial?

We will assume that all clinicians are familiar with the concept of a controlled clinical trial in which the investigator assesses the relative effectiveness of competing treatments (typically, chemotherapies). Arguments in favour of the controlled trial will not be rehearsed here. According to Spitzer *et al* (1975, p. 161): 'The research strategy of the controlled clinical trial has been a powerful scientific tool that can avoid or minimize the errors produced either by the fashions of authoritarian pronouncement or by the oversimplifications of socio-political zealotry'. The randomised controlled trial is the 'gold standard' (in terms of methodological rigour) against which other forms of evaluation are to be assessed.

In a traditional clinical trial, the experimental conditions are usually competing therapies and the participants are individual patients. In a healthcare trial, the experimental conditions are competing ways of providing a healthcare service and the participants may be patients, but are not necessarily so. They might, for example, be care providers, managers or units of healthcare provision (clinics, wards or hospitals, for example). Spitzer *et al* (1975) distinguish two types of healthcare trial: a *health service trial*, in which one assesses the mechanisms (or records) of healthcare provision; and a *patient care trial*, in which one assesses conventional therapies but the clinical outcome variables are augmented by socio-personal data. The patient care trial is distinguished from the traditional clinical trial by the use of non-clinical outcome measures. The latter may include use of medical and other services, administrative problems, family burden, days of confinement to bed and absence from work or school. They may also include estimates of cost. The health service trial may include socio-personal data among the variables under assessment, but not always.

Experiment, quasi-experiment or survey?

In his discussion of the methodology of clinical trials in psychiatry, Johnson (1989) starts with a quotation from one of the founders of clinical trial methodology, Sir Austin Bradford Hill. He describes a clinical trial as a carefully, and ethically, designed experiment with the aim of answering some precisely framed question. In its most rigorous form it demands equivalent groups of patients concurrently treated in different ways. These groups are constructed by the random allocation of patients to one or other treatment. In some instances patients may form their own controls, different treatment being applied to them in random order and the effect compared. In principle the method is applicable to any disease and any treatment (Hill, 1955).

The key component of a trial of this type is *random allocation of patients (or clusters of patients) to treatments*. Randomisation serves three important roles. First, it is an impartial method of allocation of patients to the competing treatments. Second, it will tend to balance the treatment groups in terms of the effects of extraneous variables that may influence the outcome of treatment. One might argue that it would be more effective to match or stratify on the basis of the extraneous variables. Stratification can be an important component of trial design, but it cannot cope with the extraneous variable(s) that no one has thought of. A stratified trial should still have random allocation within the strata. The third role of randomisation is that it guarantees the validity of a subsequent statistical test of significance. If there are no treatment effects (i.e. the null hypothesis is true) then, apart from unforeseen or uncontrolled biases, the observed treatment differences must be the result of randomisation (chance). One can simply ask 'What is the probability of the results if they have arisen solely as a result of randomisation?' and decide whether the data are consistent with the null hypothesis accordingly.

Returning to the problem of healthcare evaluation, randomised controlled trials of the type described by Johnson (1989) and Hill (1955) cannot always be conducted, for a variety of reasons, including logistics, ethics, cost and public opinion (Spitzer *et al*, 1975). The allocation of services to patients is

17

often beyond the control of the evaluator. He or she simply has to act as a neutral observer of someone else's innovation. That someone else might be an clinician, a health service administrator or manager, or a politician. This does not preclude evaluation, but it does considerably weaken the validity of any conclusions arising from it.

The type of evaluative experiment that, for whatever reason, cannot include random allocation of participants to the competing treatments or services has often been called a *quasi-experiment* (Cook & Campbell, 1979). Spitzer *et al* (1975) talk of *healthcare surveys*. Cochran (1983) uses the term *observational study*. This last phrase will be used here. We illustrate the idea of an observational study by reference to two simple alternative designs, one using historical controls and the other using concurrent ones. In the former type of observational study, we first assess the outcome of care for a cohort of patients before the introduction of the innovation. We then introduce the innovation (a reorganisation of the clinical services or the introduction of a case-management service, for example) and then monitor the outcome for a new cohort of patients receiving the new or reorganised clinical service. Comparison of the outcomes for these two cohorts will, we hope, give us an estimate of the effect of the innovation. In the second example of an observational study, we might be planning to introduce a new service in one particular clinic, hospital or health district. Prior to its introduction, however, we search for another clinic, hospital or district that is as similar as possible to ours – except that there are no immediate plans to change its healthcare services. The latter centre provides us with a concurrent control. The outcomes for a cohort of patients exposed to the innovation in one centre can be compared with the outcomes for another cohort in the centre in which the innovation has not been introduced. Again, comparison of the outcomes for the two cohorts of patients will, we hope, give us an estimate of the impact of the introduction of the innovation.

The weaknesses in both of the above designs are the very weaknesses that randomisation helps to rectify. First, there may be differences between the patients in the two arms of the study. Referral patterns may have inadvertently changed at about the same time as the introduction of the innovation, for example. There may be other differences between the innovative and the control arms of the trial. Innovation is usually managed by a newly appointed enthusiast (or even an evangelist) with commitment, drive and lots of energy. In the control situation there may be a run-down service managed by an ageing sceptic who is just looking forward to early retirement. As Buck & Donner (1982) point out, in many healthcare experiments the placebo effect falls upon the providers rather than the recipients of care. The estimate of the effectiveness is likely to be biased – that is, usually overoptimistic: the effect of the innovation *per se* is likely to be confounded with inherent patient differences, environmental and staff differences and non-specific effects of the introduction of an innovative service (the Hawthorne effect).

Finally, we have more subtle problems of statistical inference. In the absence of randomisation we have to build in more assumptions for our significance tests, and so on. We usually pretend, quite unrealistically, for example, that the innovation and control groups have been randomly selected from a much larger population of potential treatment groups. We then ask, 'What is the probability of selecting by chance two groups that are as different as these two?'

Now, the above weaknesses of observational studies have not been pointed out in an attempt to stop people carrying them out, but to point out the care that is needed in drawing valid inferences from the results. We have to try to avoid biases by carefully matching centres, for example, or by ensuring that the care staff are equally well organised and motivated, with equal access to appropriate facilities in both arms of the trial. We also have to think more carefully about the use of various methods of statistical analysis (covariate adjustment, for example) to attempt to eliminate or reduce the impact of potential sources of bias. Cochran (1983, p. 14) gives the following advice:

Control can usually be attempted on only a few of many variables that influence outcome; that control is likely to be only partially effective on these variables. Thus the investigator might do well to suppose that, in general, estimates from an observational study are likely to be biased. It is therefore worthwhile to think hard about what biases are most likely, and to think seriously about their sources, directions, and even their plausible magnitudes.

Over the last couple of decades there has been an enormous amount of progress made in the development of statistical and econometric methods that can yield valid inferences concerning causal effects of interventions using data obtained through uncontrolled or only partially controlled observational studies. Of particular importance are the use of methods based on propensity scores (see, for example, D'Agostino, 1998; Luellin *et al*, 2005; Angrist & Pischke, 2009) and instrumental variables (see, for example, Newhouse & McClellan, 1998; Greenland, 2000; Angrist & Pischke, 2009). These methods, however, do not (and cannot) supplant the need for good design (preferably involving randomisation).

In the following section we continue to discuss potential problems in the interpretation of the results of an evaluation, and return again to randomisation of experimental units to the different arms of a trial. We suggest that the experimental unit should be a group (cluster) of patients, however, rather than individuals themselves.

What are the experimental units?

In the interpretation of the outcome of an innovation, we are concerned with two threats to the validity of our inferences. These are threats to the *internal validity* of our evaluation (has the change we have seen really arisen as the result of the innovation or via some unintended mechanism?) and to the *external validity* (can we generalise our findings to other settings or services?). Interesting analogies can be drawn with the outcome of the clinical psychologist's well controlled single case study and with that of a controlled clinical trial. In the single case study, the quality of the design of the experiment might be such that it is very safe to conclude that the therapy or management given was indeed the cause of the resulting changes to the patient. But what about other patients? We cannot safely use statistical inference to predict the behaviour of future patients from this one, possibly very atypical patient, however well controlled the study was shown to be. We need an evaluation involving several patients to find out how patients respond to treatment or management in general. The single case study may have near perfect internal validity, but we cannot safely generalise from it – it has very limited or even no external validity.

The above arguments apply equally cogently to the evaluation of, say, a new clinic or clinical service. Can we infer anything about clinics in general from our knowledge of this one? Do we want to? We may simply want to demonstrate that our unique clinic works very effectively and are quite happy to leave others to evaluate their own services. If, however, we wish to generalise from our evaluation to other clinics, then we either have to acknowledge that statistical inference does not play a part in this generalisation or that we need to observe the behaviour of several similar clinics and compare it with that of a control group of services. It is vital that the correct unit of observation is identified at all stages of the evaluation: in the design, in the analysis of the results and in the interpretation of the findings.

Now consider a related but slightly more subtle problem. In both qualitative and quantitative approaches to evaluation one has to be very wary of the pitfalls of what Manly (1992), after Hurlbert (1984), calls 'pseudoreplication'. This arises when the units of measurement (patients, clinics, districts) are not independent replicates. Patients within a clinic will tend to have similar experiences of service provision, they share facilities and care staff, and may talk to each other and influence each other's views; they will have relatively similar outcomes (as compared with patients from different clinics), and so on. Patients, to some extent, will exhibit within-clinic or within-group correlations and they will thus not provide statistically independent items of information. The data obtained, whether qualitative or quantitative, should not be treated as if they had been obtained from a group of completely independent patients. The evaluator is not obtaining as much information as he or she might naively think! The problem is particularly acute with group-based therapies or activities. The group as a whole might do well, or it might fail. In either case there are likely to be fairly high within-group correlations. Often evaluators treat the individual patient as the unit for their analysis when, in fact, it should be the group, clinic, and so on. What is needed is replication of groups, not replication of individual units within the group.

The above provides reasons why we might wish to summarise and interpret the outcomes at the level of groups or, in a more sophisticated analysis, simultaneously analyse variation at the level of the group as well as at the level of the individual. There are also reasons why we might wish to *allocate clusters of patients* rather than individual patients to the competing arms of a healthcare trial, that is, to change the design of the trial. One reason is the rather obvious administrative and managerial one: it is often impossible to introduce an innovative service or change in administration to only part of a service and leave the rest as it is. These changes are usually all-or-nothing. The cost of having two competing services within a single district, for example, might be prohibitive. Sometimes it would simply be impossible not to introduce the changes at the level of the cluster rather than the individual. Outside the mental health field we simply need to think of the evaluation of the fluoridation of drinking water or the introduction of car seat-belt legislation to realise that there are often overriding practical difficulties concerning the introduction of change at the level of the individual patient. Another powerful argument in favour of cluster allocation is the fact that patients within a cluster are not isolated individuals (see the immediately preceding paragraph on pseudoreplication). However, as well as correlation within groups receiving the same service, there may also be contamination between the competing arms of the trial if they were both present within a cluster. If a trial involves the evaluation of some sort of educational activity (either at the level of the patient or that of the service providers or clinicians) then there will be contamination through 'cross-talk'. Patients might try to compensate for the perceived deficiencies in their service and might even attempt to change sides. Patient knowledge (lack of 'blindness') is likely to contribute to a placebo effect, and there is also the possibility of patient resentment if one of the competing services is perceived to be better than the other. If the innovations occur at the level of clinic, hospital or district, on the other hand, all the patients within the same cluster get the same service. They do not necessarily know that there is an alternative service being offered in a different location – there will usually be no need to inform the patients that they are part of a trial, and there may be no need to seek informed consent.

The problem of informed consent, however, does need careful thought. If a trial adds an active ingredient to the traditional service, personal counselling or case management for example, would it be necessary to consider whether it is unethical for the control groups to know what they are missing? Is it ethically justified to allocate this extra service randomly at the level of the individual patient? Buck & Donner (1982) considered this problem and decided that the situation should not be regarded as analogous to the traditional drug trial. They concluded that 'if group unawareness is ethically permissible in certain kinds of intervention and healthcare trials, it offers a means of achieving subject blindness which is attractively congruent with the method of randomisation'.

The literature on trials involving randomisation of clusters has been described in detail by Donner & Klar (2000). Let us assume that we are to allocate clusters of patients (clinics, districts, and so on) randomly to the alternative services, rather than randomly allocating the individual patients themselves. One of the major concerns of the clinical trial designer is that of statistical power: how many patients are required to have a sufficiently high probability of finding a statistically significant effect? This requires a knowledge of patient variability and a fairly clear idea of the likely difference between the effects of the competing therapies (including expert judgement on what would constitute a *clinically* significant difference between the groups). Readers who are unfamiliar with power calculations are referred to Lachin (1981), Pocock (1983) or Day & Graham (1991).

Once we acknowledge that the cluster is the unit of randomisation, rather than the individual patient, we then have to take this into account in our power calculations. The total number of patients entering the trial is the product of the number of clusters and the number of patients within each cluster (assuming for simplicity that the latter is constant). Cornfield (1978) provides a method for estimating sample size when large clusters, such as districts or hospitals, are being randomised, while Donner *et al* (1981) deal primarily with the case of small clusters, such as families. The design of a trial involving cluster randomisation can involve completely randomised clusters, stratification of clusters prior to randomisation or, as a special case of stratification, matched pairs of clusters. Outcome might be assessed by an interval-scaled measurement, or it might be binary (well versus ill, for example). Sample size formulae for intervention studies involving all these possibilities are provided by Hsieh (1988). Shipley *et al* (1989) also discuss power considerations for matched-pair studies. One of the aims of stratification of clusters prior to randomisation is to reduce the probability of lack of comparability of patients in the two (or more) arms of the trial. Stratification can be based on the demographic characteristics of the clusters' patients, geographical and social differences between the areas within which the clusters are embedded, various administrative characteristics of the clusters, and so on. Further issues concerning cluster randomisation in large public health trials are discussed by Duffy *et al* (1992).

Returning to power calculations for trials involving complete randomisation (i.e. no stratification or matching), what is the effect of randomising at the level of the cluster rather than the individual patient on required sample sizes? It should be obvious from the discussion of the problem of pseudoreplication that we need more patients in the trial, but how many more? Basically, the size of the trial (number of patients in each arm of the trial) should be increased by the following factor:

$$[1 + (m-1)Q] \tag{1}$$

where Q is the *intraclass correlation* (the within-cluster or within-group correlation or dependence) and m the number of patients per cluster (Donner & Klar, 2000), to achieve the same statistical power as would be obtained under a design with no clustering. The intraclass correlation would typically be estimated from pilot data in which several patients from a sample of clusters were assessed and the results subjected to a one-way analysis of variance (ANOVA) (i.e. outcome measure by cluster membership) – see, for example, Dunn (2004). This ANOVA will yield a between-cluster mean square (BMS) and a within-cluster mean square (WMS). The required estimate of the intraclass correlation is then given by:

$$Q = (\text{BMS} - \text{WMS}) / [\text{BMS} + (m-1)\text{WMS}] \tag{2}$$

where, as before, m is the number of patients per cluster. The estimation of intraclass correlation coefficients is discussed in the next section.

Evaluation of outcome measures

Before we proceed to evaluate outcome, we need to assess the quality of the outcome measures themselves. We need to be assured that we have adequate tools for the job in hand. The discussion will not include the development of outcome measures – for this the reader is referred to Streiner & Norman (2008) and Wright & Feinstein (1992) – nor will we be concerned with validity, this being more of a substantive problem than a statistical one. Instead, we will primarily be concerned with *reliability* estimation and even then with the most simple of situations. More complex examples can be found elsewhere (Dunn, 1992, 2004).

Perhaps the most important need in the planning of a healthcare trial is to check the consistency of the raters or interviewers who are to assess the outcome of the innovation(s). Typically, two or more raters will be asked to co-rate the problems or symptoms of a pilot sample of patients. We assume that all raters have assessed each of the sample of patients once and we wish to estimate a measure of agreement between these raters. For both quantitative and binary (yes/no) assessments we can carry out a two-way ANOVA (outcome by rater and subject) and use the resulting mean squares from the ANOVA table to estimate a form of the intraclass correlation coefficient:

$$Q = n(\text{PMS} - \text{EMS}) / [n.\text{PMS} + m.\text{RMS} + (nm - n - m)\text{EMS}] \tag{3}$$

where n is the number of patients and m the number of raters. PMS is the patient mean square, RMS is the rater mean square and EMS is the error or residual mean square. The dots (.) in this expression indicate multiplication. The derivation of this expression is beyond the scope of this chapter, but is based on the assumption that we are looking at the performance of a random selection of raters selected from a potentially much larger population of potential raters (the so-called random effects model) – see, for example, Fleiss (1987), Dunn (2004) or Streiner & Norman (2008). This intraclass correlation is a measure of reliability. In the case of a binary assessment it is also equivalent to the well-known *kappa coefficient*; in the case of an ordinal measure of outcome it is equivalent to the form of a weighted kappa coefficient (using quadratic weights) – see, for example, Dunn (2004) or Streiner & Norman (2008).

If the reliability exercise involved, say, the use of only one rater, who replicated his or her assessment of each patient m times (a simple replication study with m usually equal to 2), then the appropriate analysis would be a one-way ANOVA followed by an estimation of an intraclass correlation using equation 2 – but in this case the BMS would be the between-patient mean square and the WMS the within-patient mean square. Again, this intraclass correlation provides an estimate of reliability.

Be wary of relying on reliability coefficients provided in the literature or test manuals. They are only estimates (often based on inadequate sample sizes) and *they are not fixed characteristics of a particular outcome measure*. They are a measure of the proportion of the variability in the outcome measure that is explained by differences among the patients. They will vary as the heterogeneity of the patients changes and also as the heterogeneity (inconsistency) of the raters varies. That is, the reliability will depend on the raters using the outcome measure and on the population of patients being assessed.

What is good reliability? Basically, the higher it is the better, but there is no magic threshold for reliability above which we can relax. The key problem in the context of a healthcare trial is the power of the trial. Power can be increased by increasing the number of participants or by decreasing the variability of the measures (i.e. by increasing their precision or by using a more homogeneous group of patients), or both. The precision of the outcome measures will be improved by multiple assessments of each patient, but then the investigator needs to ask whether this is feasible and more cost-effective than simply increasing the number of patients in the trial. The final answer is bound to be a balance between the two.

Analysis of outcomes

This section is short because the statistical analysis of large healthcare trials is no more the province of amateurs than the analysis of clinical trial data. We will briefly illustrate, however, the problems that the analysis needs to address. Typically, there will be a need to adjust for potentially confounding variables. This will involve some sort of matching or analysis of covariance (either for quantitative outcome measures or for binary ones), which will involve the measured putative confounders themselves or a propensity score derived from them. These approaches will be particularly valuable for observational studies in which we are trying to convince the sceptic that we have allowed for sources of bias (Cook & Campbell, 1979; Cochran, 1983). Adjustment for potential confounders (lack of balance that has arisen by chance during the randomisation) may also be useful in the analysis of randomised trials but, here, the aim is usually to improve precision. In the analysis of a randomised clinical trial it is an illogical and pointless exercise to carry out significance tests for differences between baseline measures. Unless someone has been cheating, you know that the results have arisen by chance. Important prognostic factors should be included as covariates whether or not there are statistically significant differences on these variables across groups. If the analysis is being carried out on data arising from cluster randomisation then the covariates can be measured either at the level of the individual patient, or at the level of the cluster, or both, and the analysis will need to take this into account (Goldstein, 1987).

In recent years there has been considerable stress laid on the reporting of confidence intervals in the medical literature (Gardner & Altman, 1989). Confidence interval construction for effect measures arising from cluster randomisation trials is described by Donner & Klar (1993, 2000). More complex statistical analyses of cluster randomised trials will involve modelling of outcome data in which it is explicitly acknowledged that there are different levels of random variation in the measurements. There will be random variation of measurement errors among replications within patients, random variation between patients within clusters and random variations between clusters. Some form of random effects model will be needed for the data. Readers are referred to Goldstein (1987) for a general discussion, and to Collett (1991, pp. 279–280) for a description of random effects models for binary outcome measures.

Conclusion

It should be clear from the above that the author has a lot of misgivings about the design of many research studies that examine the effect of innovations in the provision of healthcare. What about the use of outcome measures in routine clinical practice? It would be clearly much more difficult to defend any particular interpretation put on the results. If it is so difficult to interpret the results of a carefully designed research study, of what possible use could outcome measures be in the haphazard world of routine clinical practice? The present author is clearly putting himself in the position of the devil's advocate and is accordingly putting forward a particularly strong view against the clinician routinely collecting outcome data. Nevertheless, it would be prudent of the clinician to convincingly answer this question before committing valuable resources to such an exercise.

Lest the reader is inclined to dismiss the author as a sceptical armchair theorist, he has been involved in many trials, including, for example, a trial to evaluate the effects of case management after severe head injury (Greenwood *et al*, 1994). It was a trial that exhibited many of the problems detailed in this chapter and also illustrates some of the technical solutions. The trial involved the comparison of the outcomes of care of patients from six hospitals in north London. Three of these hospitals were provided with the services of a case manager, three acted as controls. The whole point of the evaluation was *comparison*. The case managers were convinced that they were doing a good job and none of the outcome measures provided by the case-managed participants would have led them to doubt their beliefs. If there had been no control group of hospitals there would have been no reason to doubt the effectiveness of their service. Comparison of the outcomes for case-managed patients with those of the controls, however, failed to demonstrate any benefits of case management. Case management led to an increase in rates of referrals to specialist clinical services, but this did not appear to lead to any demonstrable benefits to the patients. Note that it is not the collection of outcome data as such that is important to the evaluation of a clinical service. On its own it is of very limited use. Only when they are used for comparison, and only then if that comparison is suitably controlled, do outcome data really become useful.

In conclusion, the present author has serious doubts about the benefits of routinely collected outcome data but is convinced that there is a need for large multicentred evaluations of mental healthcare services, possibly using cluster randomisation, as described by Donner & Klar (2000). In this way, care providers who wish to evaluate their services can do so within the context of a carefully controlled and properly resourced research study.

References

Angrist, J. D. & Pischke, J.-S. (2009) *Mostly Harmless Econometrics: An Empiricist's Companion*. Princeton University Press.

Buck, C. & Donner, A. (1982) The design of controlled experiments in the evaluation of non-therapeutic interventions. *Journal of Chronic Diseases*, **35**, 531–538.

Cochran, W. G. (1983) *Planning and Analysis of Observational Studies*. Wiley.

Collett, D. (1991) *Modelling Binary Data*. Chapman & Hall.

Cook, T. D. & Campbell, T. D. (1979) *Quasi-experimentation: Design and Analysis Issues for Field Settings*. Houghton-Mifflin.

Cornfield, J. (1978) Randomization by group: a formal analysis. *American Journal of Epidemiology*, **108**, 100–102.

D'Agostino, R. B. J. (1998) Propensity score methods for bias reduction in the comparison of treatment to a non-randomized control group. *Statistics in Medicine*, **17**, 2265–2281.

Day, S. J. & Graham, D. F. (1991) Sample size estimation for comparing two or more treatment groups in clinical trials. *Statistics in Medicine*, **10**, 33–43.

Donner, A. & Klar, N. (1993) Confidence interval construction for effect measures arising from cluster randomization trials. *Journal of Clinical Epidemiology*, **46**, 123–131.

Donner, A. & Klar, N. (2000) *Design and Analysis of Cluster Randomised Trials in Health Research*. Edward Arnold.

Donner, A., Birkett, N. & Buck, C. (1981) Randomisation by cluster – sample-size requirements and analysis. *American Journal of Epidemiology*, **14**, 906–914.

Duffy, S. W., South, M. C. & Day, N. E. (1992) Cluster randomization in large public health trials: the importance of antecedent data. *Statistics in Medicine*, **11**, 307–316.

Dunn, G. (1992) Design and analysis of reliability studies. *Statistical Methods in Medical Research*, **1**, 123–157.

Dunn, G. (2004) *Design and Analysis of Reliability Studies: The Statistical Evaluation of Measurement Errors* (2nd edition). Edward Arnold.

Fleiss, J. L. (1987) *Design and Analysis of Clinical Experiments*. Wiley.

Gardner, M. J. & Altman, D. G. (1989) *Statistics with Confidence*. BMJ.

Goldstein, H. (1987) *Multilevel Models in Educational and Social Research*. Griffin.

Greenland, S. (2000) An introduction to instrumental variables for epidemiologists. *International Journal of Epidemiology*, **29**, 722–729.

Greenwood, R. J., Macmillan, T. M., Brooks, D. N., *et al* (1994) An investigation into the effects of case management after severe head injury. *BMJ*, **308**, 1199–1205.

Hill, A. B. (1955) *Introduction to Medical Statistics* (5th edition). Lancet Monograph.

Hsieh, F. Y. (1988) Sample size formulae for intervention studies with the cluster as unit of randomization. *Statistics in Medicine*, **8**, 1195–1201.

Hurlbert, S. H. (1984) Pseudoreplication in the design of ecological field experiments. *Ecological Monographs*, **54**, 187–211.

Johnson, A. L. (1989) Methodology of clinical trials in psychiatry. In *Research Methods in Psychiatry* (eds C. Freeman & P. Tyrer), pp. 12–45. Royal College of Psychiatrists.

Lachin, J. M. (1981) Introduction to sample size determination and power analysis for clinical trials. *Controlled Clinical Trials*, **2**, 93–113.

Luellin, J. K., Shadish, W. R. & Clark, M. H. (2005) Propensity scores: an introduction and experiemtal test. *Evaluation Review*, **29**, 530–558.

Manly, B. F. J. (1992) *The Design and Analysis of Research Studies*. Cambridge University Press.

Newhouse, J. P. & McClellan, M. (1998) Econometrics in outcomes research: the use of instrumental variables. *Annual Reviews of Public Health*, **19**, 17–34.

Pocock, S. (1983) *Clinical Trials: A Practical Approach*. Wiley.

Shipley, M. J., Smith, P. G. & Dramaix, M. (1989) Calculation of power for matched pair studies when randomization is by group. *International Journal of Epidemiology*, **18**, 457–461.

Spitzer, W. O., Feinstein, A. R. & Sackett, D. L. (1975) What is a health care trial? *Journal of the American Medical Association*, **233**, 161–163.

Streiner, D. L. & Norman, G. R. (2008) *Health Measurement Scales: A Practical Guide to Their Development and Use* (4th edition). Oxford University Press.

Wright, J. G. & Feinstein, A. R. (1992) A comparative contrast of clinimetric and psychometric methods for constructing indexes and rating scales. *Journal of Clinical Epidemiology*, **45**, 1201–1218.

CHAPTER 3

Assessment instruments in mental health: description and metric properties

Luis Salvador-Carulla and Juan Luis González-Caballero

Evaluation and assessment are essential components of healthcare and they require assessment instruments with known metric properties. However, health metrics has been developed in a scattered way and the related knowledge is still fragmented, with uneven development in different areas. Whereas in areas concerned with tangible phenomena such as temperature or medical imaging the focus has been on the reliability of technical instruments and interviewers, the evaluation of intangible phenomena (pain, dizziness, anxiety, disability, quality of life, well-being) has raised a whole array of complex questions with regard to feasibility, consistency, validity and cultural transferability, among others. Furthermore, the solutions suggested, for example by mental health experts, has differed from those in the field of quality of life, and even within mental health and 'psychometrics' a significant variability appears across different approaches.

Nonetheless, considerable effort at harmonisation has been made and contributions from fields such as education and psychology have been significant, particularly in item analysis and the development of rating scales. This trend is shown by the number of manuals and books in the field published during the last decade or so, as well as by the increasing knowledge base. For example, McDonald (1999) reviews the main quantitative concepts, methods and computational techniques needed for the development, evaluation and application of tests in the behavioural sciences; Tinsley & Brown (2000) provide a detailed description of the multivariate approaches to the development of rating scales; and Farmer *et al* (2002) give a comprehensive review of the theory and methods related to measurement in psychopathology. Other manuals offer an analysis of outcome assessment in mental health, including the measurable domains (i.e. symptoms, functioning, quality of life, and perception of care), the standards and instruments used, quality measures (i.e. validity, reliability, feasibility, usability and comparability) and links between care provision and outcomes (Ishak *et al*, 2002; Furr & Bacharach, 2008). Last, but not least, guides describing the main scales and their metric properties provide useful tools for both clinicians and researchers (Badía, 2007; Rush *et al*, 2008).

Table 3.1 List of scales mentioned in the text

Abbreviation	Full name	Reference
ADL	Activity of Daily Living	Katz (1983)
BDI	Beck Depression Inventory	Beck *et al* (1961)
BPRS	Brief Psychiatric Rating Scale	Overall & Gorham (1962)
CASH	Comprehensive Assessment of History and Symptoms	Andreasen *et al* (1992)
CGI	Clinical Global Impression	Guy (1976)
EPQ	Eysenck Personality Questionnaire	Eysenck & Eysenck (1975)
GAF	Global Assessment of Functioning	Endicott *et al* (1976)
GHQ	General Health Questionnaire	Goldberg (1972)
HRSD	Hamilton Rating Scale for Depression	Hamilton (1960)
MPQ	McGill Pain Questionnaire	Melzack (1975)
MMPI	Minnesota Multiphasic Personality Inventory	Hathaway & McKinley (1943)
NDS	Newcastle Depression Scale	Carney *et al* (1965)
SCAN	Schedules for Clinical Assessment in Neuropsychiatry	Pull & Wittchen (1991), Vazquez-Barquero (1993)

Adapted from Bech *et al* (1993).

In this chapter we review the basic concepts, describe the types of assessment instruments and present the main metrics and quality parameters used in the mental health field. The main assessment instruments drawn upon to illustrate the discussion are listed in Table 3.1.

Assessment instruments: basic concepts

Assessment may be defined as the process of applying a systematic method to the description of phenomena or objects. Its degree of systematisation may vary widely, from merely assigning pre-established codes to algorithmic quantification systems. Assessment may be subjective or objective. Subjective assessment is characterised by the description of hypothetical or intangible elements (e.g. quality of life, depression), as opposed to the tangible entities described by the experimental sciences, such as weight or height, that is, objective assessment. In the health sciences, this differentiation is not always clear, since there is a great deal of individual discretion in the interpretation of complex complementary evidence (i.e. histology, imaging diagnosis, neurophysiology). This means that many quality norms are the same for objective and subjective instruments. Subjective assessment is less precise, and has been undervalued until recently. The growing demand for measures of intangible parameters – such as satisfaction, support, autonomy, quality of life or level of disability – has determined that the use of these instruments is currently essential in any healthcare field.

Assessment may also be qualitative or quantitative. Qualitative assessment describes in words rather than numbers the phenomena being observed, for example in unstructured interviews (Bowling, 1997). On the other hand, quantitative assessment consists of elaborating rules to assign numbers to a given phenomenon. When assessing a phenomenon, it is important to situate it within a categorical or dimensional model, and in the latter case to delimit whether it is uni- or multidimensional.

Assessment instruments for the measurement of intangible phenomena are based on items. An item is the basic information unit of an assessment instrument, and usually consists of a question – generally a closed question – and an answer, which can be assigned a code. A glossary is an additional list of explanatory notes regarding the precise definition of each item, and how to combine items in categories or dimensions (Stromgren, 1988). Rating scales are based on a variable number of items. These scales should be made using methods that prevent construct bias (Regier *et al*, 1998; Marshall *et al*, 2000; Braslow *et al*, 2005).

Classification of assessment instruments

Bech *et al* (1993) proposed a classification of assessment scales based on the scales' objectives and composition:

- assessment area – diagnostic, symptomatic and personality scales and scales for other specific purposes
- type of administration – scales for the patient, the doctor or other healthcare staff
- retrospective time access – time frame of the assessment
- selection of items – distinguishes among first-generation scales (based on clinical experience) and second-generation scales (derived from the former)
- number of items on the scale
- definition of individual items.

Other authors have since modified Bech *et al*'s original proposal to permit a more complete description of the different instruments used in mental health (Thompson, 1989; Wittchen *et al*, 1991; Ishak *et al*, 2002; Badia 2007; Streiner & Norman, 2008). In general terms, the classification is based on the instruments' complexity, purpose (condition assessed, reference population, assessment period, etc.) and construction (structure, composition of items, and the prevention of potential bias in its completion). These aspects of outcome instruments are discussed below.

Complexity

Assessment instruments may be classified according to their complexity. *Descriptive questionnaires* may be situated at the first level (e.g. socio-demographic questionnaires), as well as symptom inventories (e.g. inventories of adverse effects). The items on these instruments cannot be quantified, so they may be considered merely checklists.

On a second level are the *rating scales*. As their name indicates, their items can be accumulatively scaled, generating overall scores at the end of the assessment. They are composed of individual items, each one describing a well-defined characteristic of the phenomenon being assessed. Their accumulative nature differentiates them from data-collection questionnaires and simple symptom inventories.

On a third level are the *standardised interviews*. These are classified by their objectives (general or specific) and according to the degree of training required for their administration. The latter depends on how structured they are as far as formulating the questions and codifying the answers is concerned (the more structured the interview, the less previous experience interviewers need to administer it). Standardised interviews may be accompanied by a computerised correction system for assigning diagnostic criteria.

Standardised diagnostic systems constitute a fourth level. They provide a codification of nosological entities, with a detailed description of each in a glossary, to make diagnosis easier. Diagnostic systems are called *operational* when they provide a series of rules for diagnosis based on inclusion criteria (e.g. the presence of a minimum number of characteristics of the phenomenon for its diagnosis) and exclusion criteria (e.g. the presence of characteristics unrelated to the phenomenon). When the exclusion criteria refer to the presence of other syndrome-related entities, the system is considered hierarchical, since it imposes a hierarchical structure on the nosological entities included in the system for their differential diagnosis. If the standardised diagnostic system also allows for the codification of various related entities or aspects on different axes, it is considered a multi axial system. There are two principal systems of hierarchical and multi-axial operative diagnosis currently in use: the ICD–10 research system (World Health Organization, 1992) and the DSM–IV–TR (American Psychiatric Association, 2000). According to some authors, diagnostic systems should not be considered assessment instruments. However, in their construction and use, diagnostic systems fit into the general rules of standardised subjective evaluation (Room *et al*, 1996).

Composite assessment batteries may be placed on the next level. These are sets of different instruments (e.g. a data-collection questionnaire, assessment scales incorporated into a battery, a standardised interview covering past symptoms and/or current state, and a computerised system for multiple diagnosis, which allows for diagnostic codification according to different systems). Examples (see Table 3.1) of compound batteries are the SCAN and the CASH battery for the assessment of schizophrenia and mood disorders, as well as the Psychiatric Assessment Schedule for Adults with Developmental Disability (PAS–ADD) for the assessment of psychiatric disorders in intellectual disabilities (González-Gordon *et al*, 2002).

Clinical information systems comprise a whole array of automated instruments designed to link to databases incorporated into decision support systems. These systems and their relation to evidence-based medicine have been reviewed elsewhere (Hunsley & Mash, 2005; Salvador-Carulla *et al*, 2006*b*).

Purpose

The purpose of a scale will determine the content of its items and different aspects of its structure. A scale should always limit itself to the area for which it has been designed, at least until it can be standardised. The purpose is related to the dimension being assessed for the specific population under study, for a given assessment period; this in turn will determine how the scale is to be filled out.

Target content areas and population groups

In mental health and social care, scales are used to assess a wide range of areas, such as symptoms (clinical scales), personality, social, family, sexual and vocational functioning, disability and healthcare (Bulbena *et al*, 2000; Rush *et al*, 2008). Bech *et al* (1993) make a distinction between diagnostic scales and symptom scales. However, symptom scales have been used for diagnosis after calculating cut-off point by means of a predictive validity study (see 'Quality parameters of assessment instruments', below) and diagnostic scales have been used to rate symptoms. An operational definition of the target population is required to define, analyse and test the items as well as the overall reliability and validity of the scale (see below on these quality parameters).

Objective of the study

It is important to differentiate between general scales (e.g. those for evaluating psychiatric 'caseness') and specific scales (e.g. for the evaluation of depression). Specific scales may have different gradations (e.g. the HRSD for the assessment of major depression and the NDS for the assessment of endogenous depression). Wittchen & Essau (1990) distinguish between scales based on a 'wide' concept of mental disorder and those based on a 'restrictive' concept. The most restrictive instruments value specificity over sensitivity and vice versa (this factor is particularly important in the use of standardised diagnostic systems) (Ishak *et al*, 2002; Hermann, 2006).

Time frame

The time frame should be detailed in the instructions for administering the scale. Based on the stability of the phenomenon under assessment, we can differentiate between *trait scales* and *state scales*. Trait scales assess phenomena that are relatively stable over time (e.g. personality and locus of control) and predominantly use item response theory (IRT) for their development (Reise & Henson, 2003). State scales assess a person's current situation (e.g. the presence of depression or positive and negative symptoms), usually during the previous month, the previous week or few weeks, or during the 3 days before the assessment ('here and now' scales).

The assessment period differentiates *detection scales* (e.g. for identifying psychiatric cases, such as the GHQ) from *follow-up scales*. Non-transitional follow-up scales assess change based on the difference in score from one assessment to another (e.g. with the HRSD); transitional follow-up scales assess the degree of improvement or worsening experienced by the patient between the two assessments (e.g. the change subscale on the CGI). When using a follow-up scale, it is important to know how sensitive it is to change.

Type of administration

Self-administered scales are designed to be filled out by the participant or by an informant. Sometimes they include items to calibrate the validity of the answers based on the participant's tendency to dissimulate or simulate (e.g. with the EPQ). Bech *et al* (1993) call this group of instruments 'questionnaires'; however, this term is too general.

Interviewer-administered scales (which Bech *et al* term 'observer scales') are filled out by an examiner. Such assessment instruments require different degrees of professional training for their use (this factor is particularly important in designing and administering structured interviews). These scales require a previous standardisation of raters by means of an analysis of their agreement with a reference examiner ('interrater reliability'). Two extremes in the application of interviewer-administered scales have been pointed out: an *alpha situation* (where an expert rater carries out a closed interview and uses a scale with a few well-defined items, which include criteria for improvement and health), and a *beta situation* (where an unskilled rater conducts an open-ended interview and uses a scale with many poorly defined items, without criteria for improvement and health) (Bech *et al*, 1993).

Some clinical assessment instruments are of a mixed type; that is, they include one section for reported symptoms and another for symptoms observed during an interview.

Construction

As mentioned above, an item is the basic information unit of an assessment instrument, and generally consists of a closed question and its answer.

Number of items

Scales may be divided into unitary or global scales, composed of a single item (e.g. the CGI, GAF, analogue scales of pain or well-being); and multi-item scales. As a general rule, a phenomenon should be assessed with a minimum of 6 items (Bech *et al*, 1993). Scales generally consist of 10–90 items. Some scales are available in different versions. For example, the GHQ is available in versions with 60, 30, 28, and 12 items, and the HRSD in versions with 21 or 17 items (in addition there are other scales derived from this test).

Content of the items

Unidimensional and multidimensional scales are differentiated by their content. On a unidimensional scale, according to the model proposed by Israel *et al* (1983), more than 80% of the items evaluate a single dimension. For example, the MPQ evaluates a physical dimension (pain, and so somatic symptoms), BDI psychic dimensions (cognitive aspects) and the ADL social dimensions. With multidimensional scales, the items assess two or three of these dimensions (e.g. the GHQ and HRSD).

With interviewer-administered scales, there is also a distinction made between the items reported by the patient and those observed by the interviewer.

The item bias or its orientation refers to the part of the syndrome which appears to be best reflected in the scale. This is represented by a percentage of the maximum theoretical score for each category of symptoms (Thompson, 1989). For example, the HRSD has an item bias for the somatic symptoms of depression.

Formulation of the items

The following aspects should be considered when formulating the questions and alternative answers and when ordering the set of items which compose the scale.

Definition

The definition of each item should be exhaustive and mutually exclusive (Guilford's criteria) (Streiner & Norman, 2008).

Comprehension

The language and formulation of the questions and answers need to be adapted to the patient's sociocultural environment. For example, comprehension of linear analogues tends to be better in some cultural environments, while understanding of decimal numeric analogues is better in others. There are different indices for assessing how readily comprehensible a passage of text is (e.g. Flesch's index for English) (Thompson, 1989).

The problem of comprehension is extremely important in assessing specific populations, such as people who have an intellectual disability. Further, the translation and adaptation of a scale previously developed in another language, for another cultural context, should follow a specific procedure, including the process of back-translation. Recently, more complex systems have been applied, such as conceptual translation (see below).

Acceptability

It is fundamental that the items are acceptable to participants. Social desirability is a type of potential bias which can alter the validity of the answers given (Wittchen *et al*, 1991). This should be taken into account when formulating questions for certain items (this type of bias is important in assessing attitudes regarding certain illnesses, such as AIDS or intellectual disability, because participants tend to give the most socially acceptable answers). It is also necessary to limit the number of items, to avoid fatigue and to encourage the subject's collaboration (this problem is evident on questionnaires or batteries with more than 100 items, such as the MMPI).

Preventing bias in completion

Acquiescence (the tendency to answer a question affirmatively) requires that alternate questions be formulated 'positively' and 'negatively'. However, this may significantly diminish the participant's comprehension, and therefore the reliability of the answers. For example, an item such as 'It is untrue that Columbus discovered America – T/F' may easily confound someone with a low attention span.

The 'central tendency error' refers to people's general reluctance to choose extreme response alternatives. This problem mainly affects verbal analogue scales with three or five alternatives (e.g. None, Some, A lot).

Another type of bias is related to the tendency to answer more with the alternatives situated to the right or to the left, and this bias increases when one of the two extremes always contains the 'desirable' alternatives. This can be avoided by alternating which side the positive alternatives are on (first left, then right).

When an interviewer-administered scale is designed, different types of specific biases should be kept in mind. The *halo effect* refers to the tendency to make a judgement at the beginning of the interview (e.g. a provisional diagnosis) which influences how the following items are filled out. This can happen when completing the HRSD, which groups items directly related to depression and severity at the beginning of the interview. The halo effect is important in the assessment of comorbidity with those instruments which use a single evaluator (Buchanan & Carpenter, 1994). *Logical error* occurs in all those items which are apparently related and scored in a similar way (thus the rater could assume that a patient with a high score on 'suicidal ideation' will also have a high score on 'hopelessness'). *Proximity error* leads the rater to score adjoining items in a similar way. *Terminology variance* is due to the attribution of different meanings to the same term. This problem has a special impact on clinical scales, given the different interpretations of a term according to an evaluator's psychopathological orientation or background knowledge. This bias can be avoided by including an appendix with a glossary (as is done with the BPRS).

Selection, analysis and ordering of the items

Meehl & Golden (1982) described a series of principles or steps in the construction of a symptom assessment scale:

1   Select the items based on their clinical relevance and validity.
2   Select the items based on their internal correlation when they are applied to a mixed group of patients (one which includes patients with and without the assessed symptom).

35

3   Select items with different hierarchical weights (describing different aspects of the phenomenon assessed); that is, they should not be redundant.

4   All things being equal, select items with the greatest potential for consensus.

5   Check the results of the group of items selected based on different external criteria (age, gender, etc.), in order to assess their transferability.

6   When steps 3–5 cannot be carried out, repeat the analysis with modified items regarding definition or content.

Items can also be selected based on their usefulness. This is assessed in accordance with three criteria (Thompson, 1989):

1   *Calibration.* There must be a sufficient frequency of replies on an individual item in the population being tested in order to guarantee its inclusion in the scale. Arbitrarily this can be fixed at 10%.

2   *Ascending monotonicity.* The item should show a significant correlation with the global assessment.

3   *Dispersion.* There should be low dispersion with regard to the line of regression of the above correlation.

There are various models for the psychometric analysis of items and their related quality parameters (Furr & Bacharach, 2008). Some of them are based on simple decomposition of any observed rating into a 'true' or 'universal' rating plus an error term ($X = T + E$), while others are based on latent-structure models (Hambleton *et al*, 1991).

- The *classical test theory* (CTT) is a psychometric model which describes the influence of measurement errors on the scores observed for an individual. The true score for a given variable is defined as that which really corresponds to an individual. However, when something is measured with any instrument, a measurement error is always committed, which gives rise to a difference between the true theoretical score and the observed score, obtained by direct observation using a measurement instrument. The CTT is based on a simple and mathematically acceptable definition of the true score which is conceptually usable and makes certain basic suppositions which relate the true score to measurement error.

- The *generalisability theory* (GT) uses a set of techniques based on analysis of variance (ANOVA) to study the degree to which a series of measures from a group of subjects can be generalised and extended to a different group of subjects (Cronbach *et al*, 1972; Brennan, 2001*a*). GT takes into account the multiple factors which can produce variations in participants' scores by applying a multivariate design. This makes it possible to estimate the variance attributable to each one of them, as well as their interactions. Diversifying the measurement conditions increases the representativeness (generalisability) of the results. It also facilitates the design of measurement procedures in which the confounding factors are represented.

- *Item response theory* (IRT), or latent trait theory, attempts to specify the relationship between a participant's 'observable' score on a test and the 'latent traits', which, it is assumed, lie behind these scores. The models are uni- or multidimensional, depending on the set of latent traits which are necessary to explain the behaviour under study. Although IRT considers two more parameters to be kept in mind when studying the psychometric characteristics of a test, that is, getting the right answer by chance and false positives, the two are complementary to the analysis and construction of a test. The process of constructing an assessment scale composed of binary items may begin with the use of total–item correlation indices of the classic test model, followed by an analysis of its latent structure using Rasch's model. Thus, it is possible to establish the relationship by means of manifest answers and the latent dimension (Andersen *et al*, 1989). IRT is likely to be used to characterise items, select items for a test and perhaps even score tests. In IRT, responses are modelled at the item level, whereas, for the most part, CTT and GT focus on test scores over items.

The CTT and GT theories play an important role in the assessment of reliability and validity. Several authors have explored the inconsistencies between and similarities across these different models. For example, Feldt & Brennan (1989) discuss CTT and GT; Bechger *et al* (2003) discuss CTT and IRT; Bock *et al* (2002) relate GT to IRT; and Smith & Kulikowich (2004) relate GT to class latent models.

Apart from these psychometric models, a series of multivariate methods may be used for item analysis (Tinsley & Brown, 2000), such as multidimensional scaling, canonical analysis, multi-trait models and factor analysis (R-mode or Q-mode); these enable investigators to check the uni- or multidimensional structure of an instrument and prototypical profiles (Burger *et al*, 2005). Their application to instruments which have already been constructed or to new versions of them is discussed below, under 'Consistency'.

Answer codification system

Dichotomous categorical scale
Such a scale comprises a series of questions with two possible answers, typically yes/no or true/false. Examples include personality tests such as the EPQ and the MMPI.

Analogue scales
Five different types of system may be used for the answers of analogue scales (Fig. 3.1).

1 On a *linear analogue scale* (e.g. a pain or well-being scale), the participant marks a line of length 7–10 cm to give a score.
2 On an *analogue numerical scale*, the scoring is similar to that on an analogue scale except that numbers are used (e.g. from 0 to 9). On a thermometric unitary scale, the numbers are arranged vertically.

Analogue numerical scales may be graded from 0 to 100 (e.g. the GAF). Sometimes, visual and numerical analogues are combined to increase comprehension.

3   *Graphic scales* ask participants to make a rating with respect to drawings (e.g. a face scale for assessment of well-being). Some authors consider graphic scales to be linear.

4   On *verbal analogue scales*, the rating is done using previously calibrated verbal categories (e.g. by means of Guttman's escalation system). Generally, there are between three and seven response options; Likert considered five to be the optimal number of alternatives. Goldberg preferred to use four options, to avoid central tendency bias. It is generally agreed that above six options, the level of reliability diminishes significantly. Severity scales use more degrees than detection scales (e.g. the CGI has seven, while the GHQ has four). These scales are also called Likert scales in honour of the man who introduced them six decades ago (Bech *et al*, 1986). However,

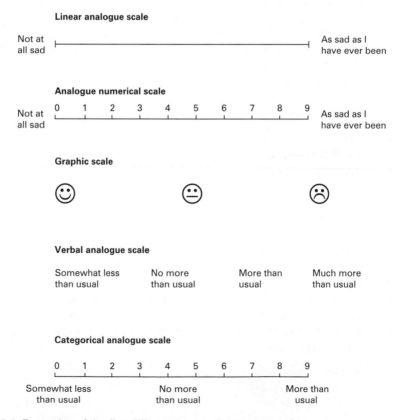

Fig. 3.1 Examples of the five different types of analogue scale.

a specific scoring system bears the same name, so this usage can be confusing.

5 Finally, *categorical analogue scales* comprise a series of responses which combine numeric and verbal ranking (as used for the CGI, GAF) (Bech *et al*, 1986). They are also known as discretised analogue scales (DISCAN).

Scoring the items

The scoring system can vary substantially from one scale to another and even within the same scale, as in the case of verbal analogue scales. Unitary non-transitional scales of severity tend to have a maximum score of 8 or 10 when they are verbal analogue in form, or of another combined form (e.g. DISCAN).

Unitary transitional global scales are generally bipolar, allowing for a positive or negative score (e.g. from greater worsening to greater improvement, or −3, −2, −1, 0, 1, 2, 3). For technical reasons, they can also be scored from 1 to 7, but then the scale's polarity may not be adequately reflected in this approach.

Multi-item verbal scales allow for different numerical assignations. Thus, the GHQ permits three different scorings: two are based on the system originally proposed by Likert in the 1930s, and the other was proposed by Goldberg himself. The HRSD is scored in accordance with the system proposed by Hamilton, which differentiates between the options of absent (0), doubtful (1) and different degrees of intensity (from 2 to 4, or sometimes 5):

- Goldberg 0–0–2–2
- Likert I   0–1–2–3
- Likert II   0–0–1–2
- Hamilton 0–1–2–3–4

Quality parameters of assessment instruments

There are four basic parameters for assessing the quality of an assessment instrument: its feasibility; its consistency or 'structural validity'; its reliability; and its validity. For follow-up scales, a fifth basic parameter should be added: sensitivity to change. Other parameters to consider are adequacy, construction, redundancy and transcultural applicability. Unfortunately, there is no consensus on a definition of these terms in epidemiology; their meaning not only varies from common use but also across different areas of study and even between authors within the same area. Furthermore, different dimensions may be assigned to more than one parameter.

Guidelines for assessing the quality of assessment instruments have been published, particularly in quality-of-life research (Burke, 1998; Marquis, 1998). Badia (2007) used an 11-item checklist which produces a global rating for assessing the level of an instrument's development (the GRAQoL index). An 'Assessment instrument quality checklist' has been included in the appendix to the present chapter.

Adequacy

Adequacy addresses a particular instrument's suitability for the purposes of a specific assessment procedure (in routine clinical practice, in research or in outcome management). Adequacy is not related to the intrinsic properties of the scale, but to its applicability to a defined purpose for a distinct condition in an specific environment. Thus, adequacy should be evaluated separately from other quality parameters.

Construction

Several aspects of the instrument's construction should be taken into consideration in appraising its overall quality. It is important to assess whether the purpose of the scale has been clearly defined, whether there is an accompanying glossary and an instruction manual which clarifies the completion process, the time frame as well as what is required of the rater (see above also on the construction of assessment instruments).

Feasibility

Feasibility has become a relevant issue owing to the increasing importance of outcome measures in routine health assessment (Salvador-Carulla, 1999). There is no consensus on how feasibility should be defined and measured, although Slade *et al* (1999) suggested a definition in the context of routine outcome assessment. However, feasibility is a relevant and frequently overlooked parameter in research-driven outcome assessment as well.

Andrews *et al* (1994) identified three dimensions of feasibility: applicability, acceptability, and practicality. The 'applicability' of a measure was defined as the degree to which a measure addresses dimensions of importance to the consumer, is useful for service providers in formulating and conducting decisions, and allows for the aggregation of data in a meaningful way to meet the purposes of service management. This aspect, defined as 'relevance' by Slade *et al* (1999), may be framed as one simple question: *Is the description meaningful to recipients (e.g. to health authorities, managers, staff, patients/families)?* The acceptability of a measure describes the ease with which a consumer or clinician can use a particular measure (i.e. user-friendliness). Practicality relates to implementation, training requirements and complexity of scoring, reporting and interpreting the data.

Efficiency may be regarded as a fourth dimension of feasibility. It may be defined as the relationship between an instrument's practicality and the costs incurred in its use.

Consistency (structural validity or internal reliability)

Consistency reflects the psychometric 'solidity' of a scale's internal structure, chiefly determined by the degree to which its different items are interrelated and the possibility of adding them up to obtain overall scores. It has been defined as that 'property which defines the level of agreement or conformity of a set of measurements among themselves' (Hernandez-Aguado *et al*, 1990). Some authors include consistency within the category of reliability (Shrout & Fleiss, 1979; Thompson, 1989; McDowell & Newell, 1996) or validity (Badia, 2007). Consistency has also been regarded as part of GT (Brennan, 2001*a*). To avoid such confusion, we distinguish here between the *internal reliability* (consistency, or structural validity) and the *external reliability* of a test (considered in the next section).

Some statistical methods, such as factor analysis, provide data both on the internal structure of a scale and on its relationship to external models. This is the case with the Scales for the Assessment of Positive and Negative Symptoms of Schizophrenia, a factor analysis of which can serve to validate, revise or even refute the models on which the construction of the instrument itself is based (Buchanan & Carpenter, 1994).

Many of the issues related to consistency have been mentioned in the context of selecting items or the hierarchy of their order. *Homogeneity* indicates the degree of agreement among the items on a scale, which determines whether it is appropriate to sum them to generate an overall score. It can be obtained by studying the correlation of the items with the total, using split-half reliability, the Kuder–Richardson formula (KR–20) or Cronbach's alpha, by factor analysis or by using Rasch's statistical objectivity models (Rasch, 1980). The split-half reliability estimates homogeneity based on the correlation between two equivalent halves of the scale (e.g. items from the first half versus items from the second half, or odd-numbered items versus even-numbered ones). Cronbach's alpha coefficient indicates the degree to which different items exhibit a positive correlation (internal consistency above 0.7 is considered adequate) (Bech *et al*, 1993), and the KR–20 is appropriate for scales with dichotomous items (for which it is in fact a particular case of Cronbach's alpha). Conceptually, both coefficients give the average of all of the possible split-half reliabilities of a scale (Streiner & Norman, 2008). Homogeneity based on factor analysis (acceptability of the global score as the sum of that obtained on each item) is confirmed if a unidimensional structure is obtained, that is, all the items show a positive load on the first factor (Thompson, 1989).

In addition to exploratory factor techniques such as principal-component analysis and principal-factor analysis, the structure of a scale can be assessed using other techniques, such as non-metric multidimensional scaling or structural equation analysis (Buchanan & Carpenter, 1994). Rasch's unidimensional model considers a scale to be homogeneous if all of its items contribute independently to the total information contained in the scale. In latent trait theory, the nexus between manifest (clinical) answers and their latent (theoretical) dimension is defined by the requirement that the answers can be combined by adding them until a total score is reached (Andersen *et al*, 1989). Rasch's model also makes it possible to study the internal hierarchy of a scale, by classifying its homogeneous items in a hierarchy ranging from the most to the least inclusive (those which measure the dimension's most to least severe symptoms).

Other quality parameters may be related to either internal or external reliability. For example the reproducibility coefficient indicates to what degree the scale reflects all of the participant's response patterns regarding the parameter measured. This concept may be also linked to the content validity (see below). 'Transferability' refers to the degree to which the scale can be applied to different population groups which present the evaluated phenomenon, independent of their age, gender or other relevant external criteria (Bech *et al*, 1993).

Formal ontology provides a new perspective on the content structure of assessment instruments, particularly in the field of classification systems. Formal ontology is an explicit specification of a conceptualisation (the objects, concepts and other entities that are assumed to exist in some area of interest and the relationships that hold among them) (Gruber, 1993). It has been applied within computer science to formalise the concepts, hierarchies and relationships between different concepts in order to enable semantic interoperability and data transfer. These techniques provide a sound method for describing the content architecture of any classification and assessment instrument, identifying internal errors and thus describing the content consistency of the instrument (see for example Héja *et al*, 2008).

Reliability (external reliability)

'Reliability' reflects the amount of error, both random and systematic, inherent in any measurement procedure (Streiner & Norman, 2008). It has been defined as the proportion of variance in a measurement that is not error variance, excluding errors related to consistency (attributable to the internal structure of the instrument). In this sense, the reliability will provide information about the reproducibility of the test's results in different situations; it also indicates the degree of the stability of the test's measures in spite of changes to external parameters (i.e. parameters not inherent in the test).

Again, there is a wide variation in the terms and methods used to assess the reproducibility or the stability of assessment instruments (i.e. accuracy, precision, agreement, dependability and consistency).

Reliability in the context of CTT

Within the CTT framework, reliability is defined as:

$$\text{reliability} = \frac{\text{participant variability}}{\text{participant variability} + \text{measurement error}}$$

It indicates the proportion of variability attributed to differences across individuals and not to differences in the measurement conditions in the assessment process. This proportion indicates the capacity of a given instrument accurately to differentiate the individuals being measured. Hence reliability depends on the instrument, the target population and the environmental conditions of the measurement (Kane, 1996). These conditions should be specified when reliability is reported (Helms *et al*, 2006).

The reliability may be given in different forms, depending on the conditions as well as on the item's content. For example, a study on the reliability of a diagnostic test should include at least an analysis of the level of agreement obtained when the same sample is assessed under the same conditions by two different raters (interrater reliability). This has also been termed 'inter-observer reliability'. The importance of having evaluators with similar experience, as far as their training and use of the assessment instrument are concerned, has been pointed out. Andersen *et al* (1989) indicated other factors which influence both inter-observer and intra-observer reliability such as the attitudes to assessment scales and therapeutic preferences.

Another measure of stability is obtained when the same sample is assessed by the same rater in different situations (test–retest reliability or intra-observer reliability). Where data are obtained from informants (as is often the case in child psychiatry or in the field of intellectual disability), it may be necessary to analyse the agreement obtained with the test using the same sample and the same evaluator, but collecting the data from two different informants (inter-informant reliability). The procedure for obtaining such information has been extensively reviewed by Costello (1994).

Coefficients for measuring reliability

The coefficients used to measure reliability depend on the characteristics of the variables to be assessed. For quantitative variables or scale scores, CTT suggests a definition of reliability based on different ANOVA models of repeated measures, which produce different types of intraclass correlation coefficient (ICC) (Fisher, 1925; Bartko, 1966; Shrout & Fleiss, 1979; McGraw & Wong, 1996). The crossed-design ANOVA between subjects and factor levels produces an ICC which can be used to analyse internal reliability or consistency, as well as to assess interrater or inter-observer, intra-observer, test–retest and inter-informants reliability.

For example, intra-observer reliability should assess the same individuals by two or more raters in order to show the proportion of variability (0–1) attributed to a single rater. Shrout & Fleiss (1979) and McGraw & Wong (1996) used this approach to assess 'consistency' and 'absolute agreement'. Consistency – ICC2(C,1) – assesses the level agreement reached by the raters in the scores obtained regardless of any existing systematic difference between these scores. On the other hand, absolute agreement – ICC2(A,1) – assesses the agreement between the scores provided by the raters where the variability attributed to those raters will appear as the denominator. Of course, $ICC2(A,1) \leq ICC2(C,1)$. Other models could be applied when raters are fixed (those who did the rating), random (a sample from a 'population' of raters) or when each participant is assessed by multiple observers or on several occasions, or completes a test with several items. Lastly, it is possible to obtain the reliability of an average rating; where items are measuring the same construct, the reliability of the average rating will provide a measure of internal consistency equivalent to Cronbach's alpha. This technique is especially useful if we wish to achieve a given reliability; then, the Spearman–Brown formula can be used to determine how long (how many items) the test should be to achieve that level of reliability (Streiner & Norman, 2008).

For qualitative variables, the use of Kendall's concordance coefficient may be appropriate (Siegel, 1966). In the case of dichotomous or binary variables, item-by-item concordance can be analysed using the percentage agreement and unweighted kappa (Kramer & Feinstein, 1981). The kappa concordance coefficient reveals the level of agreement obtained once chance concordance has been eliminated. This makes it more reliable than a simple percentage agreement. However, because the same kappa value can result from different response patterns, it is expedient to record the frequency of each item's appearance and the percentage agreement on it (Costello, 1994), as well as the confidence interval. Feinstein (1985) proposes the scheme shown in Table 3.2 for analysing kappa results. Other coefficients (Kupper & Hafner, 1989) have been suggested for assessing interrater agreement for multiple attribute responses (Salvador-Carulla *et al*, 2006*a*).

In the case of ordinal variables, analysis of item-by-item concordance can be conducted using the weighted percentage agreement and the weighted kappa. These are considered to be better than their unweighted analogues, since they give a more realistic measure of the level of agreement. This is achieved by weighting disagreement according to the number of degrees separating the score assigned by one evaluator from that assigned by another. Thus, the assigned weight can be 0 for complete agreement, 1 when there is one degree of difference, 2 when there are two, and so on (Kramer & Feinstein, 1981). Fleiss & Cohen (1973) showed that the weighted kappa value is identical to the ICC when quadratic weights are used. Quadratic weights estimate disagreement weights on the square of the amount of discrepancy.

There is currently no general agreement on the sample size required for reliability studies of scales (Bech *et al*, 1993), although several alternatives have been suggested for different coefficients of reliability (Charter, 1999).

Reliability (dependability) in the context of GT

Cronbach *et al* (1972) introduced GT as an extension of CTT. It can be used to assess a broad number of psychometric quality parameters such as accuracy and precision, validity or reliability (or 'dependability' in the terminology of GT). The reliability models and coefficients derived from GT can be used to analyse the degree of reliability attributable to all the

Table 3.2 Analysis of kappa results

Kappa value	Level of agreement
<0	Poor
0–0.20	Low
0.21–0.40	Fair
0.41–0.60	Moderate
0.61–0.80	Strong
0.81–1.0	Almost perfect

After Feinstein (1985).

factors ('facets' in GT) involved in the evaluation process at the same time, whereas CTT can analyse only one factor at a time (different periods of time, or different instruments, raters, informants, etc.). Therefore it can be used to identify the best alternative to carry out an assessment at a given level of reliability (Brennan, 2001*b*).

Also, GT allows simultaneous analysis of several coefficients of reliability (inter- and intra-observer, test–retest, inter-informant, etc.), generalised to fixed or to random conditions. For example, a questionnaire on service use could be used by different observers to collect data from different sources (clinical records, patients, family carers). Using GT, we may be able to assess the reliability of every section and of the overall questionnaire for different groupings of observers and information sources; it is then possible to select the combination of facets that gives the best reliability.

Generalisability theory was introduced in mental health measurement only recently. It has been used to analyse sources of variability and reliability in clinical trials (Vangeneugden *et al*, 2005), the accuracy and reliability of the split version of the GAF (Pedersen *et al*, 2007) and the psychometric properties of scores in a study of psychodynamic psychotherapy (Hagtvet & Hoglend, 2008). GT is still under development and needs further work. It has not been sufficiently used in mental health, probably owing to the difficulty in interpretating the ANOVA models used. For example, the analysis of reliability has to be extended to the multivariate case for complex systems with interdependent components. It is also necessary to explore the relationship with other psychometric models and different aspects related to the calculation of estimates using GT (Kane, 1996, 2002; Brennan, 2000, 2001*b*). Cronbach & Shavelson (2004) discuss the relationship between GT and classical coefficients of reliability and internal consistency such as split-half reliability, KR–20 or Cronbach's alpha.

Validity

Validity indicates which proportion of the information collected is relevant to the formulated question, and is defined by the degree to which an instrument measures what it is supposed to measure. Validity and reliability are closely connected. On the one hand, validity cannot be assessed unless the instrument is reliable. On the other, reliability and validity are related in the decomposition of the observed variance in scale scores. It includes the random error, the construct variance and the variance due to systematic errors (Judd *et al*, 1991). The construct variance has a direct influence on the validity and the reliability of any instrument, whereas systematic errors influence only the reliability. Optimising both reliability and validity requires sacrificing the maximisation of each (the 'attenuation paradox').

Validity is considered present when the measurement predicts a criterion (criterion validity); or, if there is no external criterion that can serve as a gold standard, the instrument is valid if it consistently fits a series of related constructs within the context of an accepted theory (construct validity) (Thiemann *et al*, 1987). There are multiple forms of validity, with the further complication that the same term is sometimes used to define different concepts. The six principal forms of validity can be distributed across two axes: the presence or absence of a gold standard for the dimension assessed (criterion validity *v.* construct validity); and whether mathematical techniques are used in the calculation (descriptive validity versus statistical validity). Thus, a certain type of validity can be considered of the criterion or the construct type, depending on the dimension assessed. The concurrent validity of a scale for service assessment, say, will form part of criterion validity, whereas the concurrent validity for a quality-of-life scale, for which there is no gold standard, should be considered as part of its construct validity. Likewise, estimation of discriminant validity or convergent validity may be merely descriptive or may involve the use of statistical procedures.

The absence of a conceptual framework has led to a notable degree of confusion in the definition and classification of different forms of validity. For example, concurrent and predictive validity are types of criterion validity according to some authors (Strang *et al*, 1989), while others consider them types of construct validity (Thompson, 1989). In fact, the majority of psychological attributes and mental processes are intangible parameters, which cannot be measured directly (unlike, say, height or weight); therefore, they should be considered hypothetical constructs. However, it is accepted that many psychiatric constructs are close to a gold standard (e.g. the somatic symptoms of depression, and anhedonia), while others cannot be compared with external criteria (e.g. quality of life, social integration).

Bearing in mind these considerations and exceptions, the principal types of validity of an assessment instrument are as follows:

- *Simple validity (face validity)*. This is a type of descriptive criterion validity. It reflects expert opinion. There may be a certain amount of confusion between this concept and that of applicability. However, the latter refers to the judgement of a wide-ranging group of users of the instrument, or of the information derived from it (e.g. healthcare managers or clinicians), whereas the assessment of face validity is limited to expert opinion.

- *Content validity.* This defines the degree to which the set of items on a test adequately represents the domain assessed, that is, the representativeness of the items of the set of components under assessment. In reality, this concept does not differ much from that of consistency, so that they may be considered synonymous. According to Thompson (1989), this type of validity is purely descriptive, and cannot be analysed using statistical techniques. Formal ontology has provided a new perspective to the analysis of content validity, particularly in the field of classification systems (Romá-Ferri & Palomar, 2008).

- *Commensurability.* This concept is closely linked to content validity. Commensurability is related to the 'apples and oranges' problem, where substantively disparate items have been grouped together. Classical measures of quality of life may face content validity problems related to this factor (Steel *et al*, 2008).

- *Discriminant validity.* This refers to the degree to which an instrument measures those features belonging to one domain and not to others, as well as the degree to which the features of different domains are not included within the domain examined by the instrument (inclusion and exclusion discriminant validity). Discriminant validity may be assessed either descriptively or with statistical procedures.

- *Convergent validity.* This refers to the assessment of a certain feature of a domain with two different methods (e.g. assessment of depression using an assessment scale and a biological test). This term has also been used to denote the use of two assessment instruments, each covering a different dimension, in order to find a third (e.g. the use of clinical and functioning scales to study the validity of a quality-of-life scale).

- *Concurrent validity.* This provides a measure of the association between scores on different items and the overall scores for other reference scales with an equivalent purpose and content. It is generally limited to the study of inter-score correlation. Czobor *et al* (1991) suggested the use of canonical component analysis, a method which is an extension of factor analysis for two groups of variables. Although some authors have considered this type of validity as a form of construct validity, it actually constitutes one of the strategies used to assess the validity of a test in the absence of a gold standard.

- *Predictive validity.* Predictive observation validity refers to the probability that a scale will produce a correct judgement of the observed phenomenon. The use of Bayes's analysis makes it possible to determine the predictive validity of a test, its utility and its comparability, based on an analysis of the distribution of 'cases' and 'non-cases' in a given population, as well as its relationship with the results obtained on the test under study (positive or negative). A 2×2 contingency table expresses this relationship in terms of true positives (TP), true negatives (TN), false positives (FP) and false negatives (FN). Table 3.3 defines the predictive validity coefficients obtained from the contingency table. Sensitivity (x) corresponds to the TP rate, and is defined by the rate of correct positive results on the test in relation to the total of true cases in the population assessed (TP/TP+TN). Specificity (y) corresponds to the proportion of TN on the test among all the non-cases (TN/TN+FN). Other measures related to the above are the rate of FP rate (1−y), the FN rate (1−x) and Youden's index (x + y−1).

Positive predictive value (PPV) corresponds to the proportion of TP results among all the total of positives (TP/TP+FP); negative predictive value (NPV) corresponds to the total TN as a proportion of all the negatives (TN/TN+FN). It is important to bear in mind the prevalence of the reference criteria in the population assessed, since prevalence rates above or below 50% will alter the PPV and NPV rates. Baldessarini *et al* (1988) provide a clear example of the influence of these variations. Other parameters obtainable by applying Bayes's theorem are positive and negative predictive reason, the misclassification rate of predictive values, efficiency (cases not detected by the test in relation to the total number of cases), bias (the proportion of those assessed who were considered positive or negative) and the odds ratio (Table 3.3).

These coefficients make it possible to adjust the cut-off point according to the objective of the study. If the purpose is to conduct a two-phase sampling study, we should look for a cut-off point that enables us to enrol the maximum number of cases, even though some of them may be FP (acceptable specificity with optimal sensitivity). If, on the other hand, we wish to ascertain the probable morbidity of a population with a test score, we should select a cut-off point that enables us to rule out the highest number of non-cases, even though this could mean the loss of some FN (acceptable sensitivity with optimal specificity).

Alternatively, a test's ideal cut-off point can be calculated with receiver operating characteristics (ROC) analysis. This technique was developed in the 1960s to assess radar controllers' capacity to discriminate between signals. First, a graphic representation of the TP (sensitivity) and FP (specificity) rates is obtained for each cut-off point; calculation of the area beneath the resulting curve then indicates the test's discriminatory capacity throughout the spectrum of morbidity. When discriminatory capacity is equal to that obtained randomly, the result is a diagonal line whose lower area is 0.5 (sensitivity equal to the FP rate). Although an ideal test would produce 100% TP before admitting a single FN, so that the area below the curve obtained would be 1.0, in practice the areas below the curve vary between 0.5 and 1.0. This makes it possible to produce a graphic representation of different tests' discriminatory capacities for the same dimension – with the best one being that which corresponds to the curve farthest away from the diagonal (see Thompson, 1989).

Those tests for which the standard TP deviations are very different from those of FN are called 'asymmetric' or 'eccentric'. In such cases, it may be necessary to use two cut-off points in order to differentiate between

Table 3.3 Bayes's analysis and parameters of predictive validity

Prevalence rate 50% ($P = 0.5$)

Test result	Criterion reference (e.g. diagnosis, Dx)	
	Present (P)	Absent ($1-P$)
Positive	True positive (TP) (a)	False positive (FP) (b)
Negative	False negative (FN) (c)	True negative (TN) (d)

Parameter	Definition	Computation	Symbol
Sensitivity	TP/All Dx	$a/(a+c)$	x
Especificity	TN/All no Dx	$d/(b+d)$	y
False positive rate	FP/All no Dx	$b/(b+d)$	$1-y$
False negative rate	FN/All Dx	$c/(a+c)$	$1-x$
Efficiency	TP + TN/All subjects	$(a+d)/n$	Ef
Positive predictive value	TP/TP + FP	$a/(a+b)$	PPV
Negative predictive value	TN/TN + FN	$d/(c+d)$	NPV
Error ratio	False results/TP	$(b+c)/a$	ER
Prevalence	All Dx/All subjects	$(a+c)/n$	P
'Well rate'	All no Dx/All subjects	$(b+d)/n$	$1-P$
Youden index		$x+y-1$	YI
Odds ratio (pre-test)		$P/(1-P)$	OR

Prevalence rate other than 50% ($P \neq 0.5$)

Test result	Criterion reference (e.g. diagnosis)	
	Present (P)	Absent ($1-P$)
Positive	(P) (x)	$(1-P)(1-y)$
Negative	(P)($1-x$)	$(1-P)(y)$

Parameter	Computation	Symbol
Positive predictive value	$[(P)(x) + (1-P)(1-y)]$	PPV
Negative predictive value	$[(1-P)(y)]/$ $[(1-P)(y) + (P)(1-x)]$	NPV

Adapted from Baldessarini *et al* (1988).

the 'positive' and 'negative' participants. Somoza (1996) proposed a new definition of sensitivity and specificity which takes into account the existence of asymmetric assessment instruments, and shows their properties by applying an ROC analysis.

Meta-analysis is a set of techniques used to quantify the information contained in similar studies. It is intended to produce more precise estimates of the effect being studied, and to assess consistency between different studies analysing the same variables in order to combine their results; therefore one of its principal uses is in the assessment of diagnostic examinations. In this sense, techniques for meta-analysis of scales are being used to assess the exactness of a diagnostic test and its ideal cut-off point. The different studies that assess the discriminant capacity of a test tend to present discordant results as far as the FP and FN rates are concerned, owing mainly to the use of different cut-off points and of samples of different populations. Meta-analysis generally uses the results presented in different studies that use ROC analysis to determine the ideal cut-off point: it is a matter of combining the results of these studies by presenting a summary ROC curve. Different authors have described the method (Littenberg & Moses, 1993; Midgette *et al*, 1993; Moses *et al*, 1993).

External redundancy

Generally, redundancy or overlapping of the items on a scale is assessed only when the scale is being constructed (internal redundancy). However, it is also important to investigate the possible redundancy of the items and overall scores with other, similar scales (external redundancy). This parameter is not equivalent to the association obtained in concurrent validity, as, for example, in multivariate cases it is possible to find near-zero redundancy even though there may be a perfect fit between the two tests (Czobor *et al*, 1991). The use of equivalent scales with redundant items in similar populations does not increase the amount of information obtained; however, it does raise the possibility of completion errors (due to fatigue, transcription mistakes, etc.), increase type I and type II statistical errors, and diminishes the cost–utility of administering the tests (Thiemann *et al*, 1987; Czobor *et al*, 1991).

Redundancy analysis can be considered an extension of factor analysis for two groups of separate variables. Factors are taken from a group of variables (e.g. test A) which explains the variance in another group of variables (e.g. test B). The derivation of linear criterion variates makes it possible to assess the importance of each variate in the redundancy relationship between two instruments. Thiemann *et al* (1987) expressed the opinion that, in a way, redundancy is somewhat equivalent to the instrument's inter-test reliability. In fact, redundancy has sometimes been assessed using the kappa coefficient for the agreement between items (Fenton & McGlashan, 1992; Kibel *et al*, 1993).

Sensitivity to change

Sensitivity to change can be examined in correlation studies and by analysing the principal components at the baseline and after the assessment period (e.g. after treatment) and comparing the factor structures at both points. For calculating sensitivity to change, it is useful to compare ratings with a transitional global measure (e.g. the CGI to evaluate a well-being scale's sensitivity to change). In this case, a covariance analysis can be conducted on the score obtained after treatment, taking the baseline score as a covariable and determining the factor 'change in severity' by the variation on the other scale (Salvador-Carulla *et al*, 1996).

Selection of an assessment instrument

The appropriate selection of a subjective assessment instrument is essential for any clinical research in psychiatry. In light of this, the limited number of methodological reviews of this specific area is surprising. Bech *et al* (1993) mention a series of key aspects to consider in a clinical trial:

1   Identify the purpose. Why is it necessary to use an assessment scale in the study?
2   Identify the problem. What is being assessed?
3   Identify its importance. What is the relevance of scales in relation to the hypothesis being investigated?
4   Evaluate the efficiency of potential scales. What is the utility of the information obtained by means of the instrument in relation to the cost of its use?

The last aspect is overlooked with excessive frequency in clinical research. In this case, cost–utility evaluation considers the need for training and preparation before the scale can be used, and takes into account the necessary time and requirements for statistical analysis. It is also important to evaluate whether the additional information to be obtained justifies the higher costs and the time employed both in scoring the tests and in analysing the data. The possibility of increased bias with the addition of an instrument to an assessment battery should also be considered, whether this bias is the result of participant fatigue, an increase in measurement error, or type I or II errors when using redundant scales, such as jointly administering the BPRS and the Scale for the Assessment of Negative Symptoms (Thiemann *et al*, 1987; Czobor *et al*, 1991).

Transcultural use

The use of the same questionnaire in different cultures involves a series of exceedingly complex methodological problems, two of the most important being equivalence levels and translation systems.

Transcultural equivalence

The possibility of international use is a major aspect in the selection of assessment instruments. This use involves a considerable number of problems, to the point that some authors feel it necessary to tackle this aspect in the construction of the questionnaire itself. This is rarely feasible, so other alternatives must be sought.

Flaherty *et al* (1988) proposed five levels of transcultural equivalence:

- *Content equivalence.* The content of each item on the instrument is relevant to the phenomenon in each culture.
- *Syntax equivalence.* The meaning of each item is identical in each culture after its translation into the idiomatic language (written and oral) of each culture. There are several sources of variation here (words, colloquialisms, register).
- *Technical equivalence.* The assessment method (e.g. pencil and paper, interview) is comparable in each culture with regard to the data which it produces.
- *Criterion equivalence.* The interpretation of the measurement of the variable remains the same when compared with the norm for each culture studied.
- *Conceptual equivalence.* The instrument measures the same theoretical construct in each culture. Sometimes the translation of a word can be close to the original while being extremely different on a conceptual level in the two languages.

Translation systems

The most widely used system is *back-translation*. This is different from a direct translation, in that after a first translation by one or more translators, the instrument is then 'retranslated' into the original language by another translator or team, and the two versions compared. This system, however, is not ideal, and its results are often poor as far as conceptual equivalence is concerned (Brislin, 1970). In mental health studies, investigators have tried to complement this system with techniques which enable them to turn a merely linguistic translation into a cultural one. Among these, some of the most striking are pre-test techniques (based on the congruence of the answers obtained) and different forms of translating committees. The translation of the SCAN into Spanish is a good example of the systematisation of these processes in what has been called a conceptual translation (Vazquez-Barquero, 1993; Room *et al*, 1996). A conceptual translation is one in which the essence of the experience being assessed is clearly reflected in the translated version. Concept equivalence takes precedence over syntax. The preparation of such a version is considerably more complicated than the methods discussed above. First, a literal translation is prepared, on the basis of which two independent teams make conceptual translations. Next, these translations are verified to detect problematic terms and concepts. A consensus is then sought regarding the target environment's cultural reality. This version is then back-translated, and finally the head of the project evaluates the conceptual similarity of each item.

Other tests for transcultural evaluation

There is no consensus regarding the psychometric tests required for an assessment instrument to be used in different cultures. Some authors consider that an instrument should go through the entire analytical process once again. However, this tends to be too expensive. There is generally a need to reassess reliability (Wittchen *et al*, 1991) and validity (above all in the case of screening instruments in which a cut-off point for detection has been established). The need for an exhaustive analysis of internal consistency is questionable.

Conclusion

The use of psychiatric assessment scales is well established in different areas, from clinical epidemiology to pharmacology (the purpose for which many clinical follow-up scales were originally developed). However, given their number and diversity and the fact that new ones are being developed all the time, computerised, systematic inventories are now more important than ever for the orientation of clinicians and investigators. One guide for their classification could be based on the following parameters: complexity, purpose and design. Evaluation of each instrument's quality can be based on a series of parameters related to its adequacy, construction, feasibility, consistency, reliability, validity and sensitivity to change. Lastly, it is necessary to consider an instrument's cost-effectiveness or efficiency, as well as its relationship to other instruments used in the study (redundancy). An adequate adaptation and standardisation should be performed in every different cultural setting.

References

American Psychiatric Association (2000) *Diagnostic and Statistical Manual of Mental Disorders* (4th edition, text revision) (DSM–IV–TR). APA.

Andersen, J., Larsen, J. K., Schultz, V., *et al* (1989) The Brief Psychiatric Rating Scale: dimension of schizophrenia – reliability and construct validity. *Psychopathology*, **22**, 168–176.

Andreasen, N. C., Flaum, M. & Arndt, S. (1992) The Comprehensive Assessment of Symptoms and History (CASH): an instrument for assessing diagnosis and psycho-pathology. *Archives of General Psychiatry*, **49**, 615–623.

Andrews, G., Peters, L. & Teeson, M. (1994) *Measurement of Consumer Outcome in Mental Health: A Report to the National Mental Health Information Strategies Committee.* Clinical Research Unit for Anxiety Disorders.

Badia, X. (2007) *La medida de la salud: guía de escalas de medición en español* [Health measurement: guide to rating scales in Spanish]. Tecnología y Ediciones del Conocimiento, S.L

Baldessarini, R. J., Finklestein, S. & Arana, G. W. (1988) Predictive power of diagnostic tests. In *Psychobiology and Psychopharmacology* (ed. F. Flasch), pp. 175–189. Norton.

Bartko, J. J. (1966) The intraclass correlation coefficient as a measure of reliability. *Psychological Reports*, **19**, 3–11

Bech, P., Kastrup, M. & Rafaelsen, O. J. (1986) Mini compendium of rating scales for states of anxiety, depression, mania, schizophrenia with corresponding DSM–III syndromes. *Acta Psychiatrica Scandinavica*, **73** (suppl. 326), 1–37.

Bech, P., Malt, U. F., Dencker, S. J., *et al* (eds) (1993) Scales for assessment of diagnosis and severity of mental disorders. *Acta Psychiatrica Scandinavica*, **87** (suppl. 372), 1–87.

Bechger, T., Beguin, A., Maris, G., et al (2003) *Combining Classical Test Theory and Item Response Theory*. Measurement and Research Department Reports No. 2003–4. CITO, National Institute for Educational Measurement.

Beck, A. T., Ward, C. H., Mendelson, M., *et al* (1961) An inventory for measuring depression. *Archives of General Psychiatry*, **4**, 561–571.

Bock, R. D., Brennan, R. L. & Muraki, E. (2002) The information in multiple ratings. *Applied Psychological Measurement*, **26**, 364–375.

Bowling, A. (1997) *Research Methods in Health: Investigating Health and Health Services*. Open University Press.

Braslow, J. T., Duan, N., Starks, S. L., *et al* (2005) Generalizability of studies on mental health treatment and outcomes, 1981 to 1996. *Psychiatric Services*, **56**, 1261–1268.

Brennan, R. L. (2000) Performance assessments from the perspective of generalizability theory. *Applied Psychological Measurement*, **24**, 339–353.

Brennan, R. L. (2001a) *Generalizability Theory*. Springer-Verlag.

Brennan, R. L. (2001b) An essay on the history and future of reliability from the perspective of replications. *Journal of Educational Measurement*, **38**, 295–317.

Brislin, R. W. (1970) Back-translation for cross-cultural research. *Journal of Cross-cultural Psychology*, **1**, 185–216.

Buchanan, R. W. & Carpenter, W. T. (1994) Domains of psychopathology. An approach to the reduction of heterogeneity in schizophrenia. *Journal of Nervous and Mental Diseases*, **182**, 193–204.

Bulbena, A., Berrios, G. E. & Fernandez de Larrinoa, P. (eds) (2000) *Medición clínica en Psiquiatría y Psicología* [Clinical Measurement in Psychiatry and Psychology]. Masson.

Burger, G. K., Yonker, R. D., Calsyn, R. J., *et al* (2005) Generalizability of Brief Psychiatric Rating Scale prototypical profiles and their use in evaluating treatment outcomes. *International Journal of Methods in Psychiatric Research*, **14**, 56–64.

Burke, L. B. (1998) Quality of life evaluation: the FDA experience. *Quality of Life Newsletter*, March, 8–9.

Carney, W. P., Rorn, M. & Garsider, F. (1965) The diagnosis of depressive syndromes and the prediction of ECF response. *British Journal of Psychiatry*, **111**, 659–674.

Charter, R. A. (1999) Sample size requirements for precise estimates of reliability, generalizability, and validity coefficients. *Journal of Clinical and Experimental Neuropsychology*, **21**, 559–566.

Costello, C. G. (1994) Advantages of the symptom approach to schizophrenia. In *Symptoms of Schizophrenia* (ed. C. G. Costello), pp. 1–26. John Wiley.

Cronbach, L. J. & Shavelson, R. J. (2004) My current thoughts on coefficient alpha and successor procedures. *Educational and Psychological Measurement*, **64**, 391–418.

Cronbach, L. J., Gleser, G. C., Nanda, H., *et al* (1972) *The Dependability of Behavioral Measurements: Theory of Generalizability for Scores and Profiles*. Wiley.

Czobor, P., Bitter, I. & Volavka, J. (1991) Relationship between the Brief Psychiatric Rating Scale and the Scale for the Assessment of Negative Symptoms: a study of their correlation and redundancy. *Psychiatry Research*, **36**, 129–139.

Endicott, J., Spitzer, R. L., Fleiss, J. L., *et al* (1976) The Global Assessment Scale. *Archives of General Psychiatry*, **33**, 766–771.

Eysenck, H. J. & Eysenck, S. B. G. (1975) *Manual of the Eysenck Personality Questionnaire*. Hodder and Stoughton.

Farmer, A., McGuffin, P. & Williams, J. (2002) *Measuring Psychopathology*. Oxford University Press.

Feinstein, A. R. (1985) *Clinical Epidemiology*. W. B. Saunders.

Feldt, L. S. & Brennan, R. L. (1989) Reliability. In *Educational Measurement* (3rd edition) (ed. R. L. Linn), pp. 105–146. American Council on Education and Macmillan.

Fenton, W .& McGlashan, T. H. (1992) Testing systems for assessment of negative symptoms in schizophrenia. *Archives of General Psychiatry*, **49**, 179–184.

Fisher, R. A. (1925) *Statistical Methods for Research Workers*. Oliver & Boyd.

Flaherty, J. A., Gaviria, F. M., Pathak, D., *et al* (1988) Developing instruments for cross-cultural psychiatric research. *Journal of Nervous and Mental Diseases*, **176**, 257–263.

Fleiss, J. L. & Cohen, J. (1973) The equivalence of weighted kappa and the intraclass correlation coefficient as measures of reliability. *Educational and Psychological Measurement*, **33**, 613–619.

Furr, M. & Bacharach, V. R. (2008) *Psychometrics: An Introduction*. Sage.

Goldberg, D. (1972) *The Detection of Psychiatric Illness by Questionnaire. Maudsley Monograph. No. 21*. Oxford University Press.

González-Gordon, R. G., Salvador-Carulla, L., Romero, C., *et al* (2002) Feasibility, reliability and validity of the Spanish version of Psychiatric Assessment Schedule for Adults with Developmental Disability: a structured psychiatric interview for intellectual disability. *Journal of Intellectual Disability Research*, **46**, 209–217.

Gruber, T. R. (1993) Toward principles for the design of ontologies used for knowledge sharing. *International Journal Human–Computer Studies*, **43**, 907–928.

Guy, W. (1976) *Clinical Global Impression. ECDEU Assessment Manual for Psychopharmacology*. National Institute of Mental Health, 1976.

Hagtvet, K. A. & Hoglend, P. A. (2008) Assessing precision of change scores in psychodynamic psychotherapy: a generalizability theory approach. *Measurement and Evaluation in Counseling and Development*, **41**, 162–178.

Hambleton, R. K., Swaminathan, H. & Rogers, H. J. (1991) *Fundamentals of Item Response Theory*. Sage.

Hamilton, M. (1960) A rating scale for depression. *Journal of Neurology, Neurosurgery, and Psychiatry*, **23**, 56–62.

Hathaway, S. R. & McKinley, J. C. (1943) *The Minnesota Multiphasic Personality Inventory*. The Psychological Corporation.

Héja, G., Surján, G. & Varga, P. (2008) Ontological analysis of SNOMED CT. *BMC Medical Informatics and Decision Making*, **27** (suppl. 1), S8.

Helms, S. M., Henze, K. T., Sass, T. L., *et al* (2006) Treating Cronbach's alpha reliability coefficients as data in counselling. *Counseling Psychologist*, **34**, 630–660.

Hermann, R. C. (2006) *Improving Mental Healthcare. A Guide to Measurement-Based Quality Improvement*. American Psychiatric Publishing.

Hernandez-Aguado, I., Porta, M., Miralles, M., *et al* (1990) La cuantificación de la variabilidad en las observaciones clínicas [Quantifying varibality in clinical observations]. *Medicina Clínica* (Barcelona), **95**, 424–429.

Hunsley, J. & Mash, E. J. (2005) Introduction to the special section on developing guidelines for the evidence-based assessment (EBA) of adult disorders. *Psychological Assessment*, **17**, 251–255.

Ishak, W. W., Burt, T. & Sederer, L. (eds) (2002) *Outcome Measurement in Psychiatry: A Critical Review*. American Psychiatric Publishing.

Israel, L., Kozarevic, D. & Sartorius, N. (1983) *Source Book for the Geriatric Assessment: I. Evaluation in Gerontology*. World Health Organization/Karger.

Judd, C. M., Smith, E. R. & Kidder, L. H. (1991) *Research Methods in Social Relations* (6th edition). Holt, Rinehart and Winston.

Kane, M. (1996) The precision of measurement. *Applied Measurement in Education*, **9**, 355–379.

Kane, M. (2002) Inferences about variance components and reliability–generalizability coefficients. *Journal of Educational Measurement*, **39**, 165–181.

Katz, S. (1983) Assessing self-maintenance: activities of daily living, mobility, and instrumental activities of daily living. *Journal of the American Geriatric Society*, **31**, 721–727.

Kibel, D. A., Laffont, I. & Liddle, P. F. (1993) The composition of the negative syndrome of chronic schizophrenia. *British Journal of Psychiatry*, **162**, 744–750.

Kramer, M. S. & Feinstein, A. R. (1981) Clinical biostatistics: LIV. The biostatistics of concordance. *Clinical and Pharmacological Therapy*, **29**, 111–123.

Kupper, L. L. & Hafner, K. B. (1989) On assessing interrater agreement for multiple attribute responses. *Biometrics*, **45**, 957–967.

Littenberg, B. & Moses, L. E. (1993) Estimating diagnostic accuracy from multiple conflicting reports: a new meta-analytic method. *Medical Decision Making*, **13**, 313–321.

Marquis, P. (1998) Strategies for interpreting quality of life questionnaires. *Quality of Life Newsletter*, March (special issue), 3–4.

Marshall, M., Lockwood, A., Bradley, C., *et al* (2000) Unpublished ratings scales: a major source of bias in randomised controlled trials of treatments for schizophrenia. *British Journal of Psychiatry*, **176**, 249–252.

McDonald, R. P. (1999) *Test Theory: A Unified Treatment*. Lawrence Erlbaum Associates.

McDowell, I. & Newell, C. (1996) *Measuring Health: A Guide to Rating Scales and Questionnaires*. Oxford University Press.

McGraw, K. O. & Wong, S. P. (1996) Forming inferences about some intraclass correlation coefficients. *Psychological Methods*, **1**, 30–46.

Meehl, P. & Golden, R. R. (1982) Taxonometric methods. In *Handbook of Research Methodology in Clinical Psychology* (eds P. C. Kendall & J. N. Butcher), pp. 127–181. Wiley.

Melzack, R. (1975) The McGill pain questionnaire: major properties and scoring methods. *Pain*, **1**, 275–299.

Midgette, A. S., Stukel, T. A. & Littenberg, B. (1993) A meta-analytic method for summarizing diagnostic test performances: receiver-operating-characteristic – summary point estimates. *Medical Decision Making*, **13**, 253–257.

Moses, L. E., Shapiro, D. & Littenberg, B. (1993) Combining independent studies of a diagnostic test into a summary ROC curve: data-analytic approaches and some additional considerations. *Statistics in Medicine*, **12**, 1293–1316.

Overall, J. E. & Gorham, D. R. (1962) The Brief Psychiatric Rating Scale. *Psychological Reports*, **10**, 790–812.

Pedersen, G., Hagtvetb, K. A. & Karterud, S. (2007) Generalizability studies of the Global Assessment of Functioning – split version. *Comprehensive Psychiatry*, **48**, 88–94.

Pull, C. B. & Wittchen, H.-U. (1991) The CIDI, SCAN, and IPDE: structured diagnostic interviews for ICD–10 and DSM–III–R. *European Psychiatry*, **6**, 227–285.

Rasch, G. (1980) *Probabilistic Models for Some Intelligence and Attainment Tests*. University of Chicago Press.

Regier, D. A., Kaelber, C. T., Rae, D. S., *et al* (1998) Limitations of diagnostic criteria and assessment instruments for mental disorders. *Archives of General Psychiatry*, **55**, 109–115.

Reise, S. P. & Henson, J. M. (2003) A discussion of modern versus traditional psychometrics as applied to personality assessment scales. *Journal of Personality Assessment*, **81**, 93–103.

Romá-Ferri, M. T. & Palomar, M. (2008) Analysis of health terminologies for use as ontologies in healthcare information systems [in Spanish]. *Gaceta sanitaria*, **22**, 421–433.

Room, R., Janca, A., Bennet, L. A., *et al* (1996) WHO cross-cultural applicability research on diagnosis and assessment of substance use disorders: an overview of methods and selected results. *Addiction*, **91**, 199–220.

Rush, J., First, M. B. & Blacker, D. (2008) *Handbook of Psychiatric Measures* (2nd edition). American Psychiatric Publishing.

Salvador-Carulla, L. (1999) Routine outcome assessment in mental health research. *Current Opinion in Psychiatry*, **12**, 207–210.

Salvador-Carulla, L., Huete, T., Hernan, M. A., *et al* (1996) Validación del Indice de Bienestar General en pacientes con depresión mayor [Validation of the General Wellbeing Index in patients with major depression]. In *Avances en Trastornos Afectivos* (eds M. Gutierrez, J. Ezcurra & P. Pichot), pp. 289–306. Ediciones en Neurociencias.

Salvador-Carulla, L., Poole, M., Gonzalez, J. L., *et al* (2006a) Development and usefulness of an instrument for the standard description and comparison of services for disabilities (DESDE). *Acta Psychiatrica Scandinavica*, **114** (suppl. 432), 19–28.

Salvador-Carulla, L., Haro, J. M. & Ayuso-Mateos, J. L. (2006b) A framework for evidence-based mental health care and policy. *Acta Psychiatrica Scandinavica*, **111** (suppl. 432), 5–11.

Shrout, P. E. & Fleiss, J. L. (1979) Intraclass correlation: uses in assessing rater reliability. *Psychological Bulletin*, **86**, 420–428.

Siegel, S. (1966) *Non-parametric Statistics for Behavioral Sciences*. McGraw-Hill.

Slade, M., Thornicroft, G. & Glover, G. (1999) The feasibility of routine outcome measurement. *Social Psychiatry and Psychiatric Epidemiology*, **34**, 243–249.

Smith, E. V. & Kulikowich, J. M. (2004) An application of generalizability theory and many-facet Rasch measurement using a complex problem-solving skills assessment. *Educational and Psychological Measurement*, **64**, 617–639.

Somoza, E. (1996) Eccentric diagnostic tests: redefining sensitivity and specificity. *Medical Decision Making*, **16**, 15–23.

Steel, P., Schmidt, J. & Shultz, J. (2008) Refining the relationship between personality and subjective well-being. *Psychological Bulletin*, **134**, 138–161.

Strang, J., Bradley, B. & Stockwell, T. (1989) Assessment of drug and alcohol use. In *The Instruments of Psychiatric Research* (ed. C. Thompson), pp. 211–232. Wiley.

Streiner, D. L. & Norman, G. R. (2008) *Health Measurement Scales: A Practical Guide to Their Development and Use* (4nd edition). Oxford University Press.

Stromgren, E. (1988) The lexicon and issues in the relation of psychiatric concepts and terms. In *International Classification in Psychiatry* (eds J. E. Mezzich & M. von Cranach), pp. 175–179. Cambridge University Press.

Thiemann, S., Csernansky, J. G. & Berger, P. (1987) Rating scales in research: the case of negative symptoms. *Psychiatry Research*, **20**, 47–55.

Thompson, C. (ed.) (1989) *The Instruments of Psychiatric Research*. Wiley.

Tinsley, H. E. A. & Brown, S. D. (2000) *Handbook of Applied Multivariate Statistics and Mathematical Models*. Academic Press

Vangeneugden, T., Laenen, A., Geys, H., *et al* (2005) Applying concepts of generalizability theory on clinical trial data to investigate sources of variation and their impact on reliability. *Biometrics*, **61**, 295–304.

Vazquez-Barquero, J. L. (ed.) (1993) *SCAN. Cuestionarios para la evaluación clínica en psiquiatría* [SCAN: Questionnaires for Clinical Assessment in Psychiatry]. Meditor.

Wittchen, H-U. & Essau, C. A. (1990) Assessment of symptoms and psychosocial disabilities in primary care. In *Psychological Disorders in General Medical Settings* (eds N. Sartorius, D. Goldberg, G. de Girolamo, *et al*), pp. 111–136. Hogrefe & Huber Publishers.

Wittchen, H-U., Robins, L. N., Cottler, L. B., *et al* (1991) Cross-cultural feasibility, reliability and sources of variance of the Composite International Diagnostic Interview (CIDI). *British Journal of Psychiatry*, **159**, 645–653.

World Health Organization (1992) *International Classification of Diseases* (10th revision) (ICD–10). WHO.

Appendix. Assessment Instrument Quality Checklist

- Name and acronym (if translation, note original versions, as well):

- Objective of the instrument:

- Purpose for which the rater intends to use the instrument:

- Dimensions to be evaluated:

Score the following items based on all available literature and your previous experience with the instrument. Use the information obtained in every section to score the overall ratings (do not rate sections which are not applicable for this particular instrument).

Adequacy

Is the instrument relevant to the purpose for which the rater intends to use it?
    1. Not at all   2. Insufficient   3. Acceptable   4. Excellent

Is questionnaire's complexity appropriate to the purpose for which the rater intends to use it?
    1. Not at all   2. Insufficient   3. Acceptable   4. Excellent

Does the instrument cover the dimensions to be assessed?
    1. Not at all   2. Insufficient   3. Acceptable   4. Excellent

If not, can it be 'batterised' (administered jointly with other instruments in order to assess different dimensions of the same phenomenon)?
    1. Not at all   2. Insufficient   3. Acceptable   4. Excellent

Is there information available on the instrument's standardisation in the specific cultural/group environment in which it is to be used?
    1. Not at all   2. Insufficient   3. Acceptable   4. Excellent

Overall rating:
    1. Poor   2. Fair   3. Good   4. Excellent

Construction

Is the instrument's objective defined explicitly?
    1. Not at all   2. Insufficient   3. Acceptable   4. Excellent

Is there a glossary? (Very simple instruments may be excepted)
    1. Not at all   2. Insufficient   3. Acceptable   4. Excellent

Is there an instructions manual or any equivalent within the test which clearly specifies instructions for filling it out, the time frame, and rater requirements?
    1. Not at all   2. Insufficient   3. Acceptable   4. Excellent

Overall rating:
    1. Poor   2. Fair   3. Good   4. Excellent

Feasibility

Is the description given in the questionnaire meaningful for its recipients (e.g. investigators, healthcare professionals, users, managers) (applicability)?
    1. Not at all   2. Insufficient   3. Acceptable   4. Excellent

Is the instrument user-friendly in relation to its comprehensibility, ease of filling out, completion time (acceptability)?
    1. Not at all   2. Insufficient   3. Acceptable   4. Excellent

Are the instrument's data coding and data handling practical (practicality)?
    1. Not at all   2. Insufficient   3. Acceptable   4. Excellent

What is the usefulness of the information obtained in relation to its costs (completion time and personnel) (efficiency)?
    1. Not at all   2. Insufficient   3. Acceptable   4. Excellent

Overall rating:
    1. Poor   2. Fair   3. Good   4. Excellent

Consistency

Has the consistency analysis been carried out on a sufficient number of subjects?
    1. Not at all   2. Insufficient   3. Acceptable   4. Excellent

If the questionnaire generates global ratings, has its internal consistency been analysed?
    1. Not at all   2. Insufficient   3. Acceptable   4. Excellent

If so, name the statistical test(s) used:

Has its factor structure been analysed?
    1. Not at all   2. Insufficient   3. Acceptable   4. Excellent

Overall rating:
    1. Poor   2. Fair   3. Good   4. Excellent

Reliability

Has the reliability analysis been carried out on a sufficient number of participants?
    1. Not at all   2. Insufficient   3. Acceptable   4. Excellent

Has test–retest reliability been analysed?
    1. Not at all   2. Insufficient   3. Acceptable   4. Excellent

If applicable, has interrater reliability been analysed?
    1. Not at all   2. Insufficient   3. Acceptable   4. Excellent

If applicable, has inter-informant reliability been analysed?
    1. Not at all   2. Insufficient   3. Acceptable   4. Excellent

Overall rating:
    1. Poor   2. Fair   3. Good   4. Excellent

Validity

Has the validity analysis been carried out on a sufficient number of participants?
    1. Not at all   2. Insufficient   3. Acceptable   4. Excellent

Are the results obtained significant and relevant to the expert rater (simple validity)?
    1. Not at all   2. Insufficient   3. Acceptable   4. Excellent

To what extent does the questionnaire describe the different characteristics of the phenomenon to be observed, in the expert rater's opinion (content validity)?
    1. Not at all   2. Insufficient   3. Acceptable   4. Excellent

If applicable, to what extent are similar characteristics included in the same group, and divergent ones in different groups (precision/discriminant validity)?
    1. Not at all   2. Insufficient   3. Acceptable   4. Excellent

If applicable, is information on convergent validity available?
    1. Not at all   2. Insufficient   3. Acceptable   4. Excellent

If applicable (i.e. instrument of reference available), is information on concurrent validity available?
    1. Not at all   2. Insufficient   3. Acceptable   4. Excellent

If applicable, is information on predictive validity available?
    1. Not at all   2. Insufficient   3. Acceptable   4. Excellent

If so, name the statistical test(s) used:

If applicable, is information on factorial or dimensional validity available? (Use of exploratory factor analysis should be considered insufficient, unless the data are based on extensive coinciding literature, in which case it should be rated Acceptable.)
    1. Not at all   2. Insufficient   3. Acceptable   4. Excellent

Overall rating:
    1. Poor   2. Fair   3. Good   4. Excellent

Sensitivity to change

If it is a follow-up questionnaire, what is the quality of available information on sensitivity to change?
    1. Not at all   2. Insufficient   3. Acceptable   4. Excellent

Overall rating:
    1. Poor   2. Fair   3. Good   4. Excellent

Redundancy avoidance

If the questionnaire is being used within a battery of instruments, what is the quality of available information on redundancy?
    1. Poor   2. Fair   3. Good   4. Excellent

Overall rating:
    1. Poor   2. Fair   3. Good   4. Excellent

Generalisability

To what extent has the usefulness of the instrument been analysed using different populations and settings?
    1. Not at all   2. Insufficient   3. Acceptable   4. Excellent

To what extent do data on the instrument's psychometric properties come from studies other than the original?
    1. Not at all   2. Insufficient   3. Acceptable   4. Excellent

Overall rating:
    1. Poor   2. Fair   3. Good   4. Excellent

Transcultural equivalence

What is the quality of the available data on the instrument's transcultural standardisation? (Unless the instrument has been validated in more than three different major languages/cultures, it should not be rated Excellent.)

    1. Poor   2. Fair   3. Good   4. Excellent

Overall rating:

    1. Poor   2. Fair   3. Good   4. Excellent

Assessment Instrument Quality Checklist (AIQC) index (%)

$$\text{AIQC index} = \frac{\text{Sum of all applicable 'Overall' ratings}}{\text{Maximum score among applicable sections}} \times 100$$

CHAPTER 4

Using outcomes in routine clinical practice to support recovery

Mike Slade, Lindsay Oades and Bernd Puschner

The term 'recovery' is at the heart of a debate about the *raison d'être* of mental health services. For example, empirical research into outcome in schizophrenia demonstrates that the rate of recovery in the sense of cure – what we will call *clinical recovery* – is higher than is consistent with the traditional view of schizophrenia as a chronic and degenerative disorder. We illustrate this by reviewing all studies with long-term follow-up (i.e. of more than 20 years) in Table 4.1. This highlights the first use of outcomes in relation to recovery: challenging some accepted but under-researched beliefs held by clinicians.

However, some consumers report themselves as having recovered even when they experience ongoing symptoms. This new understanding of recovery – which we call *personal recovery* (Slade, 2009a) – leads to the use of outcome measures in the service of actively supporting recovery.

In this chapter we outline the distinction between clinical and personal recovery, describe some measures which relate to recovery, and then identify specific ways in which using outcome measures in routine mental health services can support recovery.

Table 4.1 Recovery rates in long-term follow-up studies of psychosis

Reference	Location	Sample size	Mean length of follow-up (years)	% recovered or significantly improved
Huber *et al* (1975)	Bonn	502	22	57
Ciompi & Muller (1976)	Lausanne	289	37	53
Bleuler (1978)	Zurich	208	23	53–68
Tsuang *et al* (1979)	Iowa	186	35	46
Harding *et al* (1987)	Vermont	269	32	62–68
Ogawa *et al* (1987)	Japan	140	23	57
Marneros *et al* (1989)	Cologne	249	25	58
DeSisto *et al* (1995)	Maine	269	35	49
Harrison *et al* (2001)	18 sites	776	25	56

Outcomes and recovery

An evolution in the use of outcome measures has become apparent, paralleling developments within wider mental health services. Clinical recovery is a staff-rated characteristic, which has emerged from professional-led research. Clinical recovery has four key features:

1   It is an outcome or a state, generally dichotomous.
2   It is observable – in clinical parlance, it is objective, not subjective.
3   It is rated by the expert clinician, not the patient.
4   The definition of recovery is invariant across individuals.

Various definitions of recovery have been proposed by mental health professionals. For example, Torgalsbøen (1999) proposes that recovery in schizophrenia be defined as meeting the following five criteria:

1   a reliable previous diagnosis of schizophrenia
2   criteria for diagnosis not fulfilled at present
3   out of hospital for at least 5 years
4   present psychosocial functioning within a 'normal' range (e.g. scores > 65 on the General Assessment of Function scale)
5   not on antipsychotic medication or only on a low dosage (less than half 'defined daily doses').

The intention with this definition is that it be operationalisable (i.e. suitable for use in empirical research). It contains diagnostic, service use, functioning and treatment elements. Each of these can vary for reasons not related to the individual and whether he or she has recovered. Diagnostic criteria change. Hospitals close and home treatment teams operate in the deinstitutionalisation era, so admission thresholds alter. Functioning is dependent on the opportunities in the environment. Medication regimens are influenced by prescriber beliefs and current clinical guidelines.

A more socially focused definition of recovery has been proposed by Libermann & Kopelowicz (2002):

1   full symptom remission
2   full or part-time work or education
3   independent living without supervision by informal carers
4   having friends with whom activities can be shared
5   all sustained for at least 2 years.

Their conclusion, consistent with Table 4.1, is that 'it is now realistic to set as a goal the feasibility of recovery from schizophrenia for half or more individuals with first episode'. This conclusion challenges the applicability of a chronic disease model to mental illness, with its embedded assumption that conditions like schizophrenia are necessarily lifelong and have a deteriorating course. A recent collation of all long-term follow-up studies included over 1000 patients between 12 and 26 years after initial assessment

(Hopper *et al*, 2007). Commenting on the results, Richard Warner (2007) concluded:

What do we learn of the lives of people with schizophrenia from this fascinating study...? Most importantly, Kraepelin's view that a deteriorating course is a hallmark of the illness just isn't true. Heterogeneity of outcome, both in terms of symptoms and functioning, is the signature feature ... bad outcome is not a necessary component of the natural history of schizophrenia; it is a consequence of the interaction between the individual and his or her social and economic world.

When we read the accounts of people who actually use mental health services, we learn that sometimes this recovery has been in spite of, rather than because of, mental health services. For example, one such person, Coleman (1999), states:

The psychiatric system far from being a sanctuary and a system of healing was ... a system of fear and continuation of illness for me. Like so many others recovery was a process that I did not encounter within the system, indeed ... it was not until I left the system that the recovery process really got underway in my life.

Perhaps this problem arises from treating recovery as an outcome. Although this allows prevalence questions to be addressed, it also implicitly involves deep assumptions about normality. As Ralph & Corrigan (2005, p. 5) put it:

This kind of definition begs several questions that need to be addressed to come up with an understanding of recovery as outcome: How many goals must be achieved to be considered recovered? For that matter, how much life success is considered 'normal'?

The people who use mental health services have called for a new approach. For instance, Ridgway (2001) argues that:

The field of psychiatric disabilities requires an enriched knowledge base and literature to guide innovation in policy and practice under a recovery paradigm. We must reach beyond our storehouse of writings that describe psychiatric disorder as a catastrophic life event.

The second meaning of 'recovery' – personal recovery – provides this enriched knowledge base. People personally affected by mental illness have become increasingly vocal in communicating both what their life is like with the mental illness and what helps them to move beyond the role of a patient with mental illness. Early accounts were written by individual pioneers (e.g. Deegan, 1988; Davidson & Strauss, 1992; Fisher, 1994; O'Hagan, 1996; Coleman, 1999; Ridgway, 2001). These brave, and sometimes oppositional and challenging, voices provide ecologically valid pointers to what recovery looks and feels like from the inside.

Once individual stories had become more visible, compilations and syntheses of these accounts began to emerge from around the (especially Anglophone) world, for example from Australia (Andresen *et al*, 2003), New

Zealand (Mental Health Commission, 2000; Lapsley *et al*, 2002; Goldsack *et al*, 2005; Barnett & Lapsley, 2006), Scotland (Scottish Recovery Network, 2006, 2007), the USA (Spaniol & Koehler, 1994; Ridgway, 2001; Davidson *et al*, 2005) and England (McIntosh, 2005; Barker *et al*, 1999; Chandler & Hayward, 2009). The understanding of recovery which has emerged from these accounts has a different focus from clinical recovery, for example in emphasising the centrality of hope, identity, meaning and personal responsibility (Ralph, 2000; Spaniol *et al*, 2002; Andresen *et al*, 2003). We refer to this consumer-based understanding of recovery as *personal recovery*, to reflect its individually defined and experienced nature (Slade, 2009*a*).

Many definitions of recovery have been proposed by those who are experiencing it:

Recovery refers to the lived or real life experience of people as they accept and overcome the challenge of the disability ... they experience themselves as recovering a new sense of self and of purpose within and beyond the limits of disability. (Deegan, 1988)

For me, recovery means that I'm not in hospital and I'm not sitting in supported accommodation somewhere with someone looking after me. Since I've recovered, I've found that in spite of my illness I can still contribute and have an input into what goes on in my life, input that is not necessarily tied up with medication, my mental illness or other illnesses. (Sottish Recovery Network, 2006)

This chapter will use the most widely cited definition, that by Bill Anthony:

Recovery is a deeply personal, unique process of changing one's attitudes, values, feelings, goals, skills, and/or roles. It is a way of living a satisfying, hopeful, and contributing life even within the limitations caused by illness. Recovery involves the development of new meaning and purpose in one's life as one grows beyond the catastrophic effects of mental illness. (Anthony, 1993)

It is consistent with the less widely cited but more succinct definition proposed by Retta Andresen and colleagues:

[recovery involves the] establishment of a fulfilling, meaningful life and a positive sense of identity founded on hopefulness and self determination. (Andresen *et al*, 2003)

For those who value succinctness, the definition we use in our local service in London is:

Recovery involves living as well as possible. (South London and Maudsley NHS Foundation Trust, 2007)

Ralph & Corrigan (2005, pp. 4–5) propose three definitions of recovery:

1. Recovery is a naturally occurring phenomenon.
Some people who meet diagnostic criteria for a serious mental illness are able to overcome their disabilities and fully enjoy a life in which their life goals are accomplished without any kind of treatment.

2. As with other medical illnesses, people can recover from mental illness with proper treatment.
Others who do not enjoy spontaneous recovery from mental illness are able to achieve a similar state of goal attainment and life satisfaction as a result of participating in a variety of services.

3. Recovery reintroduces the idea of hope in understanding serious mental illness.
It means that even though a person is diagnosed with schizophrenia or other serious psychiatric disorder, his or her life need not be limited to institutions.

They note that mental health professionals gravitate towards the second definition (clinical recovery), whereas consumers typically find more value in the first (spontaneous recovery) and third (personal recovery).

These three definitions are also used in the joint statement on recovery issued by the Care Service Improvement Partnership, the Royal College of Psychiatrists and the Social Care Institute for Excellence in the UK. Each definition is valued:

Many concerns about engaging with a recovery approach arise from thinking that these different conceptions are in competition with one another, whereas they are complementary and synergistic.... Adopting a recovery approach harnesses the value of current treatments but is directed at living with and beyond these continuing limitations. (Care Services Improvement Partnership, *et al*, 2007, p. 2)

Personal recovery encompasses the three types of recovery listed above. Spontaneous recovery occurs for some people, when the individual's biological, psychological, social and spiritual self-righting skills and supports combine to manage the mental illness. Personal recovery occurs for some people through receiving evidence-based treatments, so treatment is an important element of mental health services. But, crucially, personal recovery is underpinned for all people by hope, meaning, identity and personal responsibility.

Recovery and outcome measurement

How can outcome measures be used to support recovery? Addressing this question involves considering a broader challenge of developing and evaluating empirically supported and recovery-focused services. From a scientific perspective, this will involve three areas: identification and prevalence; outcome measures and evaluation methodologies; and interventions and cost-effectiveness (Slade & Hayward, 2007).

First, the active ingredients of recovery-focused mental health services need to be established. As well as working practices, the ingredients will include staff attitudes, values and beliefs. This represents a change from the current modernist approach to describing services (i.e. they are fully characterised by what they do), in recognising that mental health services involve people, both using them and working in them, so how staff work also matters (Bracken & Thomas, 2005). Once identified, the active ingredients will inform the development of fidelity scales, which assess adherence by the service to the active ingredients required for a mental health service to be recovery focused. This is a standard approach to identifying whether a service model is actually implemented (Teague et al, 1998), a necessary element of evaluation (Campbell *et al*, 2000). Some recovery-focused measures – such as the Fidelity Assessment Common Ingredients Tool (FACIT; Johnsen *et al*, 2005) – and quality standards (Higgins, 2008; Davidson *et al*, 2009) are now available. These fidelity scales can then be used to establish national baseline prevalence estimates of the extent to which services are recovery focused.

Second, there is a need to develop recovery outcome measures. Some measures are already available, mainly from the USA (Wowra & McCarter, 1999) and Australia (Andresen *et al*, 2006), and some are now being evaluated in the UK (Dinniss *et al*, 2007; Slade *et al*, 2009). Most promisingly, compendia of outcome measures have been published which focus on recovery outcome measures either in whole (Campbell-Orde *et al*, 2005; National Social Inclusion Programme, 2009) or in part (National Institute for Mental Health in England, 2008). Assessment of recovery as an outcome needs to be sensitive to the fact that individuals experience recovery as a process, and to the idiosyncratic nature of what recovery means to different people. It is likely to be necessary to integrate both qualitative and quantitative methods into recovery-focused evaluations (Slade & Priebe, 2006) and to include the use of established user-led methods such as User-Focused Monitoring (Rose *et al*, 1998) or Strategies for Living (Faulkner & Layzell, 2000).

Finally, there is a need to develop and evaluate interventions to promote recovery-focused working. For example, increased visibility of recovered service users in teams may combat a clinician's illusion that no one gets better (Cohen & Cohen, 1984). Indeed, an eight-site randomised controlled trial across the USA investigated the impact of participation in patient-run service programmes (Rogers *et al*, 2007). The study found that participants experienced more empowerment in services which implemented the active ingredients, and that a dose–effect relationship was present at the participant level.

Using outcome measures routinely to support recovery

We now present three case studies of approaches to the routine use of outcome measures to improve the lives of people using mental health services.

Case study 1. The collaborative recovery model (CRM) and AIMhi study

Notwithstanding the increasing interest in personal recovery and recovery-oriented services, there are few practice models that seek to combine personal recovery principles and evidence-based practices in mental health. Moreover, a review of research into case management (Marshall *et al*, 2007) demonstrated that only one of 13 outcome studies investigated user perspectives at all. The collaborative recovery model (CRM) (Oades *et al*, 2005; Crowe *et al*, 2006), developed in Australia by a combination of mental health researchers, practitioners and service users, seeks to combine key skills that are supportive of personal recovery and clinical recovery. The development and implementation of the model required all six parts of the model to be operationalised and to include the potential for quantitative measurement as part of routine clinical practice. A key aim of this approach was to bridge the previously assumed dichotomy between personal recovery and evidence-based practice (Frese *et al*, 2001). The components of the model and its operationalisation and measurement are illustrated in Table 4.2.

As one part of the Australian Integrated Mental Health Initiative (AIMhi), the CRM was trialled across four states of Australia in 12 different community-based adult service settings, from government and non-government organisations in metropolitan, regional and rural sites. Inclusion criteria for consumer participants were a diagnosis of schizophrenia, schizoaffective disorder or bipolar disorder of at least 6 months' duration and high support needs, with six or more needs identified using the Camberwell Assessment of Need Short Appraisal Schedule (CANSAS; Andresen *et al*, 2000). Individuals with dementia, severe mental retardation or brain injury were excluded. Comorbid substance misuse or personality disorders were

Table 4.2 Components of the collaborative recovery model (CRM) and quantitative measurement as part of routine clinical practice

Component of CRM	Protocol and outcome measurement
1. Recovery as an individual process	Stages of Recovery Instrument (STORI; Andresen *et al*, 2006)
2. Collaboration and autonomy support	Working Alliance Inventory (WAI; Horvath & Greenberg, 1989)
3. Change enhancement	Decisional balance worksheets
4. Needs identification	Camberwell Assessment of Need Short Appraisal Schedule (CANSAS; Andresen *et al*, 2000)
5. Collaborative goal striving	Collaborative Goal Technology (CGT; Clarke *et al*, 2006)
6. Collaborative homework and monitoring	Homework assignment work-sheets

not excluded. Following baseline, data collection was at 3-monthly intervals, consistent with national routine data collection. Measures included the Health of the Nation Outcome Scales (HoNOS), Life Skills Profile (16-item) and Kessler–10, and the Recovery Assessment Scale.

The AIMhi focused on the use of the Collaborative Goal Technology and homework assignment worksheets as part of routine clinical practice. The goal-striving component is described here to demonstrate the role of routine outcome measurement in directly supporting personal recovery and indirectly supporting clinical recovery. The personal recovery process involves personal choice and growth, in which goal striving is ubiquitous. Goals are linked to the aforementioned key aspects of recovery: hope, meaning, identity and personal responsibility (Andresen *et al*, 2003). That is, collaborative goals, when set appropriately, are a key part of the personal recovery process. Hope and goals are closely linked. Personal meaning and identity are often expressed via personal goals. The act of setting and working towards a goal is indeed related to personal responsibility.

The Collaborative Goal Technology (CGT; Clarke *et al*, 2006) was used to operationalise the collaborative goal setting, striving and review process between staff and pairs of service users. Derived in part from Goal Attainment Scaling, the CGT involved staff and service user collaboratively identifying up to three goals, which were reviewed after 3 months. Three-month periods of review were set to be consistent with the routine collection of other outcome measurements. Based on a utility (value) model, service users were asked to rate the relative importance of each goal by assigning a total of 10 points across the goals sets. Upon review each goal was rated for its level of attainment across three levels defined previously by staff member and service user. This is illustrated in Fig. 4.1.

This enables an idiographic measurement of goal attainment to be calculated, which is weighted by values set by the service user. We call this score the Collaborative Goal Index. Two points are awarded for attainment of a goal at the highest level, one point for the middle level, and no points for the lowest level. The Collaborative Goal Index is a percentage score, calculated as five times the sum of each attainment × importance score. Hence from Fig. 4.1 the Collaborative Goal Index is $5((2 \times 5) + (1 \times 3) + (0 \times 2)) = 65$. The score is a function of level of goal attainment, anchored by perceived difficulty, then weighted by subjective importance.

In addition to calculating the index, staff members and service users were asked to discuss and identify issues that may have affected or even thwarted their goal attainment. Sixteen options were provided, such as: 'I found a better goal', 'Goal was too difficult', 'People criticised me for having this goal'. This qualitative component added to the clinical utility of the routine instrument, by informing the next goal-setting cycle.

While many staff and service users are familiar with goal setting, the routine use of the full cycle of goal striving, in which individual goals are set and then their attainment is systematically and quantitatively reviewed, is less common. Training in the use of the CGT demonstrated a transfer effect for staff members in using evidence-based goal-setting principles in their general case notes and documentation. In a related study (Clarke *et al*, 2009), an audit tool, the Goal Instrument for Quality (Goal–IQ), was used to review 122 goal records in several eastern Australian mental health services as part of AIMhi. Seventy-four per cent of people in recovery had a documented goal record and these had 54% of the evidence-based goal-setting principles measured by the Goal–IQ. It was demonstrated that staff trained in goal setting showed significantly higher frequency and quality of documenting goals.

Routine use of tools such as the CGT are likely to provide useful empirical linkages between nomothetic clinical definitions of recovery and idiographic aspects of personal recovery. While goal setting is often conceptualised as an intervention or a process, goal attainment by definition is quintessentially an outcome. At the time of writing, further research is investigating both the relationship between the level of goal attainment and symptom distress, and the types of goals service users are setting with staff members and how they relate to stage of recovery.

	My personal recovery vision is: To stand on my own two feet			
Stage 1 Meaningful vision and goals	**Attain**	**Goal 1** To do my own shopping	**Goal 2** To find a job	**Goal 3** Improve taking of medication
	Point allocation must total 10	Perceived importance points = **5**	Perceived importance points = **3**	Perceived importance points = **2**
	Awesome	To do my shopping at least once by myself ✓	Go to the return-to-work programme ☐	Complete a medication diary more than 3 times per week ☐
Stage 2 Manageable goals	**Success** >70% confident	To do my shopping at least once with a friend ☐	Go to first appointment with employment assistance service ✓	Complete a medication diary more than 3 times per week ☐
	Keep going	To do my shopping with my case worker ☐	Continue discussing employment goal with case manager ☐	Remember to take medication ✓

Fig. 4.1 Example of completed Collaborative Goal Technology.

Case study 2. The NODPAM study

Our second case study involves an intervention at the point of discharge from hospital. There is broad consensus that relapse prevention is one of the major aims of aftercare. However, the success of attempts to reduce high re-hospitalisation rates for people with severe mental illness has been limited so far. Insufficient discharge planning and follow-up are considered one of the main reasons for limited community tenure and unfavourable clinical outcomes (Olfson et al, 1998; Boyer et al, 2000; Steffen et al, 2009). There is a lack of specific interventions targeting the needs of high utilisers of mental health services (Kent et al, 1995; Lucas et al, 2001; Roick et al, 2002).

The study Effectiveness of Needs-Oriented Discharge Planning and Monitoring for High Utilisers of Psychiatric Services (NODPAM) tests such an intervention. NODPAM is a multicentre randomised controlled trial (ISRCTN59603527) carried out in five psychiatric hospitals in Germany (Puschner et al, 2008). Consecutive recruitment started in April 2006. Inclusion criteria were having given informed consent, adult age, diagnosis of schizophrenia or affective disorder, and a defined high utilisation of mental healthcare. Over 18 months, comprehensive outcome data on 491 participants were collected at baseline (i.e. discharge from psychiatric in-patient treatment) and at three follow-up measurement points.

Measures completed by the research worker during patient interview included the Camberwell Assessment of Need (CAN–EU; McCrone et al, 2000; Kilian et al, 2001), the Brief Psychiatric Rating Scale (BPRS; Lukoff et al, 1986), the Hamilton Rating Scale for Depression (HRSD; Hamilton, 1967) and the Manchester Short Assessment of Quality of Life (MANSA; Priebe et al, 1999). Patient-rated measures included the Symptom Check-List (SCL–90–R; Derogatis, 1986; Franke, 1995), the patient version of the Scale to Assess the Therapeutic Relationship in Community Mental Healthcare (STAR–P; McGuire-Snieckus et al, 2006) and the German version of the Client Satisfaction Questionnaire (ZUF–8; Attkisson & Zwick, 1982; Schmidt et al, 1989). Staff-rated measures included the Global Assessment of Functioning Scale (GAF; Sass et al, 1996) and the clinician version of the STAR (STAR–C; McGuire-Snieckus et al, 2006). Satisfaction with therapeutic work in the out-patient setting was measured with the ZUF–THERA (Puschner et al, 2005), which consists of six rephrased items of the ZUF–8.

Each site had a NODPAM research worker in charge of recruitment and data collection, and a NODPAM intervention worker responsible for carrying out the intervention. Hypotheses are that participants receiving the intervention will show fewer hospital days and readmissions to hospital (primary), and show better compliance with aftercare as well as better clinical outcome and quality of life (secondary).

The manualised intervention focuses on the in-patient–out-patient transition and is based upon principles of needs-led care (Kunze et al, 2004) and critical time intervention (Hermann et al, 2000; Dixon et al, 2009). The manual describes the tasks of the intervention worker and delineates

Table 4.3 Excerpt of a NODPAM discharge plan

Need	Problem	Objective	Time	Responsible	Contact	Compromise/ dissent
12. Alcohol	Peter tends to drink too much when in a crisis	Concurrent treatment of mental illness and alcohol problem	Immedi- ately	Peter	Dr Smith	–

the structure and content of the intervention sessions. A central part of the manual was to complement each of the 22 needs of the Camberwell Assessment of Need (Kilian *et al*, 2001; McCrone *et al*, 2000) by pragmatic, evidence-based recommendations on what to do in case of an unmet need. Intervention workers invited the 240 participants allocated to the intervention group to attend two sessions (of 45 minutes each). Core participants in these sessions were patient, clinician and intervention worker. Furthermore, patients were asked to invite carers to take part. One week before discharge, patient and in-patient clinician talked about needs after discharge in a discussion moderated by the intervention worker. This session resulted in a NODPAM discharge plan, a copy of which went to the out-patient clinician named by the patient as being in charge of his or her treatment after discharge. Three months after discharge, goals as outlined in the discharge plan were discussed by the patient and out-patient clinician. The result of this session was the NODPAM out-patient needs plan, which consisted of a list of the remaining unmet needs and description of measures on how to contribute to reducing need in the near future.

As shown in Table 4.3, a NODPAM discharge plan has a predefined format, including detailed content of the needs, in plain language, objectives and measures for how to achieve them, when to act, the responsible person(s), and who to contact for further implementation if applicable. The last category was filled in where there was disagreement between patient and clinician on how to proceed.

Recruitment ended in July 2007, and follow-up data collection was completed in February 2009. At discharge, the highest ratings for needs by patients were in the domains of psychological distress, company and daytime activities. The three needs with the lowest ratings were drugs, safety to others and telephone. Patient behaviour during the first intervention session as rated by the intervention worker was cooperative for the most part, and rarely passive, hostile or suspicious. These first results indicate that the intervention was well accepted and feasible. Acceptance by staff was also remarkable, as indicated by high participation rates among in-patient and out-patient clinicians. Unfortunately, carers rarely attended the intervention sessions, which can be considered a problem since carer burden after hospital discharge is obviously heavy. Anecdotal evidence based on researcher impressions from patient meetings suggests that a number of patients wished for additional effort, including actual involvement of NODPAM staff in carrying out the discharge plan, for example as realised in the brief critical time intervention (Dixon *et al*, 2009). The approach has promise as a feasible manualised intervention, based on an established instrument comprehensively to assess the needs of people with mental illness.

Case study 3. The FOCUS study

Our final case study uses an evidence-based approach to choosing and using outcome measures to improve subjective outcomes and to reduce crisis through earlier intervention. In the Feedback of Outcomes to Users and Staff (FOCUS) study, an intervention to investigate the routine collection and feedback of important process and outcome information was evaluated in a randomised controlled trial (Slade *et al*, 2006*a*). The intervention was based on a predefined model (Slade, 2002*a*), which in turn was based on a systematic review of outcome domains and implementation strategies (Slade, 2002*b*). The model proposed that assessing and providing feedback to staff and services users would lead to improved outcome, both through direct changes to content of care and through the mediator of process variables.

Staff measures chosen assessed helping alliance, using the Helping Alliance Scale (Priebe & Gruyters, 1993), needs, using the Camberwell Assessment of Need (Slade *et al*, 1999) and severity, using the Threshold Assessment Grid (Slade *et al*, 2002). Service user measures were helping alliance and needs using the patient-rated version of the same measures, and quality of life (using the Manchester Short Assessment (Priebe *et al*, 1999). The intervention involved asking staff and pairs of service users separately to complete a monthly postal questionnaire, with identical feedback provided to each person after 3 months. The trial took place in London between 2001 and 2003, and involved 160 staff–patient pairs (101 intervention, 59 control).

No effect was shown on patient-rated unmet needs or on quality of life (the primary outcome measures) for the full participant group, but service users with lower premorbid IQ did differentially benefit from the intervention (Slade *et al*, 2006*b*). Patients in the top quarter (premorbid IQ > 110) differentially improved in relation to patient-rated unmet need (adjusted difference 3.4, 95% CI 0.8 to 5.9, $P = 0.012$) and in the top half (premorbid IQ > 99) in quality of life (adjusted difference 0.6, 95% CI 1.1 to 0.1, $P = 0.02$). The top quarter result remained when controlling for the influence of baseline ($P = 0.004$) and baseline plus follow-up variables ($P = 0.047$). Furthermore, the intervention led to earlier intervention and averted crisis and hospitalisation (Slade *et al*, 2006*a*). Intervention-group patients had reduced hospital admissions, with admissions in the 6 months before follow-up being both fewer (means 0.13 versus 0.33, bootstrapped 95% CI –0.46 to –0.04) and tending to be shorter (mean 3.5 days versus 10.0 days, bootstrapped 95% CI –16.4 to 1.5). Hence service use costs were £2586 (95% CI £102 to £5391) less for intervention-group patients, and net benefit analysis indicated that the intervention was cost-effective. Overall, there was evidence that carefully choosing the outcome measures to assess and feedback can lead to improved pro-recovery outcomes.

Conclusion

If recovery is to be fully supported by mental health services, then the choice and use of outcome measures is central. More focus needs to be put on assessing and basing care on the service user's perspective than on the staff perspective (Lasalvia *et al*, 2007) and developing methods which recognise the uniqueness of individuals and their life goals – an important outcome to one person may not be as important to another. Therefore, evaluation of personally valued goals is central (Slade, 2009*b*). Scientific and clinical developments will be needed to increase the focus on outcome while also individualising care to support each person's unique recovery journey.

Acknowledgements

We are grateful to Sabine Steffen and Thomas Becker for their contribution to case study 2.

References

Andresen, R., Caputi, P. & Oades, L. G. (2000) Interrater reliability of the Camberwell Assessment of Need Short Appraisal Schedule. *Australian and New Zealand Journal of Psychiatry*, 34 ,856–861.

Andresen, R., Oades, L. & Caputi, P. (2003) The experience of recovery from schizophrenia: towards an empirically-validated stage model. *Australian and New Zealand Journal of Psychiatry*, 37, 586–594.

Andresen, R., Caputi, P. & Oades, L. (2006) The Stages of Recovery Instrument: development of a measure of recovery from serious mental illness. *Australian and New Zealand Journal of Psychiatry*, 40, 972–980.

Anthony, W. A. (1993) Recovery from mental illness: the guiding vision of the mental health system in the 1990s. *Innovations and Research*, 2, 17–24.

Attkisson, C. C. & Zwick, R. (1982) The Client Satisfaction Questionnaire. *Evaluation and Program Planning*, 5, 233–237.

Barker, P. J., Davidson, B. & Campbell, P. (eds) (1999) *From the Ashes of Experience*. Whurr.

Barnett, H. & Lapsley, H. (2006) *Journeys of Despair, Journeys of Hope. Young Adults Talk About Severe Mental Distress, Mental Health Services and Recovery*. Mental Health Commission.

Bleuler, M. (1978) *The Schizophrenic Disorders*. Yale University Press.

Boyer, C. A., McAlpine, D. D., Pottick, K. J., *et al* (2000) Identifying risk factors and key strategies in linkage to outpatient psychiatric care. *American Journal of Psychiatry*, 157, 1592–1598.

Bracken, P. & Thomas, P. (2005) *Postpsychiatry. Mental Health in a Postmodern World*. Oxford University Press.

Campbell, J., Fitzpatrick, R., Haines, A., *et al* (2000) Framework for design and evaluation of complex interventions to improve health. *BMJ*, **321**, 694–696.

Campbell-Orde, T., Chamberlin, J., Carpenter, J., *et al* (2005) *Measuring the Promise: A Compendium of Recovery Measures. Vol. II*. Human Services Research Institute.

Care Services Improvement Partnership, Royal College of Psychiatrists & Social Care Institute for Excellence (2007) *A Common Purpose: Recovery in Future Mental Health Services*. Care Services Improvement Partnership.

Chandler, R. & Hayward, M. (eds) (2009) *Voicing Psychotic Experiences. A Reconsideration of Recovery and Diversity*. Pavilion.

Ciompi, L. & Muller, C. (1976) *The Life-Course and Aging of Schizophrenics: A Long-Term Follow-Up Study into Old Age*. Springer.

Clarke, S. P., Oades, L. G., Crowe, T., *et al* (2006) Collaborative Goal Technology: theory and practice. *Psychiatric Rehabilitation Journal*, **30**, 129–136.

Clarke, S., Crowe, T., Oades, L., *et al* (2009) Do goal setting interventions improve the quality of goals in mental health services? *Psychiatric Rehabilitation Journal*, **32**, 292–299.

Cohen, P. & Cohen, J. (1984) The clinician's illusion. *Archives of General Psychiatry*, **41**, 1178–1182.

Coleman, R. (1999) *Recovery – An Alien Concept*. Hansell.

Crowe, T., Deane, F., Oades, L. G., *et al* (2006) Effectiveness of a collaborative recovery training program in Australia in promoting positive views about recovery. *Psychiatric Services*, **57**, 1497–1500.

Davidson, L. & Strauss, J. (1992) Sense of self in recovery from severe mental illness. *British Journal of Medical Psychology*, **65**, 131–145.

Davidson, L., Sells, D., Sangster, S., *et al* (2005) Qualitative studies of recovery: what can we learn from the person? In *Recovery in Mental Illness. Broadening Our Understanding of Wellness* (eds R. O. Ralph & P. W. Corrigan), pp. 147–170. American Psychological Association.

Davidson, L., Tondora, J., Lawless, M. S., *et al* (2009) *A Practical Guide to Recovery-Oriented Practice Tools for Transforming Mental Health Care*. Oxford University Press.

Deegan, P. (1988) Recovery: the lived experience of rehabilitation. *Psychosocial Rehabilitation Journal*, **11**, 11–19.

Derogatis, L. R. (1986) SCL–90–R: self report symptom inventory. In *Internationale Skalen für Psychiatrie* (ed. Collegium Internationale Psychiatriae Scalarum). Beltz.

DeSisto, M. J., Harding, C. M., McCormick, R. V., *et al* (1995) The Maine and Vermont three-decades studies of serious mental illness: II. Longitudinal course. *British Journal of Psychiatry*, **167**, 338–342.

Dinniss, S., Roberts, G., Hubbard, C., *et al* (2007) User-led assessment of a recovery service using DREEM. *Psychiatric Bulletin*, **31**, 124–127.

Dixon, L., Goldberg, R., Iannone, V., *et al* (2009) Use of a critical time intervention to promote continuity of care after psychiatric inpatient hospitalization. *Psychiatric Services*, **60**, 451–458.

Faulkner, A. & Layzell, S. (2000) *Strategies for Living. A Report of User-Led Research into People's Strategies for Living with Mental Distress*. Mental Health Foundation.

Fisher, D. V. (1994) Health care reform based on an empowerment model of recovery by people with psychiatric disabilities. *Hospital and Community Psychiatry*, **45**, 913–915.

Franke, G. H. (1995) *Die Symptom-Checkliste von Derogatis – Deutsche Version*. [Derogatis' Symptom Checklist – German version.] Beltz.

Frese, F. J., Stanley, J., Kress, K., *et al* (2001) Integrating evidence-based practices and the recovery model. *Psychiatric Services*, **52**, 1462–1468.

Goldsack, S., Reet, M., Lapsley, H., *et al* (2005) *Experiencing a Recovery-Oriented Acute Mental Health Service: Home Based Treatment from the Perspectives of Services Users, Their Families and Mental Health Professionals*. Mental Health Commission.

Hamilton, M. (1967) Development of a rating scale for primary depressive illness. *British Journal of Social and Clinical Psychology*, **6**, 278–296.

Harding, C. M., Brooks, G., Ashikage, T., *et al* (1987) The Vermont longitudinal study of persons with severe mental illness II: long-term outcome of subjects who retrospectively met DSM–III criteria for schizophrenia. *American Journal of Psychiatry*, **144**, 727–735.

Harrison, G., Hopper, K., Craig, T., *et al* (2001) Recovery from psychotic illness: a 15- and 25-year international follow-up study. *British Journal of Psychiatry*, **178**, 506–517.

Hermann, D., Opler, L., Felix, A., *et al* (2000) A critical time intervention with mentally ill homeless men: Impact on psychiatric symptoms. *Journal of Nervous and Mental Disease*, **188**, 135–140.

Higgins, A. (2008) *A Recovery Approach Within the Irish Mental Health Services. A Framework for Development*. Mental Health Commission.

Hopper, K., Harrison, G., Janca, A., *et al* (2007) *Recovery from Schizophrenia: An International Perspective. A Report from the WHO Collaborative Project, the International Study of Schizophrenia*. Oxford University Press.

Horvath, A. O. & Greenberg, L. S. (1989) Development and validation of the Working Alliance Inventory. *Journal of Counseling Psychology*, **36**, 223–233.

Huber, G., Gross, G. & Schuttler, R. (1975) A long-term follow-up study of schizophrenia: Psychiatric course and prognosis. *Acta Psychiatrica Scandinavica*, **52**, 49–57.

Johnsen, M., Teague, G. B. & Herr, E. M. (2005) Common ingredients as a fidelity measure for peer-run programs. In *On Our Own, Together: Peer Programs for People with Mental Illness* (eds S. Clay, B. Schell, P. Corrigan, *et al*), pp. 213–238. Vanderbilt University Press.

Kent, S., Fogarty, M. & Yellowlees, P. (1995) A review of studies of heavy users of psychiatric services. *Psychiatric Services*, **46**, 1247–1253.

Kilian, R., Bernert, S., Matschinger, H., *et al* (2001) The standardized assessment of the need for treatment and support in severe mental illness: the development and testing of the German version of the Camberwell Assessment of Need-EU. *Psychiatrische Praxis*, **28** (suppl. 2), 79–83.

Kunze, H., Becker, T. & Priebe, S. (2004) Reform of psychiatric services in Germany: hospital staffing directive and commissioning of community care. *Psychiatric Bulletin*, **28**, 218–221.

Lapsley, H., Nikora, L. W. & Black, R. (2002) *Kia Mauri Tau! Narratives of Recovery from Disabling Mental Health Problems*. Mental Health Commission.

Lasalvia, A., Bonetto, C., Salvi, G., *et al* (2007) Predictors of changes in needs for care in patients receiving community psychiatric treatment: a 4-year follow-up study. *Acta Psychiatrica Scandinavica*, suppl. 437, 31–41.

Libermann, R. P. & Kopelowicz, A. (2002) Recovery from schizophrenia: a challenge for the 21st century. *International Review of Psychiatry*, **14**, 242–255.

Lucas, B., Harrison-Read, P., Tyrer, P., *et al* (2001) Costs and characteristics of heavy inpatient service users in outer London. *International Journal of Social Psychiatry*, **47**, 63–74.

Lukoff, D., Nuechterlein, K. H. & Ventura, J. (1986) Manual for expanded Brief Psychiatric Rating Scale (BPRS). *Schizophrenia Bulletin*, **12**, 594–602.

Marneros, A., Deister, A., Rohde, A., *et al* (1989) Long-term outcome of schizoaffective and schizophrenic disorders, a comparative study, I: Definitions, methods, psychopathological and social outcome. *European Archives of Psychiatry and Clinical Neuroscience*, **238**, 118–125.

Marshall, S. L., Crowe, T., Oades, L., *et al* (2007) A review of consumer involvement in evaluations of case management: consistency with a recovery paradigm. *Psychiatric Services*, **58**, 396–401.

McCrone, P., Leese, M., Thornicroft, G., *et al* (2000) Reliability of the Camberwell Assessment of Need – European Version: EPSILON Study 6. *British Journal of Psychiatry*, **177**, 34–40.

McGuire-Snieckus, R., McCabe, R., Catty, J., *et al* (2006) A new scale to assess the therapeutic relationship in community mental health care: STAR. *Psychological Medicine*, **37**, 85–95.

McIntosh, Z. (2005) *From Goldfish Bowl to Ocean: Personal Accounts of Mental Illness and Beyond*. Chipmunka Publishing.

Mental Health Commission (2000) *Three Forensic Service Users and Their Families Talk About Recovery*. Mental Health Commission.

National Institute for Mental Health in England (2008) *Outcomes Compendium*. NIMHE.

National Social Inclusion Programme (2009) *Outcomes Framework for Mental Health Services*. NSIP.

Oades, L., Deane, F., Crowe, T., *et al* (2005) Collaborative recovery: an integrative model for working with individuals who experience chronic and recurring mental illness. *Australasian Psychiatry*, **13**, 279–284.

Ogawa, K., Miya, M., Watarai, A., *et al* (1987) A long-term follow-up study of schizophrenia in Japan, with special reference to the course of social adjustment. *British Journal of Psychiatry*, **151**, 758–765.

O'Hagan, M. (1996) Two accounts of mental distress. In *Speaking Our Minds* (eds J. Read & J. Reynolds), pp. 44–50. Macmillan.

Olfson, M., Mechanic, D., Boyer, C. A., *et al* (1998) Linking inpatients with schizophrenia to outpatient care. *Psychiatric Services*, **49**, 911–917.

Priebe, S. & Gruyters T. (1993) The role of the helping alliance in psychiatric community care: a prospective study. *Journal of Nervous and Mental Disease*, **181**, 552–557.

Priebe, S., Huxley, P., Knight, S., *et al* (1999) Application and results of the Manchester Short Assessment of Quality of Life (MANSA). *International Journal of Social Psychiatry*, **45**, 7–12.

Puschner, B., Bauer, S., Kraft, S., *et al* (2005) Zufriedenheit von Patienten und Therapeuten mit ambulanter Psychotherapie. [Patient and therapist satisfaction in out-patient psychotherapy.] *Psychotherapie, Psychosomatik, medizinische Psychologie*, **55**, 517–526.

Puschner, B., Steffen, S., Gaebel, W., *et al* (2008) Needs-oriented discharge planning and monitoring for high utilisers of psychiatric services (NODPAM): design and methods. *BMC Health Services Research*, **8**, 152.

Ralph, R. O. (2000) Recovery. *Psychiatric Rehabilitation Skills*, **4**, 480–517.

Ralph, R. O. & Corrigan, P. W. (eds) (2005) *Recovery in Mental Illness. Broadening Our Understanding of Wellness*. American Psychological Association.

Ridgway, P. (2001) Restorying psychiatric disability: learning from first person narratives. *Psychiatric Rehabilitation Journal*, **24**, 335–343.

Rogers, E. S., Teague, G. B., Lichenstein, C., *et al* (2007) Effects of participation in consumer-operated service programs on both personal and organizationally mediated empowerment: results of multisite study. *Journal of Rehabilitation Research and Development*, **44**, 785–800.

Roick, C., Gärtner, A., Heider, D., *et al* (2002) Heavy User psychiatrischer Versorgungsdienste: Ein Überblick über den Stand der Forschung. [Heavy users of psychiatric care: a review of the state of research.] *Psychiatrische Praxis*, **29**, 334–342.

Rose, D., Ford, R., Lindley, P., *et al* (1998) *In Our Experience: User-Focussed Monitoring of Mental Health Services*. Sainsbury Centre for Mental Health.

Sass, H., Wittchen, H-U. & Zaudig, M. (1996) Skala zur Globalbeurteilung des Funktionsniveaus für DSM–IV. [Global Assessment of Functioning Scale.] In *Diagnostisches und Statistisches Manual psychischer Störungen*. Hogrefe.

Schmidt, J., Lamprecht, F., Wittmann, W. W. (1989) Zufriedenheit mit der stationären Versorgung: Entwicklung eines Fragebogens und erste Validitätsuntersuchungen. [Satisfaction with in-patient management: development of a questionnaire and initial validity studies.] *Psychotherapie, Psychosomatik, medizinische Psychologie*, **39**, 248–255.

Scottish Recovery Network (2006) *Journeys of Recovery. Stories of Hope and Recovery from Long Term Mental Health Problems*. Scottish Recovery Network.

Scottish Recovery Network (2007) *Routes to Recovery. Collected Wisdom from the SRN Narrative Research Project*. Scottish Recovery Network.

Slade, M. (2002a) Routine outcome assessment in mental health services. *Psychological Medicine*, **32**, 1339–1343.

Slade, M. (2002b) What outcomes to measure in routine mental health services, and how to assess them: a systematic review. *Australian and New Zealand Journal of Psychiatry*, **36**, 743–753.

Slade M. (2009a) *Personal Recovery and Mental Illness. A Guide for Mental Health Professionals*. Cambridge University Press.

Slade, M. (2009b) *100 Ways to Support Recovery*. Rethink.

Slade, M. & Hayward, M. (2007) Recovery, psychosis and psychiatry: research is better than rhetoric. *Acta Psychiatrica Scandinavica*, **116**, 81–83.

Slade, M. & Priebe, S. (eds) (2006) *Choosing Methods in Mental Health Research*. Routledge.

Slade, M., Loftus, L., Phelan, M., *et al* (1999) *The Camberwell Assessment of Need*. Gaskell.

Slade, M., Cahill, S., Kelsey, W., *et al* (2002) Threshold 2: the reliability, validity and sensitivity to change of the Threshold Assessment Grid (TAG). *Acta Psychiatrica Scandinavica*, **106**, 453–460.

Slade, M., McCrone, P., Kuipers, E., *et al* (2006a) Use of standardised outcome measures in adult mental health services: randomised controlled trial. *British Journal of Psychiatry*, **189**, 330–336.

Slade, M., Leese, M., Gillard, M., *et al* (2006b) Pre-morbid IQ and response to routine outcome assessment. *Psychological Medicine*, **36**, 1183–1191.

Slade, M., Luke, G. & Knowles, L. (2009) Methodologies for evaluating recovery training. *Clinical Psychology Forum*, **193**, 10–15.

South London and Maudsley NHS Foundation Trust (2007) *Social Inclusion, Rehabilitation and Recovery Strategy 2007–2010*. South London and Maudsley NHS Foundation Trust.

Spaniol, L. & Koehler, M. (eds) (1994) *The Experience of Recovery*. Center for Psychiatric Rehabilitation.

Spaniol, L., Wewiorski, N., Gagne, C., *et al* (2002) The process of recovery from schizophrenia. *International Review of Psychiatry*, **14**, 327–336.

Steffen, S., Kösters, M., Becker, T., *et al* (2009) Discharge planning in mental health care: a systematic review of the recent literature. *Acta Psychiatrica Scandinavica*, **120**, 1–9.

Teague, G. B., Bond, G. R. & Drake, R. E. (1998) Program fidelity in assertive community treatment: development and use of a measure. *American Journal of Orthopsychiatry*, **68**, 216–232.

Torgalsbøen, A. K. (1999) Full recovery from schizophrenia: the prognostic role of premorbid adjustment, symptoms at first admission, precipitating events and gender. *Psychiatry Research*, **88**, 143–152.

Tsuang, M. T., Woolson, R. F. & Fleming J. (1979) Long-term outcome of major psychosis. *Archives of General Psychiatry*, **36**, 1295–1301.

Warner, R. (2007) Review of 'Recovery from Schizophrenia: An International Perspective. A Report from the WHO Collaborative Project, the International Study of Schizophrenia'. *American Journal of Psychiatry*, **164**, 1444–1445.

Wowra, S. A. & McCarter, R. (1999) Validation of the empowerment scale with an outpatient mental health population. *Psychiatric Services*, **50**, 959–961.

Part II
Domains of outcome measurement

CHAPTER 5

Global functioning scales

Emese Csipke and Til Wykes

Mental health professionals have increasingly come to view mental illness not simply as a sum of its symptoms, a reduction in which will translate to an independent, successful individual with a high quality of life. This is especially true in the case of schizophrenia, but applies to virtually all neuropsychiatric/mental health conditions. Both patients and their families have repeatedly identified social and occupational functioning as equally important to them as symptom reduction. Individuals often have difficulties with employment, education, fulfilling basic roles such as spouse or parent and even everyday tasks like negotiating a transport system. In this chapter, we review assessment schedules used among psychiatric populations that are intended to provide a measure of a person's level of functioning in all or nearly all areas of life.

Global functioning is now seen as a legitimate target for clinical interventions, both psychosocial and pharmacological. However, global functioning itself is a rather vague and abstract concept that tries to encompass a broad canvas of behaviour and abilities, but can include social functioning, vocational functioning and independent living skills. There is a close and complex relationship between mental illness and impairment of global functioning. Cognitive deficits, such as in memory, attention and psychomotor speed, all contribute to poor functioning. At the same time, the overt symptoms of mental illness such as delusions or depression can also contribute directly to poor functioning, for instance through negative social interactions or the inability to maintain a job. Although impairment of functioning is usually viewed as a consequence of mental illness, it may at times be a significant causal or maintaining factor in specific disorders. Measuring this construct is further complicated by 'real world' restrictions such as limited financial resources, disincentives to seek employment and restricted housing options, which can all prevent someone achieving their full potential.

One model helpful in the conceptualisation of global function is reported by McKibben *et al* (2004). It is a threefold concept:

1   *impairments* – body level (e.g. brain structure, cognitive and psychiatric deficits)
2   *limitations* – person as a whole (e.g. difficulty with mental calculations such as fluid speech)
3   *participation restrictions* – person in social contexts (e.g. no opportunities in job market).

Although beyond the remit of this chapter, Harvey & Bellack (2009) provide a comprehensive, up-to-date, in-depth discussion of global functioning/ functional recovery. In a demonstration of how important this area is becoming to clinicians and researchers alike, the National Institute of Mental Health (NIMH) convened a workshop to discuss how the lack of valid and reliable measures for assessing global functioning is hampering progress in developing interventions to address these difficulties, which resulted in a 'white paper' (Bellack *et al*, 2007).

The measurement of global functioning

The most common methods of measuring global function are self-report, direct observation, informant reports, clinician ratings, and performance-based assessments, each of which has is advantages and drawbacks.

Self-report

A major advantage of self-report is that it can tap worries, feelings, thoughts and behaviours that only the individuals themselves can know about. However, these reports are limited by a lack of objectivity, aspirations, personal values, comparison to previous states, their current situation and the possibility that they do not always recognise problems, especially if they lack insight.

Direct observation

Direct observations are more objectively valid and reliable if done by trained assessors. It involves shadowing people either throughout their daily routine or during specific observational periods. Shadowing someone is not only labour and time intensive but also raises the possibility of the Hawthorne effect, where behaviour changes as a result of observation. Observing only during specific periods limits the types of behaviour that can be observed and may miss less-frequent behaviours.

Informant reports

Informant observation may provide a more accurate picture, as informants can often be counted on to have more insight and a better memory, but in many cases people with severe mental illness may not have any key informants. Furthermore, family members or other informants are limited in their knowledge, may have different standards to base their criteria on, may attribute inability to attitude (e.g. not being able to hold a job versus laziness) and can vary greatly in the amount of time spent with the individual they are rating, leading to underreporting or insensitivity to change.

Clinician/researcher ratings

Clinician ratings can be more objective and consistent than other methods but vary greatly depending on what information is available and how well the individual knows the person being rated. The amount of observed and reported behaviour is limited and this may lead to underestimates of functioning. However, certain ratings, such as those based on DSM or ICD criteria, are widely used, and this allows comparisons of diverse populations.

Performance-based measures

Performance-based measures typically involve asking individuals to perform a task and rating them according to strict guidelines. This has the advantage that it can eliminate response bias and be objective/specific about what is being measured. However, there is a difference between what one *does* do, and what one *can* do in a laboratory or doctor's office and threatens external validity. Even conducting it at the individual's own home is artificial, and typically excludes the complex range of behaviours that occur simultaneously in the real world, such as answering a ringing telephone while cooking. Furthermore, the focus on skills does not take into account the fact that, for example, someone may be able to demonstrate how to get a prescription when prompted, but outside of the test setting may not realise the importance of not running out of medication and fail to do so.

A gold standard measure

As the NIMH white paper (Bellack *et al*, 2007) stated, until we have nuanced, reliable and valid measures of functioning, testing the efficacy of interventions will be a challenge. The measures presented in this chapter all have their strengths and weaknesses, but a gold standard scale does not exist currently. An *ideal* scale would cover a broad range of areas to ensure it is as global as possible, while having an acceptable administration time, with clearly described administrator instructions and rating guidelines. It would be applicable to a wide range of difficulties and cover as wide an array of mental health problems as possible. It would also be appropriate for people from a wide range of cultural and ethnic backgrounds, and all age groups.

It would be reliable and valid. Involving the potential patient population in the creation of the measure would ensure that a service user perspective is included, rather than simply basing it on expert opinion, which has largely been the case with current measures. In addition, the perfect global functioning scale would produce a total rating that accurately and equally reflects all aspects of a patient's functioning. An ideal scale would also have 'adaptive testing' so that the item pool can cover a range of levels and be tailored to specific individuals. This could help eliminate floor and ceiling effects, as well as taking into consideration real-life limits on functioning (e.g. a person might be highly capable of a job, but stigma might prevent him or her from being appointed). Finally, such a measure should be judgement free and take into consideration that different individuals have different goals and hopes and different opinions of what good functioning means.

The scales presented in this chapter were chosen either because they try to summarise global functioning in a single rating, or because they are social functioning scales which cover a broad enough area to be considered measures of global functioning. We excluded those which are inappropriate for use with a psychiatric population. We briefly review some of the early scales that have contributed to the development of the ones currently being used, but our main focus is on those that have been more widely used in the past few decades. The main characteristics of each scale are summarised in Table 5.1.

Early global rating scales

Health Sickness Rating Scale and Global Assessment Scale

The earliest published global rating scale is the Health Sickness Rating Scale (HSRS; Luborsky, 1962). Luborsky proposed seven factors that were important domains of global health: autonomous functioning, symptom severity, discomfort, effect upon the environment, utilisation of abilities, quality of interpersonal relationships, and breadth and depth of interests. A scale of 0–100 was used, and it was intended to measure changes over time. Attempts to improve upon the HSRS resulted in the development of the Global Assessment Scale (GAS; Endicott *et al*, 1976). While maintaining the same basic structure, the authors introduced a number of changes in an attempt to simplify the scale and provided guidelines on difficult rating decisions. Neither the HSRS nor the GAS is widely used any more.

Psychiatric Status Schedule and Psychiatric Evaluation Form

The Psychiatric Status Schedule (PSS; Spitzer *et al*, 1970) covers 15 areas of psychopathology and five social roles (wage earner, housekeeper, student or trainee, spouse and parent) in a scale of over 300 items. Scores discriminate between in-patients, out-patients and non-patients, and are correlated with other measures of psychopathology, such as the Brief Psychiatric Rating Scale and the Beck Depression Inventory. The Psychiatric Evaluation Form (PEF; Endicott & Spitzer, 1972) is a 28-item schedule that was designed in tandem with the PSS, with considerable overlap. The PEF is designed to be completed by experienced clinicians using information from a variety of sources, rather than from a direct patient interview.

Denver Community Mental Health Questionnaire

The Denver Community Mental Health Questionnaire (DCMHQ; Ciarlo & Riehman, 1977) was designed to assess a wide range of mental health problems in an out-patient population. The authors deemed psychological distress, interpersonal isolation from friends, interpersonal isolation from family, productivity at work, productivity at home, dependency on public agencies, alcohol misuse, soft drug use, hard drug use, client satisfaction with services, interpersonal aggression with friends, and legal difficulties as the domains to assess. The time frame is between 24 hours and 1 month.

Current global rating scales

Disabilities Assessment Schedule

The Disability Assessment Schedule (DAS; Schubert *et al*, 1986) was developed by the World Health Organization (WHO) to assess disabilities. It is specifically to be used in tandem with ICD (WHO, 1988, 1992). It was updated in 2000 (WHO, 2000) with recent ICD–10 revisions. Cognition, mobility, self-care, social interactions and roles are covered, but symptoms and subjective well-being are excluded from the ratings. Unlike the other measures discussed here, it covers physical functioning that might prevent wider functioning. It has demonstrated good test–retest reliability, yet is reported to be sensitive to change. It also has good convergent reliability and high internal consistency.

Social Behaviour Schedule

The Social Behaviour Schedule (SBS; Wykes & Sturt, 1986) was designed specifically to assess the functioning of people with severe and long-lasting psychiatric disabilities, and in particular to identify behaviours that result in dependence on psychiatric care. It is based on the Wing Ward Behaviour Scale, which was published over 30 years ago. It is a 21-item schedule, with most items rated on a five-point scale, on which 0 represents no problems in this area and 5 signifies major problems, so the total item score ranges from 0 to 105. All items except for one (inappropriate sexual

Table 5.1 Summary of schedules suitable for the assessment of global functioning

Schedule	Description	Strengths/Weaknesses	Uses
Disability Assessment Schedule (DAS; WHO, 1988)	11-item scale, covering social roles and disabilities	Appears to be valid and reliable, but only a few published studies describe its use; difficult for untrained staff	Clinical and research, but users need training
Social Behaviour Schedule (SBS; Wykes & Sturt, 1986)	21-item schedule; emphasis on observable behaviours	Easy to use, no training required; good reliability and validity; suitable for more severely ill patients	Clinical and research
Global Assessment of Functioning (GAF; American Psychiatric Association, 1987) and Social and Occupational Functioning Assessment Scale (SOFAS)	Scale of 0–100 for one global rating on the GAF; separate symptom functioning ratings on the SOFAS	Easy to learn and use; widely used	Clinical and research
REHAB (Baker & Hall, 1988)	23-item schedule, covering general and deviant behaviour	Easy to use; impressive psychometric properties; suitable only for patients in residential or hospital setting	Clinical and research
Life Skills Profile (LSP; Rosen et al, 1989)	39-item schedule covering disability and functioning	Easy to use; free of jargon; currently few published studies	Clinical and research
Health of the Nation Outcome Scales (HoNOS; Wing et al, 1998)	12 domains covering clinical and social areas	Extensive trials and routine use in recent years. Quick to use and suitable for wide range of patients	Clinical and research
Social Functioning Scale (SFS; Birchwood et al, 1990)	7 areas of social functioning covered; designed originally for family intervention studies	Appears to have good psychometric properties, and to be acceptable to patients	Clinical and research

Scale	Description	Comments	Use
Maryland Assessment of Social Competence (MASC; Bellack et al, 1994)	Role-play-based measure covering four domains, with video coding	Good reliability, but lengthy assessment requiring trained confederates and raters	Owing to length and video facility requirements not suitable for clinical
Social Skills Performance Assessment (SSPA; Patterson et al, 2001b)	Drawn from the MASC, but uses only 2 role-plays	Takes 5–10 minutes to administer. Has good reliability but has not been widely used	Clinical and research
University of California Performance Based Skills Assessment (UPSA; Patterson et al, 2001a)	Five areas assessed via role-play, designed for non-clinicians	Good reliability and validity; requires many props, making it difficult to transport. It is vulnerable to ceiling effects	Research, but brief version more suitable if used for clinical work
Test of Adaptive Behavior in Schizophrenia (TABS; Velligan et al, 2007)	Performance-based measure of 5 domains, designed to assess the ability to identify the existence of a problem	Shows reliability and validity but needs further testing	Clinical and research
Functional Assessment for Comprehensive Treatment of Schizophrenia (FACT–Sz; Suzuki et al, 2008)	Clinician-rated scale of 0–100. Designed to be better able to differentiate between types of patients than the GAF	Has shown ability to differentiate between patients but needs further testing	Clinical and research
Social Functioning Schedule (SFS; Remington & Tyrer, 1979)	12-item schedule designed specifically for people with non-psychotic illness	Few published studies; only limited psychometric data but shown to be appropriate for different cultural groups and a variety of settings	Clinical and research

behaviour) are those exhibited by at least 5% patients who have a long history of dependence on psychiatric care. Inappropriate sexual behaviour was added because although not frequent, it was a characteristic which would impede progress towards community independence. The scale covers communication difficulties, social relationships, risk or unacceptable behaviours (suicide and aggression), behaviours associated with positive symptoms (e.g. acting on delusions), personal appearance and hygiene, underactivity and slowness.

The scale scores discriminate between patients living in accommodation with differing levels of support. Reliability studies have provided data on interrater and test–retest reliability for different settings and informants, with kappa coefficients ranging from 0.67 to 0.94. Internal consistency for the two total problem scores is 0.71 and 0.75. It has been used in numerous studies with patients in institutions and in the community, as well as across different cultures. It has also been translated into a number of languages and has had separate assessments in these languages (Morejon & Garciaboveda, 1994; Lima *et al*, 2006). The studies have been extensive and it has been used in the evaluation of both services and treatments (psychological and medication), as well as being used in routine care. The scale has been in frequent use as it provides some sensitivity to change over relatively short periods but has also been used to assess predictions of outcome in studies lasting as long as 6 years (Wykes *et al*, 1990). The outcome assessed can include the overall score as well as two measures of problems (mild and severe problems or severe problems), which allows some further flexibility in use. The scale has been factor analysed to provide four factors (thought disturbance, social withdrawal, depressed behaviour and antisocial behaviour), which distinguished between the patient subgroups and had significant differential relationships to symptoms and social functioning variables (Harvey *et al*, 1996).

Diagnostic and Statistical Manual (DSM) – Global Assessment of Functioning and the Social and Occupational Functioning Assessment Scale

The Global Assessment of Functioning (GAF) scale was designed as part of the fifth axis on DSM–III–R (American Psychiatric Association, 1987), with the hope that it would increase the usefulness of the axis, used to measure 'a person's psychological, social, and occupational functioning'. The GAF itself is a modified version of the GAS (see above) and produces a single score of 0–100 (0 itself is rated to indicate insufficient information). Ratings generally reflect the current need for treatment or care, with most out-patients scoring between 31 and 70, while in-patients typically score between 1 and 40 (Williams, 2007). The major limitation of the GAF is that symptoms and functioning are combined to produce a single rating. There is also concern that the interrater reliability usually reported is between members of study teams, but that only inadequate reliability between centres, or clinicians and researchers can be achieved (Vatnaland *et al*, 2007). There were proposals (see Goldman *et al*, 1992) that these two factors (symptoms and functioning) be rated separately for DSM–IV (American Psychiatric Association, 1994). When this approach became used routinely by mental health practitioners, satisfactory reliability was obtained for the total GAF score and for the separate symptom and disability measures. Jones *et al* (1995) demonstrated differences in the relationships between the three scores and medication and support needs, indicating the usefulness of this separation. Additionally, it has been criticised for the ratings not being operationally defined (Juckel *et al*, 2008).

In DSM–IV the GAF is still included as the major axis V assessment. However, an alternative assessment is also included – the Social and Occupational Functioning Assessment Scale (SOFAS), which is similar to the GAF but with no mention of psychiatric symptoms. It is suggested that SOFAS may be useful in certain settings to monitor social and occupational disability independent of the severity of psychological symptoms, but doubt has been cast on its validity (Roy-Byrne *et al*, 1996). Williams *et al* (2008) found that cognitive deficits are related to scores on the SOFAS, in that they have a detrimental effect, as can be expected.

Both the measures continue to be used quite widely.

REHAB

This is a schedule specifically designed to assess people with long-term or disabling psychiatric handicap who at the time of assessment are 'living in, or attending, a residential or day care institutional setting' (Baker & Hall, 1983, 1988). One of the aims of the authors was to design a scale that could correctly identify patients who have the potential for living outside hospital. There are 23 items, 7 covering deviant behaviour and 16 covering general behaviour. Each item is measured along a visual analogue scale. The psychometric properties have been extensively studied, and norms for over 800 patients are available. Interrater reliability of the individual items ranges from 0.61 to 0.92, and total scores discriminate day-hospital patients, long-stay in-patients and in-patients selected for a predischarge training programme (Baker & Hall, 1988). The REHAB is easy to use, is suitable for patients with a high level of disability, and provides a broad measure of behaviour. It is particularly suitable as a repeated measure during the routine evaluation of a treatment plan. A user's guide and other training materials are available.

Life Skills Profile

The Life Skills Profile (LSP; Rosen *et al*, 1989) addresses five domains (self-care, non-turbulence, social contact, communication and responsibility) with 39 individual items that are rated on a four-point scale, but does not include symptoms. It was specifically designed for use with people who have schizophrenia. Reported internal consistency ranges from 0.67 to 0.88, and the mean interrater reliability coefficient is 0.68. This is a carefully developed schedule, which, although specifically designed for people with schizophrenia, can be used for other serious psychiatric disorders. It is suitable for routine use by a range of professional staff and has been translated into numerous languages. Since its inception, two brief forms have also been developed, the LSP–16 and LSP–20 (Rosen *et al*, 2001). It is suggested the LSP–16 be used primarily with populations in which psychosis is not present. The LSP–20 was specifically developed to be used with those with psychosis in particular. The correlation with the original LSP–39 is 0.92 and its test–retest and interrater reliability are comparable with those of the original, but it takes half the time to complete (Rosen *et al*, 2001).

Health of the Nation Outcome Scales

The Health of the Nation Outcome Scales (HoNOS; Wing *et al*, 1998) cover 12 domains, which are rated on a scale of 0 (no problem) to 4 (severe problem), and the sum of the ratings is the total score. They were designed to be used in routine clinical settings, and therefore are clinician rated. Eight of the items concern behavioural problems that have an impact on self or others (violence, self harm and drug/alcohol use), deficits in basic functions (cognitive impairments), distressing mental experiences, and environmental problems (e.g. housing). It has specific versions for children, adolescents, elderly people, forensic populations and people with intellectual disability. One of the drawbacks is that symptoms are included in the ratings. Salvi *et al* (2005) recommend its use in epidemiological studies to categorise patients' problems or in a clinical setting to highlight the specific problem areas patients may have. HoNOS are quick to use, and their reliability and validity were established during development (Wing *et al*, 1998). Subsequent use in routine practice has indicated that, as with so many other scales, reliability is less good when completed by clinical staff (Bebbington *et al*, 1999) and that although routine use is feasible, the information obtained is of limited value for care planning (Sharma *et al*, 1999). The HoNOS continue to be used in mental health services in the UK and Australia and where ratings are typically made at the start and end of periods of care. They have also been more recently taken up in North America, where clinicians carried out an acceptability (to clinicians) and validity/reliability trial in Canada, with promising results (Kisely *et al*, 2007).

Social Functioning Scale

The Social Functioning Scale (SFS; Birchwood *et al*, 1990) was devised to measure social functioning in patients with schizophrenia. The scale covers seven areas: social engagement/withdrawal; interpersonal behaviour;

pro-social activities; recreation; independence–competence; independence–performance; and employment/occupation. The authors of the scale have shown its reliability, validity and sensitivity, and state that it is acceptable to patients and their families, and requires little time to complete. A study examining theory of mind found that those with better functioning according to the SFS performed better on theory of mind tasks, which lends further support for the validity of these scales (Bora *et al*, 2006). Aside from being used in evaluations of family interventions with schizophrenia, it has been used in studies assessing a variety of treatments and disorders, and has been translated into a number of languages. The only difficulty observed in its use in randomised trials is that it is not very sensitive to change.

Maryland Assessment of Social Competence

The Maryland Assessment of Social Competence (MASC; Bellack *et al*, 1994; Sayers *et al*, 1995) was designed as part of a larger battery, the Social Problem Solving Assessment Battery for chronic psychiatric populations. The MASC is a measure based on role-play that is completed with a confederate trained to respond in a standardised way. The resulting patient behaviours are then coded by trained raters who watch the assessment on video. It covers four skill domains: problem-solving in an interpersonal context; response generation to social problem situations; the evaluation of response effectiveness; and evaluating one's own problem-solving abilities. Dickinson *et al* (2007) found that good MASC scores were positively correlated with having been competitively employed in the previous 2 years. Sayers *et al* (1995) reported good interrater and test–retest reliability. However, the lengthy assessment and video requirements may make it unsuitable for some settings.

Social Skills Performance Assessment

The Social Skills Performance Assessment (SSPA; Patterson *et al*, 2001*b*) was drawn from the MASC, but only uses two role-plays (meeting a new neighbour and reporting a problem to a landlord) after a simple practice scene. The role-plays are scored 1–5 on eight or nine dimensions. The measure requires about 5–10 minutes to administer. Patterson *et al* reported interrater reliability coefficients of 0.91 and test–retest reliability scores at 0.92 over a 2-week interval. The measure appears to have good discriminant and convergent validity. Lower symptom severity has been found to be associated with better performance on the SSPA (Sitzer *et al*, 2007). However, it has not been widely used.

University of California Performance Based Skills Assessment

The University of California Performance Based Skills Assessment (UPSA; Patterson *et al*, 2001*a*) was constructed to assess the skills necessary

93

for everyday living among older people with schizophrenia, and was designed to be used by non-clinicians. It consists of role-plays in five areas (household chores, communication, finance, transportation and planned recreational activities) and has been found to be correlated with personal care skills, interpersonal skills, neurocognitive functioning and activities in the community. The interrater reliability coefficients has been reported to be 0.91, while the 2-week test–retest coefficient was reported to be 0.93 (Harvey *et al*, 2007). Comparison of the level of independence and social circumstances to UPSA scores also points to high validity. One of the limitations, however, is that it is vulnerable to ceiling effects, especially with younger individuals (Harvey *et al*, 2007). Indeed, Heinrichs *et al* (2006) found that in a sample with ages ranging from 18 to 65 years, some domains (household chores and transportation) had very skewed scores, with patients and normal controls scoring indistinguishably.

Mausbach *et al* (2007) modified the UPSA to develop the UPSA–Brief in order to cut down on the number of stage props, to make it more portable. (One of the biggest disadvantages of the UPSA is the large number of props required, which can make administration a challenge and which limits portability between sites.) After factor analysis, the authors concluded that the financial and communication subscales achieved high correlations with other measures of overall functioning and are able to predict whether individuals can live independently. The scale is sensitive to change. Support has been found for the UPSA–Brief's consistency across two samples in rural Sweden and urban New York, with two very different healthcare and social systems (Harvey *et al*, 2009). This measure has been used quite extensively recently, although the authors account for much of the literature.

Test of Adaptive Behavior in Schizophrenia

The Test of Adaptive Behavior in Schizophrenia (TABS; Velligan *et al*, 2007), a performance-based measure, was designed to assess functional capacity across five domains (basic hygiene, independent living skills, medication/treatment compliance, social skills and work/ability to work). These domains generated six assessment area tasks, each of which is scored as 'percentage correct', leading to a final score of 0–100. One of the key features of the TABS is that it was designed to address the limitation of measures that do not allow for the assessment of the ability to identify problems spontaneously. That is, it is one thing to be asked how one would solve a problem, quite another to be able to see that there is a problem to be solved, something the TABS addresses (e.g. noticing that one has been short-changed at a shop). The developers report internal consistency (a Cronbach alpha score of 0.84) and a 3-month test–retest correlation of 0.80, and give preliminary reports of convergent and discriminant validity. Velligan *et al* (2007) recommend using the total score, rather than individual task scores.

Functional Assessment for Comprehensive Treatment of Schizophrenia

The Functional Assessment for Comprehensive Treatment of Schizophrenia (FACT–Sz; Suzuki *et al*, 2008) was a response to the GAF – an attempt to increase the ability to differentiate patients. The authors argued that the GAF lumps together many dissimilar individuals, which limits its use in evaluating whether a treatment goal has been reached. Like the GAF, it is a clinician-rated scale of 0–100, with anchor points clearly defined. In the development study, the FACT–Sz was able to differentiate between in-patients and out-patients, and out-patients rated on both the FACT–Sz and GAF scored significantly higher on the FACT–Sz, providing initial support that it is better able to differentiate between patient groups. The Spearman correlation coefficient of 0.90 indicated good interrater reliability. Considering that one of the motivations behind it was to give clinicians a tool that would better detect change, a cross-sectional study is not sufficient. This test is newly developed and needs further independent testing.

Instruments for patients who do not have psychosis

Social Functioning Schedule

The Social Functioning Schedule (SFS; Remington & Tyrer, 1979) is primarily designed to measure the level of social functioning in people with a non-psychotic psychiatric disorder. Twelve main areas of functioning are included, and these are rated along a 10 cm visual analogue scale. Symptoms are not included. The time frame is the last month. Interrater reliability for the different sections ranges from 0.45 to 0.81 (mean 0.62) when audiotaped interviews are used, and from 0.50 to 0.80 with independent interviews. The scale discriminates between people with personality disorders and those with other psychiatric disorders.

The Social Functioning Questionnaire (SFQ) was developed from the SFS. It is a short, robust questionnaire that is suitable for a variety of settings, and appropriate across different cultural groups (Tyrer *et al*, 2005).

Conclusion

Each of the measures reviewed in this chapter is designed to be suitable for the population and purposes of some studies and only a few have been widely disseminated (e.g. the GAF and SBS). There are various methods of assessment, each with its advantages and disadvantages. However, the use of, and further development of, global functioning scales has a vital role in the evaluation of both psychosocial and pharmacological interventions.

Indeed, drug regulatory bodies are now requiring that global functioning be considered when evaluating the efficacy of novel treatments. In routine clinical work they can serve as a marker against which to measure improvements, and point to areas that need further work.

Despite the inherent difficulties in evaluating global functioning, alongside the limitations of the measures themselves, continuing to improve the scales is an important task. For the time being, the research or clinical questions need to be precisely specified and the most appropriate measure used. The population and level of expected disability need to be taken into account, as well as floor and ceiling effects, which will reduce an instrument's sensitivity to treatment effects. Finally, we must continue to work on developing the understanding of what global functioning/functional recovery actually encompasses and continue to improve the way that it can be measured.

References

American Psychiatric Association (1987) *Diagnostic and Statistical Manual of Mental Disorders* (3rd edition, revised) (DSM–III–R). APA.

American Psychiatric Association (1994) *Diagnostic and Statistical Manual of Mental Disorders* (4th edition) (DSM–IV). APA.

Baker, R. & Hall, J. N. (1983) *Rehabilitation Evaluation of Hall and Baker (REHAB)*. Vine Publishing.

Baker, R. & Hall, J. N. (1988) REHAB: a new assessment instrument for chronic psychiatric patients. *Schizophrenia Bulletin*, **14**, 95–113.

Bebbington, P., Brugha, T., Hill, T., *et al* (1999) Validation of the Health of the Nation Outcome Scales (HoNOS). *British Journal of Psychiatry*, **174**, 389–394.

Bellack, A. S., Sayers, M., Mueser, K. T., *et al* (1994). Evaluation of social problem solving in schizophrenia. *Journal of Abnormal Psychology*, **103**, 371–378.

Bellack, A. S., Green, M. F., Cook, J. A., *et al* (2007) Assessment of community functioning in people with schizophrenia and other severe mental illnesses: a white paper based on an NIMH-sponsored workshop. *Schizophrenia Bulletin*, **33**, 805–822.

Birchwood, M., Smith, J., Cochrane, R., *et al* (1990) The Social Functioning Scale. The development and validation of a new scale of social adjustment for use in family intervention programmes with schizophrenic patients. *British Journal of Psychiatry*, **157**, 853–859.

Bora, E., Eryavuz, A., Kayahan, B., *et al* (2006) Social functioning, theory of mind and neurocognition in outpatients with schizophrenia; mental state decoding may be a better predictor of social functioning than mental reasoning. *Psychiatry Research*, **145**, 95–103.

Ciarlo, J. A. & Riehman, J. (1977) The Denver Community Mental Health Questionnaire: development of a multidimensional program evaluation. In *Program Evaluation for Mental Health: Methods, Strategies and Participants* (eds R. D. Coursey, G. A. Specter, S. A. Murrell, *et al*), pp. 131–167. Grune and Stratton.

Dickinson, D., Bellack, A. S. & Gold, J. M. (2007) Social/communication skills, cognition and vocational functioning in schizophrenia. *Schizophrenia Bulletin*, **33**, 1213–1220.

Endicott, J. & Spitzer, R. L. (1972) What another rating scale? The Psychiatric Evaluation Form. *Journal of Nervous and Mental Disease*, **154**, 88–104.

Endicott, J., Spitzer, R. L., Fleiss, J. L., *et al* (1976) The Global Assessment Scale. *Archives of General Psychiatry*, **33**, 766–771.

Goldman, H. H., Skodol, A. E. & Lave, T. R. (1992) Revising axis V for DSM–IV: a review of measures of social functioning. *American Journal of Psychiatry*, **149**, 1148–1156.

Harvey, C. A., Curson, D., Taylor, C. J., *et al* (1996) Four behavioural syndromes of schizophrenia. *British Journal of Psychiatry*, **168**, 562–570.

Harvey, P. D. & Bellack, A. S. (2009) Toward a terminology for functional recovery in schizophrenia: is functional remission a viable concept? *Schizophrenia Bulletin*, **35**, 300–306.

Harvey, P. D., Velligan, D. I. & Belack, A. S. (2007) Performance based measures of functional skills: usefulness in clinical treatment studies. *Schizophrenia Bulletin*, **33**, 1138–1148.

Harvey, P. D., Helldin, L., Bowie, C. R., *et al* (2009) Performance-based measurement of functional disability in schizophrenia: a cross national study in the United States and Sweden. *American Journal of Psychiatry*, **166**, 821–827.

Heinrichs, R. W., Statucka, M., Goldber, J., *et al* (2006) The University of California Performance Skills Assessment (UPSA) in schizophrenia. *Schizophrenia Research*, **88**, 134–141.

Jones, S. H., Thornicroft, G., Coffey, M., *et al* (1995) A brief mental health outcome scale. Reliability and validity of the Global Assessment of Functioning (GAF). *British Journal of Psychiatry*, **166**, 654–659.

Juckel, G., Schaub, D., Fuchs, N., *et al* (2008) Validation of the Personal and Social Performance (PSP) scale in a German sample of acutely ill patients with schizophrenia. *Schizophrenia Research*, **104**, 287–283.

Kisely, S., Campbell, A. A., Corssman, D., *et al* (2007) Are the Health of the Nation Outcomes Scales a valid and practical instrument to measure outcomes in North America? A three-site evaluation across Nova Scotia. *Community Mental Health Journal*, **43**, 91–107.

Lima, L. A. & Bachrach, H. (1974) Factors influencing clinician's judgements of mental health. *Archives of General Psychiatry*, **31**, 292–299.

Lima, L. A., Goncalves, S., Pereira, B. B., *et al* (2006) The measurement of social disablement and assessment of psychometric properties of the Social Behaviour Schedule (SBS–BR) in 881 Brazilian long-stay psychiatric patients. *International Journal of Social Psychiatry*, **52**, 101–109.

Luborsky, L. (1962) Clinicians' judgements of mental health. A proposed scale. *Archives of General Psychiatry*, **7**, 407–417.

Mausbach, B. T., Harvey, P. D., Goldman, S. R., *et al* (2007) Development of a brief scale of everyday functioning in persons with serious mental illness. *Schizophrenia Bulletin*, **33**, 1364–1372.

McKibben, C. L., Brekke, J. S., Sires, D., *et al* (2004) Direct assessment of functional abilities: relevance to persons with schizophrenia. *Schizophrenia Research*, **72**, 53–67.

Morejon, J. V. & Garciaboveda, R. J. (1994) Social Behavior Schedule – reliability and validity as an instrument for evaluating chronic mental patients. *Actas Luso Espanoles de Neurologia Psiquiatria y Ciencias Afines*, **22**, 34–39.

Patterson, T. L., Goldman, S., McKibbin, C L., *et al* (2001*a*) UCSD performance-based skills assessment: development of a new measure of everyday functioning for severely mentally ill adults. *Schizophrenia Bulletin*, **27**, 235–245.

Patterson, T. L., Moscona, S., McKibben, C. L., *et al* (2001*b*) Social skills performance assessments among older patients with schizophrenia. *Schizophrenia Research*, **48**, 351–360.

Remington, M. & Tyrer, P. (1979) The Social Functioning Schedule – a brief semi structured interview. *Social Psychiatry*, **14**, 151–157.

Rosen, A., Hadzi-Pavlovic, D. & Parker, G. (1989) The Life Skills Profile: a measure assessing function and disability in schizophrenia. *Schizophrenia Bulletin*, **15**, 325–337.

Rosen, A., Trauer, T., Hazdi-Pavlovic, D., *et al* (2001) Development of a brief form of the Life Skills Profile: the LSP–20. *Australian and New Zealand Journal of Psychiatry*, **35**, 677–683.

Roy-Byrne, P., Dagadakis, C., Unutzer, J., *et al* (1996) Evidence for limited validity of the revised global assessment of functioning scale. *Psychiatric Services*, **47**, 864–866.

Salvi, G., Leese, M. & Slade, M. (2005) Routine use of mental health outcome assessments: choosing the measure. *British Journal of Psychiatry*, **186**, 146–152.

Sayers, M. D., Bellack, A. S., Wade, J. H., *et al* (1995) An empirical method for assessing social problem solving in schizophrenia. *Behaviour Modification*, **19**, 267–289.

Schubert, C., Krumm, B., Biehl, H., *et al* (1986) Measurement of social disability in a schizophrenic patient group: definition, assessment and outcome over two years in a cohort of schizophrenic patients of recent onset. *Social Psychiatry*, **21**, 1–9.

Sharma, V. K., Wilkinson, G. & Fear, S. (1999) Health of the Nation Outcome Scales. A case study in general psychiatry. *British Journal of Psychiatry*, **174**, 395–398.

Sitzer, D. I., Twamley, E. W., Patterson, T. L., *et al* (2007) Multivariate predictors of social skills performance in middle aged and older out-patients with schizophrenia spectrum disorders. *Psychological Medicine*, **38**, 755–763.

Spitzer, R. L., Endicott, J., Fleiss, J. L., *et al* (1970) The Psychiatric Status Schedule: a technique for evaluating psychopathology and impairment in role functioning. *Archives of General Psychiatry*, **23**, 41–55.

Suzuki, T., Hiroyuki, U., Nomura, K., *et al* (2008) Novel rating scales for schizophrenia – Targeted Inventory on Problems in Schizophrenia (TIP–Sz) and Functional Assessment for Comprehensive Treatment of Schizoprenia (FACT–Sz). *Schizophrenia Research*, **106**, 328–336.

Tyrer, P., Nur, U., Crawford, M., *et al* (2005) The Social Functioning Questionnaire: a rapid and robust measure of perceived functioning. *International Journal of Social Psychiatry*, **51**, 265–275.

Vatnaland, T., Vatnaland, J., Friid, S., *et al* (2007) Are GAF scores reliable in routine clinical use? *Acta Psychiatrica Scandinavica*, **115**, 326–330.

Velligan, D. I., Diamond, P., Glahn, D. C., *et al* (2007) The reliability and validity of the Test of Adaptive Behavior in Schizophrenia (TABS). *Psychiatry Research*, **151**, 55–66.

WHO (1988) *WHO Psychiatric Disability Assessment Scale (WHO/DAS)*. World Health Organization.

WHO (1992) *International Classification of Diseases (10th edn) (ICD–10)*. World Health Organization.

WHO (2000) *International Classification of Diseases (10th edn) (ICD–10) Updates 2000*. World Health Organization.

Williams, J. (2007) Mental health status, functioning, and disabilities measures. In *Handbook of Psychiatric Measures* (eds A. J. Rush, M. B. First & D. Blacker), pp. 83–105. American Psychiatric Publishing.

Williams, L. M., Whitford, T. J., Flynn, G., *et al* (2008) General and social cognition in first episode schizophrenia: identification of separable factors and prediction of functional outcome using the IntegNeuro test battery. *Schizophrenia Research*, **99**, 182–191.

Wing, J. K., Beevor, A. S., Curtis, R. H., *et al* (1998) Health of the Nation Outcome Scales: research and development. *British Journal of Psychiatry*, **172**, 11–18.

Wykes, T. & Sturt, E. (1986) The measurement of social behaviour in psychiatric patients: an assessment of the reliability and validity of the SBS schedule. *British Journal of Psychiatry*, **148**, 1–11.

Wykes, T., Sturt, E. & Katz, R. (1990) The prediction of rehabilitative success after three years: the use of social, symptom and cognitive variables. *British Journal of Psychiatry*, **157**, 865–870.

CHAPTER 6

Satisfaction with mental health services

Mirella Ruggeri

In routine psychiatric practice, clinicians, patients and carers are all involved in the care process and their perspectives should all be considered when assessing mental health outcome. The fact that their views may markedly differ (Gunkel & Priebe, 1993; Ellwood, 1998; Walter *et al*, 1998; Priebe *et al*, 2007; Brown *et al*, 2008) is confirmation that taking into account multiple perspectives and integrating these views are necessary steps when evaluating mental health outcomes.

The subjective appraisals made by patients who are mentally ill had been neglected for a long time, in both clinical practice and research, due to the view (or the prejudice) that they were unable, by the nature of their illness, to appreciate their need for treatment or to make the 'correct' decisions about how to conduct their lives. Therefore, for many years, the mental health system took a paternalistic stance and controlled the lives of people diagnosed with severe mental disorder, and the only form of 'involvement' of service users was as passive recipients of decisions made by others (Chamberlain, 2005).

The idea of patients' involvement in the planning and evaluation of mental healthcare has been growing over the last 20 years, especially in those countries where institutional service provision has been transformed into a community-oriented model of care (Beresford, 2005; Chamberlain, 2005; Thornicroft & Tansella, 2005). This represents a major challenge for mental health services, since the so-called 'users' movement' advocates a shift towards a modern 'shared model' or 'partnership model' between health professionals and service users, based on mutual respect for each other's skills and competencies and recognition of the advantages of combining these resources to achieve beneficial outcomes (Simpson & House, 2002; Crawford *et al*, 2003; Bramesfeld *et al* 2007; Brimblecombe *et al*, 2007; Killaspy *et al*, 2008; Stringer *et al*, 2008).

Within this methodological framework, it is particularly important not only to combine optimal measures of both the 'service level' and the 'patient level' (Thornicroft & Tansella 1999) but also to pay attention to (in addition to the traditional outcome dimensions such as clinician-rated symptoms and disability) patients' self-perceived outcomes, such as self-rated needs for care, subjective quality of life, carer burden and satisfaction with care (Jenkins, 1990; Mirin & Namerow, 1991; Attkisson *et al*, 1992; Ruggeri & Tansella, 1995; Smith *et al*, 1997).

Satisfaction with services has been given increasing attention in the field of mental health service research and evaluation. In the USA, large-scale studies of satisfaction have been performed since the early 1960s, both in medicine and in psychiatry, following the principles of 'consumerism' (Attkisson & Pascoe, 1983). In Europe, interest in satisfaction with services grew later, and achieved widespread diffusion in psychiatry only in the mid-1990s. More than from consumerism, this interest derives from developments in social psychiatry and specifically in the field of outcome assessment. In this regard, *multidimensionality* (i.e. assessing several domains) and *multi-axiality* (i.e. assessing outcomes in these domains according to different perspectives) have been increasingly recognised to be key requirements; in both cases, satisfaction with services, being a major dimension of outcome, one that may involve multiple axes, contributes to a fuller depiction of the performance of a system of care.

This chapter should be read as a supplement to the review chapters that appeared in the first and second editions of this book (Ruggeri, 1996, 2001), which summarised the psychometric properties of satisfaction rating scales published until 2000 and which discussed their methodological limitations, and to other papers (Lasalvia & Ruggeri, 2007).

The role of satisfaction in service evaluation

As early as 1966, Donabedian had stated that 'the effectiveness of care in achieving and producing health and satisfaction, as defined for its individual members by a particular society or subculture, is the ultimate validator of the quality of care' (Donabedian, 1966: pp. 166–203). Later, Locker & Dunt (1978: pp. 283–292) suggested that, particularly in long-term care, 'quality of care can become synonymous with quality of life and satisfaction with care an important component of life satisfaction'. Overall in service evaluation, satisfaction may be viewed as a dependent variable which is a *measure of outcome and quality per se* and/or an independent variable which is *a factor* in the process of care.

As an outcome variable, satisfaction has been hypothesised to be the consequence of various factors, including: expectations of services, attitudes to life, self-esteem, illness behaviour, previous experience with services and service characteristics (Svensson & Hansson, 1994; Barker *et al*, 1996). Conflicting results have been obtained on the relationships between patients' satisfaction and their socio-demographic characteristics, type of diagnosis and severity of illness (Larsen *et al*, 1979; Hansson, 1989; Kelstrup *et al*, 1993; Leavey *et al*, 1997; Greenwood *et al*, 1999; Perreault *et al*, 1999) and several studies in this area have had methodological shortcomings. The Epsilon

Study of Schizophrenia conducted in five European sites (Amsterdam, London, Copenhagen, Santander, Verona) using a cross-culturally validated set of instruments confirmed that demographic characteristics of people with schizophrenia have a very small effect not only on total satisfaction but also on satisfaction in the various domains, and that this finding is likely to have cross-cultural stability. Moreover, the same study found that illness severity, as measured by score on the Brief Psychiatric Rating Scale (BPRS), is cross-culturally associated with lower service satisfaction, especially in domains assessing involvement of relatives and self-perceived efficacy, although the amount of variance explained is relatively low (Ruggeri et al, 2003a).

The main variable shown to be clearly and consistently associated with service satisfaction is self-perceived quality of life. A 6-month follow-up study of the outcome of care, for a group of patients with full spectrum of psychiatric disorders in the Verona community-based psychiatric service, used graphical chain models and reported that the best predictor of patient satisfaction is subjective quality of life (Ruggeri et al, 1998a,b). Another study conducted in Verona, on a larger sample of psychiatric patients, including individuals with schizophrenic and non-schizophrenic disorders, also showed that service satisfaction is closely related to subjective quality of life (Ruggeri et al, 2001, 2002). These findings have been confirmed in other studies (Rohland et al, 2000; Berghofer et al, 2001; Druss et al, 2001). In the Epsilon Study of Schizophrenia, among all the explanatory variables considered, high satisfaction with life had, after study site, the strongest and most positive association with service satisfaction. Interestingly, domains which are very likely to be affected by severe mental illness, such as quality of social relations and quality of health, are those with the larger effects on satisfaction with services.

All these consistent findings tend to confirm the statement made by Locker & Dunt (1978), quoted above. The cross-cultural stability of this association, and its predominance over the other associations tested, offers the appealing perspective that improvements in patients' subjective quality of life can be achieved by providing adequate and individualised care. However, for the time being, caution is needed in interpreting these findings, as conflicting results have been obtained on possible confounders. On the one hand, it has been shown that subjective and objective quality of life have different latent constructs (Ruggeri et al, 2001), and that self-rated symptoms, subjective quality of life, self-rated needs and patients' assessments of treatments are all substantially correlated (Priebe et al, 1998). On the other hand, it has been found that mood and personality interfere with ratings of quality of life, but have a small influence on satisfaction with care (Atkinson & Caldwell, 1997; Ruggeri et al, 2003b). Finally, there is little consensus on the factors which influence subjective quality of life in the general population and results from national surveys do not provide reliable information on cross-cultural differences (Veenhoven, 1993).

In contrast, service characteristics do seem to play a clear role in determining service satisfaction. For example, studies have consistently reported that patients treated in community-based mental health services express higher levels of satisfaction than those receiving hospital-based mental healthcare (Hoult & Reynolds, 1984; Elbeck & Fecteau, 1990; Merson *et al*, 1992; Dean *et al*, 1993; Audini *et al*, 1994; Marks *et al*, 1994; Leese *et al*, 1998; Boardman *et al*, 1999; Henderson *et al*, 1999). A study conducted in England on an epidemiologically representative sample of patients with psychosis reported that having more unmet needs for care is correlated with lower service satisfaction (Leese *et al*, 1998). Another study has shown that availability of community beds results in significant reduction of unmet needs and better satisfaction with services (Boardman *et al*, 1999). In the Epsilon Study, a significant association was found between unmet needs and satisfaction, with lower satisfaction when more unmet needs were detected. This association maintained its significance after cross-site variability was accounted for, and in the separate domains of satisfaction. The biggest effect was found in the domain of patients' satisfaction with the involvement of relatives in care. This might suggest that one of the major problems that services have to face, when caring for people with schizophrenia who are more disabled, is to find an appropriate strategy to support their relatives (Ruggeri *et al*, 2003*a*).

As an *independent* variable, satisfaction can influence various behaviours of consumers, such as compliance and service utilisation. According to Ware & Davies (1983), satisfaction influences *care-seeking behaviour* (e.g. whether consumers seek care during an illness episode and the number of visits), *adherence behaviour* (whether patients do the things they are supposed to do while in care, for example adherence to regimens, compliance with follow-up visits and referrals) and *reactive behaviour* (actions initiated by consumers specifically to express their satisfaction or dissatisfaction, such as recommending a particular provider or facility, changing providers, registering formal complaints). Rossi *et al* (2002, 2008) found that (lack of) patient satisfaction was a significant predictor of both a change of doctor and dropping out of a health plan, and that relatively small differences in satisfaction ratings had noteworthy consequences for patient behaviour.

It has been shown that patients with a more negative assessment of treatment tend to have less improvement of psychopathology and longer hospital stays, in both the short and the long term (Gunkel & Priebe, 1993; Priebe & Bröker, 1999). Various findings highlight the relevance of the subjective view of users in understanding treatment effectiveness. In fact, when users are given a role as 'consumers', as opposed to passive service recipients, a disparity between the intended purposes of various treatments and the results as described by patients themselves may emerge and greatly enlighten data based on professional evaluations alone. Already in the 1980s, some findings pointed to a strong relationship between clients' satisfaction and their reports of outcome; a less strong relationship was found between reported satisfaction and outcome as rated by therapists (Lebow, 1983*b*). Later studies confirmed the relevance of the subjective perspective of users in assessing treatment outcome (Hansson, 1989; Merson *et al*, 1992; Dean *et* *al*, 1993; Dincin *et al*, 1993; Gomez Carrion *et al*, 1993; Kelstrup *et al*, 1993; Diamond & Factor, 1994; Leavey *et al*, 1997; Perreault *et al*, 1999; Lester *et al*, 2003; Garety *et al*, 2006; Kessing *et al*, 2006; Van Schaick *et al*, 2007; Taylor *et al*, 2009).

Service satisfaction and clinical routine

Service satisfaction seems to be a key variable both in *determining* the efficacy of interventions and in *understanding* the effect of interventions from the patient perspective. Thus, high satisfaction with mental health services is a valid goal for providers, and its measurement is relevant to those who evaluate services. Irrespective of this, clinicians tend to ignore the views of users about their own treatment. 'Transference distortions', 'manipulative behaviour', 'aggressivity', 'secondary advantages from illness' and 'defence mechanisms' are the reasons professionals commonly give for users' dissatisfaction (if they perceive it). The assessment of service satisfaction on the part of patients with a severe mental illness has been relatively neglected due to a view, held by many clinicians and researchers, that a lack of insight may compromise the validity of self-reported outcomes. While these difficulties should not be discounted, a growing body of evidence has shown that the self-reports of people suffering from psychotic disorders are reliable and convey valid and useful information (Naber *et al*, 1994; Awad *et al*, 1995; Voruganti *et al*, 1998; Awad & Voruganti, 2000; Lasalvia & Ruggeri, 2007) and suggests that the severity of illness in itself does not necessarily undermine the ability of patients to report their views and experiences. Overall, empirical data disconfirm the prejudice that patients are not capable of judging the care they receive. Andrews *et al* (1986) demonstrated that most requests for a change of therapist in an out-patient psychotherapy service result from patient–therapist mismatch and the majority of patients who changed therapists remained in treatment with the new therapist and reported being satisfied with the change.

Various studies have found that patients are sensitive to verbal and non-verbal elements of the healthcare process, are fairly accurate in distinguishing the quality of provider behaviours, such as courtesy and competence, and base their satisfaction ratings on these discriminations. Satisfaction ratings of patients have also been found to correlate with criteria for physician excellence customarily used by health providers, such as more years of training, positive motivation of the physician towards patients and peer supervision of physicians (for a review of these data see Lebow, 1983*a*). Sheppard (1993) has correlated patients' satisfaction with the nature of the intervention and the quality of some skills used by practitioners in extended interventions in a community mental health centre. Considerable differences were identified between 'satisfied' and 'not satisfied' clients in the service received and their perception; satisfaction was clearly related to the use of interpersonal skills such as communication, empathy, listening, openness and genuineness. This paper both indicates that the concept of satisfaction does meaningfully represent the client's experience and provides considerable support for the fundamental importance of the acquisition and use of these skills in practice.

On the other hand, especially in psychiatric patients who are severely ill, awareness of clients' problems may be incomplete and their capacity to judge reliably the care they receive is not guaranteed. A careful analysis of the components of care which may be properly assessed by users is needed (for a discussion of perception by users of the technical and non-technical components of care, see Hornstra & Lubin 1974; Brody *et al*, 1989; Salmon *et al*, 1994; Bjørngaard *et al*, 2007a,b; Hansson *et al*, 2007). But, despite these difficulties, assessing the subjective perspective of users is an opportunity not to be missed in either service evaluation or routine clinical practice.

When considering the impact of satisfaction on care, short-term and long-term dissatisfaction should be differentiated. It is obvious that there may be times when fulfilling clients' requests may prove too difficult or too costly, or may not be clinically indicated. Short-term dissatisfaction in some cases can be legitimately considered a side-effect of a therapeutic intervention which changes the patient's perspective (e.g. a shift from institutional to community care, or pursuing a change in the relationship of the patient with significant others). Apart from the risk of early drop-out from treatment, dissatisfaction itself may not be a worry here. More importance should be attached to consumers' dissatisfaction in the long term. Long-term dissatisfaction, in fact, may indicate that the planned change did not contribute to an improvement in the client's life. In this case the value of the intervention should be seriously reconsidered. Dissatisfaction here may indicate that the client did not have enough personal resources to appreciate the advantages of the intervention. In such a case, if not a change in the therapeutic strategy, at least an improvement in communication between client and professionals is necessary.

Short-term dissatisfaction can easily become satisfaction in the long run if professionals perceive it correctly, communicate their perception to the consumer, and discuss with any problems. Moreover, it should be stressed that different perspectives do not necessarily result in dissatisfaction. In fact, when consumers feel that their viewpoint has been taken into account and an acceptable therapeutic management plan has been worked out through a process of mutual negotiation, they may still feel satisfied, even if their initial requests are not fully met.

Methodological issues in measuring satisfaction

That the issue of patient satisfaction has elicited contradictory data and radically divergent opinions among experts is a fact. What has not been stated clearly enough is that the contradictory findings are a consequence of the poor quality of the research in the field, especially in relation to study design and instrument development and validation. Efforts to measure satisfaction with services have varied widely in method, and knowledge within this area has been scattered rather than systematic (Ruggeri, 1994). Inadequate study design or implementation and a lack instruments with sufficient psychometric data play a major role in producing biased or flattened responses from patients, as does lack of confidentiality.

Users' views have often been solicited using qualitative methods, such as records of their spontaneous reports, but, owing to lack of sensitivity, this method is not considered to be the approach of choice in measuring satisfaction (Ruggeri, 1996). A combination of quantitative and qualitative methods can be useful for gaining a deeper understanding of the reasons for dissatisfaction (Everett & Boydell, 1994), but is not a substitute for quantitative assessments.

When quantitative methods are used in satisfaction research, researchers may be tempted to adopt questionnaires composed of either a few broad questions about satisfaction or unstandardised, single-item subscales that tap reactions to one or two dimensions of what is known to be a multifaceted construct (Ruggeri, 1996). This happens notwithstanding the fact that the majority of findings reported in the literature support the idea that satisfaction is a multidimensional concept; the dimensions include professionals' skills and behaviour, access, information, efficacy and type of interventions (Ware & Snyder 1976; Ware & Davies, 1983; Attkisson & Greenfield, 1994). Thus, enquiries based on overall satisfaction not only may fail to detect dissatisfaction but are also inherently destined *not* to detect the reasons for dissatisfaction. No wonder such measures give highly skewed distributions with little variance. This leads to lack of knowledge about the causes of dissatisfaction or to high ratings despite other evidence to the contrary.

Scales for measuring satisfaction with services

While in the past, researchers conducting satisfaction studies tended to develop their own instruments, since the 1990s the need for research that develops and refines measures of client satisfaction and establishes their psychometric properties has been considered a priority in service evaluation by a growing number of authors (Steinwachs *et al*, 1992; Ruggeri, 1994).

Some scales were developed in the 1970s and the 1980s for assessing psychiatric out-patient treatment (Love *et al*, 1979; Deiker *et al*, 1981; Slater *et al*, 1981). Several excellent scales were developed that assess satisfaction with medical care (Hulka *et al*, 1970; Ware & Snyder, 1976) and these could readily be adapted to assess mental health treatment.

A major contribution in this field was made by Attkisson, Greenfield and their colleagues at the University of California at San Francisco (Attkisson & Greenfield, 1994, 1996; Attkisson *et al*, 1995; Greenfield & Attkisson, 2004). They first developed the Client Satisfaction Questionnaire (CSQ; Larsen *et al*, 1979). The CSQ, which, in its 31- and 8-item versions, assesses a general satisfaction factor, uses a four-point Likert scale, and has been developed through a careful sequential process to enhance reliability and validity. It is the only instrument for measuring patients' satisfaction which has had widespread use. It has been applied in many types of service setting, including mental health services (Dyck & Azim, 1983; Greenfield, 1983; Azim & Joyce, 1986; Sishta *et al*, 1986; Huxley & Warner, 1992), and has been translated into Spanish, Dutch and French (de Brey, 1983; Roberts *et al*, 1984; Sabourin *et al*, 1987). However, the monodimensionality of the CSQ constitutes a limit to its sensitivity and content validity, other than as a global measure.

Based on the experience with the CSQ, Greenfield & Attkisson (1989) later developed another instrument, the Service Satisfaction Scale (SSS–30), specifically designed as a multidimensional measure which, on a five-point Likert scale, assesses several components of satisfaction with either medical health or mental health out-patient services (practitioner manner and skill, perceived outcome, office procedures and access), and has been used in a range of service settings (Attkisson & Greenfield, 1994; Greenfield & Attkisson, 2000). The SSS–30 can be considered an excellent instrument for cross-setting studies or studies in general practice but, although it is a substantial improvement on previous questionnaires, it still lacks validity for studies specific to mental health settings.

The Verona Service Satisfaction Scale (VSSS) is an attempt to combine cross-setting and setting-specific items for measuring satisfaction with community-based mental health services. It is a setting-specific, validated, multidimensional scale for measuring patients' satisfaction with mental health services. It was first developed in an 82-item version (Ruggeri & Dall'Agnola, 1993): a set of 37 cross-setting items for health services and a set of 45 items specific to mental health services. The former group of items involved aspects meant *a priori* to be relevant across a broad array of both medical and psychiatric settings, and was derived from the SSS–30 (Ruggeri & Greenfield, 1995); the latter group of items involved aspects relevant specifically in mental health settings, particularly in community-based services, such as social skills and types of intervention (e.g. admissions, psychotherapy, rehabilitation), and its development was informed in part by family and community-residential versions of the SSS–30 (Ruggeri & Greenfield, 1995). The original VSSS–82, in its versions for patients and relatives, was developed by the author of this chapter at the University of Verona in the early 1990s and has been tested for acceptability, content validity, sensitivity and test–retest reliability, and it shows good psychometric properties (Ruggeri *et al*, 1994). Factor analysis has also been performed (Ruggeri *et al*, 1996). The combination of results obtained in the validation study and factor analysis gave rise to an intermediate (VSSS–54) and a short version (VSSS–32), two reliable instruments that are easy to use in everyday clinical settings.

The European version (EU version) of the questionnaire was developed from the VSSS–54, between 1997 and 2000, in the context of the Epsilon Study (Becker *et al*, 1999), which produced standardised versions of a series of key instruments, one of which was the VSSS–EU, in four languages (Spanish, Italian, English, Danish). VSSS versions are available also in French (Corbiere *et al*, 2003), Spanish, Portuguese, German (Mory *et al*, 2001), Norwegian, Greek, Sloven, Polish, Chinese, Japanese, Farsi and Kuwaiti. The VSSS is being used in a growing number of studies in many countries (Tonelli & Merini, 1995; Artal *et al*, 1997; Parkman *et al*, 1997; Leese *et al*, 1998; Boardman *et al*, 1999; Clarkson *et al*, 1999; Merinder *et al*, 1999; Chiappelli & Berardi, 2000; Ruggeri *et al*, 2001, 2002, 2003*a,b*, 2004, 2005, 2006, 2007; Perez de los Cobos *et al*, 2002, 2004, 2005; Rossi *et al*, 2002, 2008; Henderson *et al*, 2003; Lester *et al*, 2003; Lora *et al*, 2003; Garety *et al*, 2006; Kessing *et al*, 2006; Ayton *et al*, 2007). Details of the instrument development process, including translation, cross-cultural adaptation and reliability testing, are given by Ruggeri *et al* (2000).

Conceptually, the items in VSSS–EU cover seven dimensions exploring various aspects of satisfaction with services:

1   the overall satisfaction dimension comprises three items which cover general aspects of satisfaction with mental health services
2   the professionals' skills and behaviour dimension comprises 24 items which cover various aspects of satisfaction with the professionals' behaviour such as technical skills, interpersonal skills, cooperation between service providers, respect of patients' rights, and so on (psychiatrists, psychologists, nurses and social workers are assessed in separate items)
3   the information dimension comprises three items which cover aspects related to satisfaction with information on services, disorders and therapies
4   the access dimension comprises two items which cover aspects related to satisfaction with service location, physical layout, and costs
5   the efficacy dimension comprises eight items which cover aspects related to satisfaction with overall efficacy of the service, and service efficacy on specific aspects such as symptoms, social skills and family relationships
6   the types of intervention dimension comprises 17 items which cover various aspects of satisfaction with mental health care, such as drug prescription, response to emergencies, psychotherapy, rehabilitation, domiciliary care, admissions, housing, recreational activities, work, benefits and so on
7   the relative's involvement dimension comprises six items which cover various aspects of patients' satisfaction with help given to their closest relative, such as listening, understanding, advice, information, help coping with the patient's problems, and so on.

The VSSS–EU is thus a reliable instrument for use in comparative cross-national research projects as well as in routine clinical practice. It has been specifically designed for community-based mental health services run by multidisciplinary teams of psychiatrists, psychologists, social workers and nurses. These services are assumed to have various treatment options (e.g. hospitalisation, day care, rehabilitation, psychotherapy, home help, out-patient visits) available (either directly or through various services which closely cooperate). The VSSS–EU may be easily adapted to community settings which differ slightly from this model (e.g. fewer treatment options in the service or different composition of the care personnel), but caution should be used if the service organisation is radically different from the model assumed.

Conclusion

The process of evaluating mental health services is a timely, long term, and complex process, and different strategies, as well as various techniques, need to be used (Tansella 1989, 1991; Ruggeri *et al*, 1998*a*; Thornicroft & Tansella, 1999). Developing a comprehensive model for the assessment of the outcome of psychiatric care has been a great challenge for service evaluators, but major progress has been made in the last 20 years (Lasalvia & Ruggeri, 2007) and an increasing number of researchers and clinicians are using a multidimensional and multi-axial model for the assessment of outcome in both naturalistic and experimental studies.

Integration of data from randomised trials assessing the efficacy or potential of a treatment under experimental conditions, and naturalistic studies assessing the effectiveness or result of treatment as provided in the 'real world', should be encouraged. Community surveys that incorporate multidimensional measurement of the outcome of mental healthcare, with the use of standardised instruments, administered as part of routine clinical activities within community-based psychiatric services, should be planned. The South-Verona Outcome Project (Lasalvia & Ruggeri, 2007) has been a successful attempt to standardise information that clinicians collect and record, in periodic reviews of cases in treatment in their everyday clinical practice, and to employ for service evaluation the same professionals involved in the clinical work. Results obtained so far confirm both the feasibility of this kind of study and its contribution to service evaluation and planning, and constitutes a comprehensive example of the potential of such an approach (Thornicroft, 2008).

From this perspective, users' satisfaction plays an important role and is one of the most promising areas. Sustained effort is required to spread the use of well validated instruments and to discourage continual recourse to *ad hoc* measures. Content validity in capturing users' views, acceptability to users and the use of instruments which have established psychometric properties and a norm base should be the rule. Comparability between studies should be pursued vigorously in order both to allow the refinement of existing instruments and to advance our theoretical and substantive understanding of satisfaction with psychiatric services and its relationships with care provided and with the other indicators of outcome.

References

Andrews, S., Leavy, A., DeChillo, N., *et al* (1986) Patient–therapist mismatch: we would rather switch than fight. *Hospital and Community Psychiatry*, **37**, 918–922.

Artal, J., Vazquez-Barquero, J. L., Rodriguez-Pulido, F., *et al* (1997) Evaluacion de la satisfaccion con los servicios de salud mental: la escala de Verona (VSSS–54) [Evaluation of satisfaction with mental health service: the Verona Scale (VSSS-54)]. *Archivos de Neurobiologia*, **60**, 185–200.

Atkinson, M. J. & Caldwell, L. (1997) The differential effects of mood on patients' ratings of life quality and satisfaction with their care. *Journal of Affective Disorders*, **44**, 169–175.

Attkisson, C. C. & Greenfield, T. K. (1994) The Client Satisfaction Questionnaire–8 and the Service Satisfaction Questionnaire–30. In *Psychological Testing: Treatment Planning and Outcome Assessment* (ed. M. Maruish), pp. 404–420. Lawrence Erlbaum Associates.

Attkisson, C. C. & Greenfield, T. K. (1996) The Client Satisfaction Questionnaire (CSQ) scales and the Service Satisfaction Scale–30 (SSS–30). In *Outcomes Assessment in Clinical Practice* (eds L. I. Sederer & B. Dickey), pp. 120–127. Williams & Wilkins.

Attkisson, C. C. & Pascoe, G. C. (eds) (1983) *Patient Satisfaction in Health and Mental Health Services*. Evaluation and Program Planning 6, Special Issue. Pergamon Press.

Attkisson, C., Cook, J., Karno, M., *et al* (1992) Clinical services research. *Schizophrenia Bulletin*, **18**, 627–668.

Attkisson, C. C., Greenfield, T. K. & Melendez, D. (1995) The Client Satisfaction Questionnaire (CSQ) scale and Service Satisfaction Scale (SSS): a history of scale development and a guide for users. Department of Psychiatry, University of California, San Francisco. See http://www.ucsf.edu/csq/CSQMANU.htm (accessed 29 May 2005).

Audini, B., Marks, I. M., Lawrence, R. E., *et al* (1994) Home-based versus out-patient/in-patient care for people with serious mental illness. Phase II of a controlled study. *British Journal of Psychiatry*, **165**, 204–210.

Awad, A. G. & Voruganti, L. N. P. (2000) Intervention research in psychosis: issues related to the assessment of quality of life. *Schizophrenia Bulletin*, **26**, 557–564.

Awad, A. G., Hogan, T. P., Voruganti, L. N. P., *et al* (1995) Patients' subjective experiences on antipsychotic medications: implications for outcome and quality of life. *International Clinical Psychopharmacology*, **10** (suppl. 3), 123–133.

Ayton, A. K., Mooney, M. P., Sillifant, K., *et al* (2007) The development of the child and adolescent versions of the Verona Service Satisfaction Scale (CAMHSSS). *Social Psychiatry and Psychiatric Epidemiology*, **42**, 892–901.

Azim, H. F. A. & Joyce, A. S. (1986) The impact of data-based program modifications on the satisfaction of outpatients in group psychotherapy. *Canadian Journal of Psychiatry*, **31**, 119–122.

Barker, D. A., Shergill, S. S., Higginson, I., *et al* (1996) Patients' views towards care received from psychiatrists. *British Journal of Psychiatry*, **168**, 641–646.

Becker, T., Knapp, M., Knudsen, H. C., *et al* (1999) The Epsilon study of schizophrenia in five European countries: design and methodology for standardising outcome measures and comparing patterns of care and service costs. *British Journal of Psychiatry*, **175**, 514–521.

Beresford, P. (2005) Developing the theoretical basis for service user/survivor-led research and equal involvement in research. *Epidemiologia e Psichiatria Sociale*, **14**, 4–9.

Berghofer, G., Lang, A., Henkel, H., *et al* (2001) Satisfaction of inpatients and outpatients with staff, environment, and other patients. *Psychiatric Services*, **52**, 104–106.

Bjørngaard, J. H., Ruud, T. & Friis, S. (2007*a*) The impact of mental illness on patient satisfaction with the therapeutic relationship. A multilevel analysis. *Social Psychiatry and Psychiatric Epidemiology*, **42**, 803–809.

Bjørngaard, J. H., Ruud, T., Garratt, A., *et al* (2007*b*) Patients' experiences and clinicians' ratings of the quality of outpatient teams in psychiatric care units in Norway. *Psychiatric Services*, **58**, 8.

Boardman, A. P., Hodgson, R. E., Lewis, M., *et al* (1999) North Staffordshire Community Beds Study: longitudinal evaluation of psychiatric in-patient units attached to community mental health centres. *British Journal of Psychiatry*, **175**, 70–78.

Bramesfeld, A., Klippel, U., Seidel, G., *et al* (2007) How do patients expect the mental health service system to act? Testing the WHO responsiveness concept for its appropriateness in mental health care. *Social Science and Medicine*, **65**, 880–889.

Brimblecombe, N., Tingle, A. & Murrells, T. (2007) How mental health nursing can best improve service users' experiences and outcomes in inpatient settings: responses to a national consultation. *Journal of Psychiatric and Mental Health Nursing*, **14**, 503–509.

Brody, D. S., Miller, S. M., Lerman, C. E., *et al* (1989) The relationship between patients' satisfaction with their physicians and perceptions about interventions they desired and received. *Medical Care*, **27**, 1027–1035.

Brown, C., Rempfer, M. & Hamera, E. (2008) Correlates of insider and outsider conceptualizations of recovery. *Psychiatric Rehabilitation Journal*, **32**, 23–31.

Chamberlain, J. (2005) User/consumer involvement in mental health service delivery. *Epidemiologia e Psichiatria Sociale*, **14**, 10–14.

Chiappelli, M. & Berardi, S. (2000) Pattern of intervention and patients' satisfaction with community mental health services in Bologna [in Italian]. *Epidemiologia e Psichiatria Sociale*, **9**, 272–281.

Clarkson, P., McCrone, P., Sutherby, K., *et al* (1999) Outcomes and costs of a community support worker service for the severely mentally ill. *Acta Psychiatrica Scandinavica*, **99**, 196–206.

Corbiere, M., Lesage, A., Lauzon, S., *et al* (2003) French validation of the Verona Service Satisfaction Scale – VSSS–54F [in French]. *Encephale*, **29**, 110–118.

Crawford, M. J., Aldridge, T., Bhui, K., *et al* (2003) User involvement in the planning and delivery of mental health services: a cross-sectional survey of service users and providers. *Acta Psychiatrica Scandinavica*, **107**, 410–414.

Dean, C., Philipps, J., Gadd, E. M., *et al* (1993) Comparison of community based service with hospital based service for people with acute, severe psychiatric illness. *BMJ*, **307**, 473–476.

de Brey, H. (1983) A cross-national validation of the client satisfaction questionnaire: the Dutch experience. *Evaluation and Program Planning*, **6**, 395–400.

Deiker, T., Osborn, S. M., Distefano, M. R., *et al* (1981) Consumer accreditation: development of a quality assurance patient evaluation scale. *Hospital and Community Psychiatry*, **32**, 565–567.

Diamond, R. J. & Factor, R. M. (1994) Taking issue. Treatment-resistant patients or a treatment-resistant system? *Hospital and Community Psychiatry*, **45**, 197.

Dincin, J., Wasmer, D., Witheridge, T. F., *et al* (1993) Impact of assertive community treatment on the use of state hospital inpatient bed-days. *Hospital and Community Psychiatry*, **44**, 833–838.

Donabedian, A. (1966) Evaluating the quality of medical care. *Milbank Memorial Fund Quarterly*, **44**, 166–203.

Druss, B. G., Schlesinger, M. & Hallen, H. M. (2001) Depressive symptoms, satisfaction with health care, and 2-year work outcomes in an employed population. *American Journal of Psychiatry*, **5**, 731–734.

Dyck, R. J. & Azim, H. F. (1983) Patient satisfaction in a psychiatric walk-in clinic. *Canadian Journal of Psychiatry*, **28**, 30–33.

Elbeck, M. & Fecteau, G. (1990) Improving the validity of measures of patient satisfaction with psychiatric care and treatment. *Hospital and Community Psychiatry*, **41**, 998–1001.

Ellwood, P. (1998) A technology of patient experience. *New England Journal of Medicine*, **318**, 1549–1556.

Everett, B. & Boydell, K. (1994) A methodology for including consumers' opinions in mental health evaluation research. *Hospital and Community Psychiatry*, **45**, 76–78.

Garety, P. A., Craig, T. K. J., Dunn, G., *et al* (2006) Specialised care for early psychosis: symptoms, social functioning and patient satisfaction. *British Journal of Psychiatry*, **188**, 37–45.

Gomez Carrion, P., Swann, A., Kellert-Cecil, H., *et al* (1993) Compliance with clinic attendance by outpatients with schizophrenia. *Hospital and Community Psychiatry*, **44**, 764–767.

Greenfield, T. K. (1983) The role of client satisfaction in evaluating university counselling services. *Evaluation and Program Planning*, **6**, 315–327.

Greenfield, T. K. & Attkisson, C. C. (1989) Steps toward a multifactorial satisfaction scale for primary care and mental health services. *Evaluation and Program Planning*, **12**, 271–278.

Greenfield, T. K. & Attkisson, C. C. (2000) Service Satisfaction Scale–30 (SSS–30). In *Handbook of Psychiatric Measures* (eds A. J. Rush, H. A. Pincus, M. B. First, *et al*), pp. 188–191. American Psychiatric Association.

Greenfield, T. K. & Attkisson, C. C. (2004) The UCSF Client Satisfaction Scales: II. The Service Satisfaction Scale–30. In *Psychological Testing: Treatment Planning and Outcome Assessment, Vol. 3. Instruments for Adults* (ed. M. Maruish), pp. 813–837. Lawrence Erlbaum Associates.

Greenwood, N., Key, A., Burns, T., *et al* (1999) Satisfaction with in-patient psychiatric services. Relationship to patient and treatment factors. *British Journal of Psychiatry*, **174**, 159–163.

Gunkel, S. & Priebe, S. (1993) Different perspectives of short-term changes in the rehabilitation of schizophrenic patients. *Comprehensive Psychiatry*, **34**, 352–359.

Hansson, L. (1989) Patient satisfaction with in-hospital psychiatric care. A study of 1-year population of patients hospitalised in a sectorised care organisation. *European Archives of Psychiatry and Neurological Sciences*, **239**, 93–100.

Hansson, L., Björkman, T. & Priebe, S. (2007) Are important patient-rated outcomes in community mental health care explained by only one factor? *Acta Psychiatrica Scandinavica*, **116**, 113–118.

Henderson, C., Phelan, M., Loftus, L., *et al* (1999) Comparison of patients' satisfaction with community-based vs. hospital psychiatric services. *Acta Psychiatrica Scandinavica*, **99**, 188–195.

Henderson, C., Hales, H. & Ruggeri, M. (2003) Cross-cultural differences in the conceptualisation of patients' satisfaction with psychiatric services: content validity of the English version of the Verona Service Satisfaction Scale. *Social Psychiatry and Psychiatric Epidemiology*, **38**, 142–148.

Hornstra, R. K. & Lubin, B. (1974) Relationship of outcome of treatment to agreement about treatment assignment by patients and professionals. *Journal of Nervous and Mental Disease*, **158**, 420–423.

Hoult, J. & Reynolds, I. (1984) Schizophrenia. A comparative trial of community orientated and hospital orientated psychiatric care. *Acta Psychiatrica Scandinavica*, **69**, 359–372.

Hulka, B., Zyzansky, L., Cassel, J., *et al* (1970) Scale for the measurement of attitudes toward physicians and primary health care. *Medical Care*, **8**, 429–430.

Huxley, P. & Warner, R. (1992) Case management, quality of life, and satisfaction with services of long-term psychiatric patients. *Hospital and Community Psychiatry*, **43**, 799–803.

Jenkins, R. (1990) Toward a system of outcome indicators for mental health care. *British Journal of Psychiatry*, **157**, 500–514.

Kelstrup, A., Lund, K., Lauridsen, B., *et al* (1993) Satisfaction with care reported by psychiatric inpatients. *Acta Psychiatrica Scandinavica*, **87**, 374–379.

Kessing, L. V., Hansen, H. V., Ruggeri, M., *et al* (2006) Satisfaction with treatment among patients with depressive and bipolar disorders. *Social Psychiatry and Psychiatric Epidemiology*, **41**, 148–155.

Killaspy, H., Johnson, S., King, M., et al (2008) Developing mental health services in response to research evidence. *Epidemiologia e Psichiatria Sociale*, **17**, 1.

Larsen, D., Attkisson, C. C., Hargreaves, W., et al (1979) Assessment of client/patient satisfaction: development of a general scale. *Evaluation and Program Planning*, **2**, 197–207.

Lasalvia, A. & Ruggeri, M. (2007) Assessing the outcome of community-based psychiatric care: building a feedback loop from 'real world' health services research into clinical practice. *Acta Psychiatrica Scandinavica*, suppl. 437, 6–15.

Leavey, G., King, M., Cole, E., et al (1997) First-onset psychotic illness: patients' and relatives' satisfaction with services. *British Journal of Psychiatry*, **170**, 53–57.

Lebow, J. L. (1983a) Research assessing consumer satisfaction with mental health treatment: a review of findings. *Evaluation and Program Planning*, **6**, 211–236.

Lebow, J. L. (1983b) Client satisfaction with mental health treatment: methodological considerations in assessment. *Evaluation Review*, **7**, 729–752.

Leese, M., Johnson, S., Slade, M., et al (1998) User perspective on needs and satisfaction with mental health services. *British Journal of Psychiatry*, **173**, 409–415.

Lester, H., Allan, T., Wilson, S., et al (2003) A cluster randomised controlled trial of patient-held medical records for people with schizophrenia receiving shared care. *British Journal of General Practice*, **53**, 197–203.

Locker, D. & Dunt, D. (1978) Theoretical and methodological issues in sociological studies of consumer satisfaction with medical care. *Social Science and Medicine*, **12**, 283–292.

Lora, A., Rivolta, N. & Lanzara, D. (2003) Patient satisfaction with community-based psychiatric services. *International Journal of Mental Health*, **32**, 32–48.

Love, R. E., Caid, C. D. & Davis, A. (1979) The User Satisfaction Survey: consumer evaluation of an inner city community mental health center. *Evaluation and the Health Profession*, **2**, 42–54.

Marks, I. M., Connolly, J., Muijen, M., et al (1994) Home-based versus hospital-based care for people with serious mental illness. *British Journal of Psychiatry*, **165**, 179–194.

Merinder, L. B., Viuff, A. G., Laugesen, H. D., et al (1999) Patient and relative education in community psychiatry: a randomized controlled trial regarding its effectiveness. *Social Psychiatry and Psychiatric Epidemiology*, **34**, 287–294.

Merson, S., Tyrer, P., Onyett, S., et al (1992) Early intervention in psychiatric emergencies: a controlled clinical trial. *Lancet*, **339**, 1311–1314.

Mirin, S. M. & Namerow, M. J. (1991) Why study treatment outcome? *Hospital and Community Psychiatry*, **42**, 1007–1013.

Mory, C., Matschinger, H., Roick, C., et al (2001) The German adaptation of the Verona Service Satisfaction Scale: an instrument for patients' satisfaction with mental health care [in German]. *Psychiatrische Praxis*, **28** (suppl. 2), S91–96.

Naber, D., Walther, A., Kirchner, T., et al (1994) Subjective effects of neuroleptics predict compliance. In *Prediction of Neuroleptic Treatment Outcome in Schizophrenia: Concepts and Methods* (eds W. Gabel & A. G. Awad), pp. 469–473. Springer-Verlag.

Parkman, S., Davies, S., Leese, M., et al (1997) Ethnic differences in satisfaction with mental health services among representative people with psychosis in South London: PRISM Study 4. *British Journal of Psychiatry*, **171**, 260–264.

Perez de los Cobos, J., Valero, S., Haro, G., et al (2002) Development and psychometric properties of the Verona Service Satisfaction Scale for methadone-treated opioid-dependent patients (VSSS–MT). *Drug and Alcohol Dependence*, **68**, 209–214.

Perez de los Cobos, J., Fidel, G., Escuder, G., et al (2004) A satisfaction survey of opioid-dependent clients at methadone treatment centres in Spain. *Drug and Alcohol Dependence*, **73**, 307–313.

Perez de los Cobos, J., Trujols, J., Valderrama, J. C., et al (2005) Patient perspectives on methadone maintenance treatment in the Valencia region: dose adjustment, participation in dosage regulation, and satisfaction with treatment. *Drug and Alcohol Dependence*, **79**, 405–412.

Perreault, M., Paquin, G., Kennedy, S., *et al* (1999) Patients' perspective on their relatives' involvement in the treatment during a short-term psychiatric hospitalization. *Social Psychiatry and Psychiatric Epidemiology*, **34**, 157–165.

Priebe, S. & Bröker, M. (1999) Prediction of hospitalizations by schizophrenia patients' assessment of treatment: an expanded study. *Journal of Psychiatric Research*, **33**, 113–119.

Priebe, S., Kaise, W., Huxley, P. J., *et al* (1998) Do different subjective evaluation criteria reflect distinct constructs? *Journal of Nervous and Mental Disease*, **186**, 385–392.

Priebe, S., McCabe, R., Bullenkamp, J., *et al* (2007) Structured patient–clinician communication and 1-year outcome in community mental healthcare. *British Journal of Psychiatry*, **191**, 420–426.

Roberts, R., Attkisson, C. & Mendias, R. M. (1984) Assessing the Client Satisfaction Questionnaire in English and Spanish. *Hispanic Journal of Behavioural Sciences*, **6**, 385–396.

Rohland, B. M., Langbehn, D. R. & Rohrer, J. E. (2000) Relationship between service effectiveness and satisfaction among persons receiving Medicaid mental health services. *Psychiatric Services*, **51**, 248–250.

Rossi, A., Amaddeo, F., Bisoffi, G., *et al* (2002) Dropping out of care: inappropriate terminations of contact with community-based psychiatric services. *British Journal of Psychiatry*, **181**, 331–338.

Rossi, A., Amaddeo, F., Sandri, M., *et al* (2008) What happens to patients seen only once by psychiatric services? Findings from a follow-up study. *Psychiatry Research*, **157**, 53–65.

Ruggeri, M. (1994) Patient's and relatives' satisfaction with psychiatric services: the state of the art of its measurement. In *Designing Instruments for Mental Health Service Research. Part I* (eds G. Thornicroft & M. Tansella). *Social Psychiatry and Psychiatric Epidemiology*, **29**, 212–227. [Special issue.]

Ruggeri, M. (1996) Satisfaction with psychiatric services. In *Mental Health Outcomes Measures* (eds G. Thornicroft & M. Tansella), pp. 27–52. Springer-Verlag.

Ruggeri, M. (2001) Measuring satisfaction with psychiatric services: towards a multi-dimensional, multi-axial assessment of outcome. In *Mental Health Outcomes Measures* (eds G. Thornicroft & M. Tansella), pp. 34–47. Gaskell.

Ruggeri, M. & Dall'Agnola, R. (1993) The development and use of the Verona Expectations for Care Scale (VECS) and the Verona Service Satisfaction Scale (VSSS) for measuring expectations and satisfaction with community-based psychiatric services in patients, relatives and professionals. *Psychological Medicine*, **23**, 511–523.

Ruggeri, M. & Greenfield, T. (1995) The Italian version of the Service Satisfaction Scale (SSS–30) adapted for community-based psychiatric services: development, factor analysis and application. *Evaluation and Program Planning*, **18**, 191–202.

Ruggeri, M. & Tansella, M. (1995) Evaluating outcome in mental health care. *Current Opinion in Psychiatry*, **8**, 116–121.

Ruggeri, M., Dall'Agnola, R., Agostini, C., *et al* (1994) Acceptability, sensitivity and content validity of VECS and VSSS in measuring expectations and satisfaction in psychiatric patients and their relatives. *Social Psychiatry and Psychiatric Epidemiology*, **29**, 265–276.

Ruggeri, M., Dall'Agnola, R., Greenfield, T., *et al* (1996) Factor analysis of the Verona Service Satisfaction Scale–82 and development of reduced versions. *International Journal of Methods in Psychiatric Research*, **6**, 23–38.

Ruggeri, M., Biggeri, A., Rucci, P., *et al* (1998a) Multivariate analysis of outcome of mental health care using graphical chain models. The South-Verona Outcome Project 1. *Psychological Medicine*, **28**, 1421–1431.

Ruggeri, M., Riani, M., Rucci, P., *et al* (1998b) Multidimensional assessment of outcome in psychiatry: the use of graphical displays. The South-Verona Outcome Project 2. *International Journal of Methods in Psychiatric Research*, **7**, 186–198.

Ruggeri, M., Lasalvia, A., Dall'Agnola, R., *et al* (2000) Development, internal consistency and reliability of the Verona Service Satisfaction Scale – European Version. In *Reliable

Outcome Measure for Mental Health Service Research in Five European Countries: The Epsilon Study (eds G. Thornicroft, T. Becker, M. Knapp, *et al*). *British Journal of Psychiatry*, **177** (suppl. 39), 41–48.

Ruggeri, M., Warner, R., Bisoffi, G., *et al* (2001) Subjective and objective dimensions of quality of life in psychiatric patients: a factor analytical approach. The South-Verona Outcome Project 4. *British Journal of Psychiatry*, **178**, 268–275.

Ruggeri, M., Gater, R., Bisoffi, G., *et al* (2002) Determinants of subjective quality of life in patients attending community-based mental health services. The South-Verona Outcome Project 5. *Acta Psychiatrica Scandinavica*, **105**, 131–140.

Ruggeri, M., Lasalvia, A., Bisoffi, G., *et al* (2003a) Satisfaction with mental health services among people with schizophrenia in five European sites: results from the Epsilon study. *Schizophrenia Bulletin*, **29**, 229–245.

Ruggeri, M., Pacati, P. & Goldberg, D. (2003b) Neurotics are dissatisfied with life, but not with services. The South Verona Outcome Project 7. *General Hospital Psychiatry*, **25**, 338–344.

Ruggeri, M., Bisoffi, G., Lasalvia, A., *et al* (2004) A longitudinal evaluation of two-year outcome in a community-based mental health service using graphical chain models. The South-Verona Outcome Project 9. *International Journal of Methods in Psychiatric Research*, **13**, 10–23.

Ruggeri, M., Nosè, M., Bonetto, C., *et al* (2005) Changes and predictors of change in objective and subjective quality of life. A multiwave follow-up study in community psychiatric practice. *British Journal of Psychiatry*, **186**, 47.

Ruggeri, M., Salvi, G., Perwanger, V., *et al* (2006) Satisfaction with community and hospital-based emergency services amongst severely mentally ill service users. *Social Psychiatry and Psychiatric Epidemiology*, **41**, 302–309.

Ruggeri, M., Lasalvia, A., Salvi, G., *et al* (2007) Applications and usefulness of routine measurement of patients' satisfaction with community-based mental health care. *Acta Psychiatrica Scandinavica Supplementum*, **437**, 53–65.

Sabourin, S., Gendreau, P. & Frenette, L. (1987) Le neveau de satisfaction des cas d'abandon dans un service universitaire de psychologie. *Canadian Journal of Behavioral Sciences*, **19**, 314–323.

Salmon, P., Sharma, N., Valori, R., *et al* (1994) Patients' intentions in primary care: relationship to physical and psychological symptoms, and their perception by general practitioners. *Social Science and Medicine*, **38**, 585–592.

Sheppard, M. (1993) Client satisfaction, extended intervention and interpersonal skills in community mental health. *Journal of Advanced Nursing*, **18**, 246–259.

Simpson, E. L. & House, A. O. (2002) Involving users in the delivery and evaluation of mental health services: systematic review. *BMJ*, **325**, 1265.

Sishta, S. K., Rinco, S. & Sullivan, J. C. F. (1986) Clients' satisfaction survey in a psychiatric inpatient population attached to a general hospital. *Canadian Journal of Psychiatry*, **31**, 123–128.

Slater, V., Linn, M. W. & Harris, R. (1981) Outpatient evaluation of mental health care. *Southern Medical Journal*, **74**, 1217–1219.

Smith, G. R., Manderscheid, R. W., Flynn, L. M., *et al* (1997) Principles for assessment of patient outcomes in mental health care. *Psychiatric Services*, **48**, 1033–1036.

Steinwachs, D. M., Cullum, H., Dorwart, R. A., *et al* (1992) Service systems research. *Schizophrenia Bulletin*, **18**, 627–668.

Stringer, B., Van Meijel, B., De Vree, W., *et al* (2008) User involvement in mental health care: the role of nurses. A literature review. *Journal of Psychiatric and Mental Health Nursing*, **15**, 678–683.

Svensson, B. & Hansson, L. (1994) Patient satisfaction with inpatient psychiatric care. The influence of personality traits, diagnosis and perceived coercion. *Acta Psychiatrica Scandinavica*, **90**, 379–384.

Tansclla, M. (1989) Evaluating community psychiatric services. In *The Scope of Epidemiological Psychiatry* (eds P. Williams, C. Wilkinson & K. Rawnsley), pp. 386–403. Routledge.

Tansella, M. (ed.) (1991) *Community-Based Psychiatry: Long Term Patterns of Care in South-Verona*. Psychological Medicine Monograph Supplement 19. Cambridge University Press.

Taylor, T. L., Hawton, K., Fortune, S., *et al* (2009) Attitudes towards clinical services among people who self-harm: systematic review. *British Journal of Psychiatry*, **194**, 104–110.

Thornicroft, G. (2008) Multidimensional Outcomes in 'Real World' Mental Health Services. Follow-up Findings from the South Verona Outcome Project [Book review]. *Psychological Medicine*, **38**, 1516–1517.

Thornicroft, G. & Tansella, M. (1999) *The Mental Health Matrix. A Manual to Improve Services*. Cambridge University Press.

Thornicroft, G. & Tansella, M. (2005) Growing recognition of the importance of involvement in mental health service planning and evaluation. *Epidemiologia e Psichiatria Sociale*, **14**, 1–3.

Tonelli, G. & Merini, A. (1995) La valutazione del Servizio di Salute mentale della I Clinica Psichiatrica dell'Università di Bologna tramite la Verona Service Satisfaction Scale (VSSS). *Rivista Sperimentale di Frenatria*, **119**, 825–842.

Van Schaik, D. J. F., Van Marwijk, H. W. J., Beekman, A. T. F., *et al* (2007) Interpersonal psychotherapy (IPT) for late-life depression in general practice: uptake and satisfaction by patients, therapists and physicians. *BMC Family Practice*, **8**, 52.

Veenhoven, R. (1993) *Happiness in Nations. Subjective Appreciation of Life in 56 Nations 1946–1992*. RISBO, Studies in Social and Cultural Transformation No. 2, Erasmus University.

Voruganti, L., Heslegrave, R., Awad, A. G., *et al* (1998) Quality of life measurement in schizophrenia: reconciling the quest for subjectivity with the question of reliability. *Psychological Medicine*, **28**, 165–172.

Walter, G., Cleary, M. & Rey, J. M. (1998) Attitudes of mental health personnel towards rating outcome. *Journal of Quality in Clinical Practice*, **18**, 109–115.

Ware, J. E. & Davies, A. R. (1983) Behavioral consequences of consumer dissatisfaction with medical care. *Evaluation and Program Planning*, **6**, 291–298.

Ware, J. E. & Snyder, M. K. (1976) Dimensions of patients attitudes regarding doctors and medical care services. *Medical Care*, **13**, 669–683.

CHAPTER 7

Measuring family and carer burden in severe mental illness: the instruments

Bob van Wijngaarden and Aart H. Schene

Until the middle of the twentieth century, neither society nor psychiatry as the principal responsible discipline could offer people with severe mental illness much more than hospital care for periods ranging from months to years. The recognition of the detrimental effects of hospitalisation and developments in psychopharmaceutical, psychotherapeutic and social treatments gave impetus to deinstitutionalisation and opened doors to new approaches now associated with community psychiatry and community care. Over the past five decades this movement away from hospital care resulted in a great interest in the community adjustment of psychiatric patients (Weissman, 1975, 1981). Treating patients in the least restrictive environment and consumer empowerment made social functioning and social performance important concepts, not only for patients, practitioners and researchers, but certainly also for patients' family and carers (Fisher *et al*, 1990). Confronted with caring tasks that had been taken away from them since the start of institutionalism in the early nineteenth century, family members had to learn to cope again with the dysfunctional behaviour inherent in most of the severe mental illnesses.

Family and carer burden

Caring refers to the relationship between two adult individuals who are typically related through kinship. One, the carer, assumes an unpaid and unanticipated responsibility for another, the care recipient, whose mental health problems are disabling, long term in nature and essentially incurable. The care recipient is unable to fulfil the reciprocal obligations associated with normative adult relationships and the mental health problems are serious enough to require substantial amounts of care. What makes the situation particularly burdensome is the addition of the caring role to the already existing family role (Gubman & Tessler, 1987; Gubman *et al*, 1987; Gallop *et al*, 1991). Although the concept is referred to as 'family' burden, most studies have sampled 'primary carers'. Carer burden has a narrower perspective than family burden, as the latter includes the consequences for family members other than the main carer, such as the interpersonal relations within the family, the consequences for children of patients and the social network of the whole family.

Measuring burden

The adverse consequences of psychiatric disorders for relatives have been studied since the early 1950s, for different reasons: at first, to determine the feasibility of discharging patients into the community; later, to refine the concept of caring, its content and its underlying structure; and, most recently, to measure burden as an outcome variable in programme evaluations and controlled clinical trials (Schene *et al*, 1996). Reviews of instruments that measure family burden (e.g. Platt, 1985; Schene, 1990; Schene *et al*, 1996, 2001) have indicated that, although a number of instruments or scales have been developed to measure carer burden, there is still no standard, generally accepted instrument within the scientific community. Until 2000 the application of burden measures in routine clinical settings – to screen for burden, to identify individual family members at risk, and to monitor changes in burden over time – was still in its infancy.

In the previous edition of the present book, Schene *et al* (2001) reviewed 20 instruments developed and used in the previous 10 years. Some of those instruments covered a broad range of domains, while others were focused on only certain aspects of burden, for instance economic burden (Clark & Drake, 1994) or grief (Miller *et al*, 1990). All the instruments identified by Schene *et al* (2001) were assessed for their suitability for both routine clinical and research use. The protocols were described in terms of their method and comprehensiveness, precursors and theoretical foundations, and types of psychometric information available.

The question now is, how has the use of burden instruments developed over the last 10 years? Which instruments have been used in the decade and which instruments have not, and have new instruments been developed since 2000? Which instruments nowadays are most popular, and which instruments are available and validated in other countries or languages? For this purpose we reviewed the international literature since 2000. This means that only instruments that were mentioned in papers are included in this overview; this means that instruments that are used only in clinical practice may have been omitted, but their popularity and applicability are in any case not known. This review therefore is mainly aimed at the use and validation of research instruments.

Method

In the mid-1990s, when the first edition of the book was published and we prepared the chapter on measures of burden (Schene *et al*, 1996), the research was still in its infancy. Owing to a lack of suitable and well-validated instruments, many researchers started to develop their own. Many of these instruments were not tested yet, so papers or other information were scarce. Therefore, for the chapter in that edition, we contacted researchers personally to identify instruments available in English. We used our personal knowledge of researchers in the field and identified others from the literature on family burden. A letter describing our purpose asked researchers whether they were adaptors or developers of family burden instrumentation, and also to name other persons who might be working in the area. An 80-item Family Burden Researchers' Questionnaire was sent to 52 of 128 researchers whom the authors believed had developed or adapted measures that could be shared with other researchers. When possible, the original author was contacted. Researchers were *not* sent a questionnaire if they failed to respond to the first letter, if they replied that they were not developers or adaptors, or if they were using an instrument developed by someone already represented in the sample. Instruments were excluded if they had been developed primarily for use with people who were caring for someone who did not have a severe mental illness (e.g. a geriatric patient).

To update that initial review for the second edition, in 1999 we screened the 1994–99 literature with regard to the instruments included in the 1994 review (Schene *et al*, 1994). We also sent the Family Burden Researchers' Questionnaire to another three researchers who had published new scales between 1994 and 1999. With this method we found a final sample of 20 instruments.

For this third review, we screened the 2000–9 international literature again, also for new instruments. In this review we mainly focused on new information regarding validation and reliability of existing instruments, popularity in use, and translations. The reason for this focus was to see if any instruments had become commonly used in burden research, possibly inter-nationally. When instruments become standard (throughout the world), comparison between studies and countries becomes possible.

The search was done for burden instruments that were especially developed for mental healthcare. Although some instruments developed for measuring burden in, for instance, dementia, such as the Zarit Caregiver Burden Interview (Zarit *et al*, 1980), are used to measure burden resulting from psychosis, these instruments are not included here.

Results

Of the 20 instruments found for the 1999 review, only half emerged in the literature update since 2000. The other ten seem to have no or only limited use in (international) research. For this reason they were dropped from the present review. These were: the Burden on Family Interview Schedule (Pai & Kapur, 1981, 1982), the Family Distress Scale for Depression (Jacob *et al*, 1987), the Scale of Assessment of Family Distress (Gopinath & Chaturvedi, 1986, 1992), the Family Distress Scale (Birchwood & Smith, 1992), the Thresholds Parental Burden Scale (Cook & Pickett, 1987), the Texas Inventory of Grief – Mental Illness Version (Miller *et al*, 1990), the Family Caregiving of Persons with Mental Illness Survey (Biegel *et al*, 1994), the Family Burden and Services Questionnaire (Greenberg *et al*, 1993), the Family Economic Burden Interview (Clark & Drake, 1994) and the Victorian Carers Program Questionnaire (Schofield *et al*, 1997).

Our review also resulted in ten possible *new* instruments. However, four of them turned out to be an existing instrument under a slightly different name, or a translation of an existing instrument. The authors of the remaining six instruments were contacted by email with a request for information on the instrument. After one reminder, only two authors had responded. In one case there had been a study in which burden was assessed in a qualitative way, not using any instrument. Therefore, only one instrument remained to be added to the list (Östman & Hansson, 2000).

Table 7.1 lists the 11 instruments included here. To the best of our knowledge, Table 7.1 covers all of the state-of-the-art of burden measures currently in use. For brevity of presentation, the numbers shown in Table 7.1 are used to identify specific instruments throughout the text and in the other tables.

Table 7.1 Family or carer burden instruments and main references

No.[a]	Instrument	References
1	Social Behaviour Assessment Schedule	Platt *et al* (1980, 1983)
2	Family Burden Scale	Madianos *et al* (1987), Madianos & Madianou (1992)
3	Family Burden Questionnaire	Fadden (1984), Fadden *et al* (1987*a,b*)
4	Significant Other Scale	Herz *et al* (1991)
5	Family Problems Questionnaire	Morosini *et al* (1991), Magliano *et al* (1998)
6	Involvement Evaluation Questionnaire	Schene (1990), Schene & van Wijngaarden (1992)
7	Family Burden Interview Schedule	Tessler *et al* (1992)
8	Burden Assessment Scale	Reinhard *et al* (1994)
9	Experience of Caregiving Inventory	Szmukler *et al* (1996*a,b*)
10	Perceived Family Burden Scale	Levene *et al* (1996)
11	Interview Schedule for Families and Relatives of Severely Mentally Ill Persons	Östman & Hansson (2000)

[a] Reference number for purposes of the present chapter.

119

Conceptual issues and content

In the previous reviews researchers were asked to give information on the underlying dimensions of their instruments. All researchers but one (no. 10) considered burden to be a multidimensional concept (see Table 7.2). The one new instrument that was found (no. 11) is also based on a multidimensional concept. The specifications of this instrument are added to the list in Table 7.2. Some researchers consider patient symptoms and behaviours to be the origin of burden. Dysfunctional behaviour disrupts the household routine as well as the caring tasks for close relatives. Others suggest that caring may result in role strain because it is added to the culturally defined relationships between family members. Some researchers also referred to the stress research literature. They considered patients' dysfunction and its consequences as chronic stressors with which family members must learn to cope.

A major theoretical distinction made by many researchers is that between objective and subjective burden. However, definitions of objective and subjective burden are implicit rather than explicit and operationalisations

Table 7.2 Dimensions assessed by instruments

Dimension	Instrument (see Table 7.1)										
	1	2	3	4	5	6	7	8	9	10	11
Effect of patient's illness on:											
family interaction		+	+	+	+	+	+	+	+		+
family routine		+	+	+	+	+	+	+			
leisure	+	+	+	+	+	+	+	+	+		+
work/employment	+	+	+	+	+		+	+			+
mental health	+	+		+	+	+					+
physical health	+	+			+	+					
use of psychotropics		+		+		+					
social network	+	+	+	+	+	+		+	+		+
others outside household	+	+	+	+	+	+		+	+		
children	+	+	+		+	+		+	+		
Financial consequences	+	+	+	+		+	+	+			
Helping the patient with:											
activities of daily living		+	+			+	+		+		
supervising the patient		+	+	+		+	+		+		+
encouraging the patient						+	+		+		
Distress	+		+	+	+	+	+		+		+
Stigma		+	+	+		+	+	+	+		
Worrying	+	+	+	+		+	+	+	+		+
Shame		+	+		+		+	+	+		
Guilt					+		+	+	+		+
Gobal burden		+	+	+		+	+		+		
Total no. of dimensions	10	16	15	14	13	16	14	12	15		9

differ. The following approaches can be distinguished. Platt (no. 1) considers symptoms and dysfunctioning to be objective and assesses the informant's distress (subjective burden) in relation to each particular problem or difficulty associated with the patient's illness. Tessler (no. 7) also uses this approach. However, he also includes measures of subjective burden such as anger, depression and embarrassment, which are separate from objective measures of caring.

Schene (no. 6) argues that burden should be measured in terms of behaviour that can be measured objectively, which involves determining how often relatives have to perform specific caring tasks. Like Tessler, he also measures distress, tension and worrying, but not directly related to patient behaviour. Reinhard (no. 8) considers subjective burden to be affective dimensions subjectively felt, such as shame, stigma, guilt, resentment, grief and worry. The instrument developed by Szmukler (no. 9) concentrates on the cognitive and emotional experience of caring.

Table 7.2 shows that some dimensions are included in almost all instruments. Effect on leisure activities ($n = 10$), family interaction ($n = 9$), family routine ($n = 8$), social network ($n = 9$), as well as worrying ($n = 9$) and distress ($n = 8$) are most frequently included. Among the less frequently measured dimensions are use of psychotropics ($n = 3$), having to encourage the patient ($n = 3$), effects on the physical health of the carer ($n = 4$), carer's feelings of guilt ($n = 5$) and helping the patients with activities of daily living ($n = 5$).

More than half the researchers mentioned additional burden dimensions, including: positive aspects of caring and knowledge about the illness (no. 3), problems with patients using alcohol or drugs, feeling threatened (no. 6), having to change personal plans for the future and being upset about the change in the patient from his or her former self (no. 8).

Leaving the instrument without dimensions (no. 10) out of the equation, the average number of dimensions is 13.5. These may be represented by a single item or by a fully developed scale. A measure of global burden is included in six of the ten instruments. It may comprise a single general item, summary scales or cumulative indexes constructed from items or interviewer assessments.

Another way to examine the structure underlying the burden concept is to use results from factor analyses (see Table 7.4). These results show some empirical basis for the dimensions of worrying, effect on family routine/interaction (tension, familial discord, disruption), care and control (supervision, urging, ongoing responsibility), behavioural problems, economic hardship, preoccupation (also emotional overinvolvement), distress and stigma.

Specialised instruments

One instrument was developed for specific purposes, that of Fadden (no. 3). It was designed for family members of patients with depression. Other specialised instruments that were found in the previous review were removed from the list, because of a lack of information during the last decade.

Structure and psychometrics

Tables 7.3 and 7.4 give an overview of the instruments, country of origin, and most important psychometric characteristics. Three instruments are from the USA, three from the UK, and one each from Greece, Italy, the Netherlands, Canada and Norway.

Five instruments are self-administered questionnaires, of which one also can be used as a personal interview, two also as postal questionnaires, and one also as a telephone interview. Six instruments can be used as personal interviews, of which four can be used only as such; two can also be used as telephone interviews. The instruments that use an interview format almost all require trained interviewers who have knowledge of severe mental illness.

The number of questions ranges from 19 to 186, with a mean of 70. Three instruments have fewer than 30 questions and four have 95 or more. Most of the briefer instruments contain carer burden questions only. The instruments with more than 70 questions also incorporate non-burden items, such as asking about the patient, the family, the carer, social support, use of mental health services, opinions about mental health services, coping, and patients' contributions to the household.

Of the five self-administered questionnaires, three have fewer than 30 questions and take 5–15 minutes to complete. The other two self-administered questionnaires have 77 (no. 6) and 66 (no. 9) questions. These instruments also gather information about the patient, the family, the household, contact with the patient and so on. However, they also take less than 30 minutes to complete.

Of the personal and telephone interviews, two have 100 questions or more, and take between 60 and 90 minutes to complete. The completion time of the other six ranges from 30 to 90 minutes.

For the majority of instruments the time frame is the past 4 weeks or month, for one it is 8 weeks, and for another 6 months. Three instruments do not have a specific time frame.

Table 7.4 shows whether information is available about construct validity, internal consistency, interrater reliability (if applicable), test–retest reliability and sensitivity to change. For seven instruments information on construct validity and internal consistency is available, six have information about test–retest reliability, and five have information about sensitivity to change. Seven instruments produce subscale scores as well as a summary score, one only produces subscale scores. For five instruments subscale scores are associated with factor analyses.

Regarding the type of patient populations in relation to which burden was measured, researchers' descriptions in the questionnaire were used. Most

Table 7.3 General characteristics of family and carer burden instruments

Instrument	Country of origin	No. of questions	Completion time (min)	Time frame	Type of instrument
1. Social Behaviour Assessment Schedule	UK	186	90	4 weeks	Structured personal interview
2. Family Burden Scale	Greece	34	30	Not specified	Structured personal interview
3. Family Burden Questionnaire	UK	95	90	Not specified	Semi-structured personal interview
4. Significant Other Scale	USA	50	15	Last month	Structured personal interview
5. Family Problems Questionnaire	Italy	29	15	8 weeks	Self-administered questionnaire
6. Involvement Evaluation Questionnaire	Netherlands	77	30	4 weeks	Self-administered mail questionnaire
7. Family Burden Interview Schedule	USA	100	60	4 weeks	Telephone interview (structured), structured personal interview
8. Burden Assessment Scale	USA	19	5	6 months	Self-administered questionnaire, telephone interview (structured), structured personal interview
9. Experience of Caregiving Inventory	UK	66	15	4 weeks	Self-administered mail questionnaire
10. Perceived Family Burden Scale	Canada	24	Not specified	Not specified	Self-administered questionnaire
11. Interview Schedule for Families of Severely Mentally Ill Persons	Norway	95	60–90	4 weeks	Semi-structured personal interview

studied relatives of patients with severe mental illness. Neurotic patients were studied by only two researchers. Another two studied only relatives of patients with affective disorders. Parents and siblings have been most often studied, indicating a tendency to focus on the family of origin. Significant others, partners and offspring have been studied less often.

Table 7.4 Psychometric characteristics of the family and carer burden instruments

Instrument (see Table 7.1)	Information available on:					Subscale scores	Summary score	Factor analyses
	Construct validity	Internal consistency	Interrater reliability	Test–retest reliability	Sensitivity to change			
1	−	−	+	−	−	+	−	−
2	−	−	+	+	−	+	+	−
3	−	−	−	+	−	−	−	−
4	−	−	+	−	−	+	+	−
5	+	+	na	+	−	+	+	Objective burden; subjective burden; support; positive criticism of patient; positive attitude to patient
6	+	+	na	+	+	+	+	Tension, worrying; supervision; urging
7	+	+	−	−	+	+	+	Care, control; disruption
8	+	+	−	−	+	+	+	Disrupted activities; personal distress; time perspective; guilt; basic social functioning
9	+	+	na	−	+	+	+	Difficult behaviour; negative symptoms; stigma; problems with services; effects on family; need to provide back-up; dependency; loss
10	+	+	na	+	+	−	−	−
11	+	−	+	+	−	−	−	−

na, not applicable.

Individual instruments

In the following sections, a summary description of each instrument is given. Instruments are divided into two categories: those suitable for research use only and those suitable for clinical use too, according to the authors of the instruments. All instruments are considered suitable for research use, while eight are also considered suitable for clinical use.

Scales suitable for research use only

1. Social Behaviour Assessment Schedule (SBAS)

This interview, developed in the UK, is still used, although the author himself is no longer active in the field (personal communication to the senior author of this chapter). The SBAS is administered by trained interviewers, for whom a training guide is available, and information on interrater reliability is available. The instrument is comprehensive and measures social behaviour as well as burden. In the 1999 review the length of this interview (186 questions) was considered to be a possible barrier to regular use (Schene *et al*, 2001).

Despite the length of the interview, this instrument is regularly used, especially outside the UK. Since 2000 ten references were found of studies in Italy, the USA, Spain, Denmark, Canada and New Zealand. A Spanish version has been validated (Reinares *et al*, 2004), and a Danish version exists, though that has not been validated.

3. Family Burden Questionnaire

This 95-item interview, developed in the UK, concentrates on family members of patients with depression. It has been used effectively in descriptive studies. Its psychometric properties are not well established. In the 1999 review the author mentioned that the interview would probably be perceived as too long for routine clinical work.

This instrument is still in use. Four studies were found, three in Germany and one in the USA. All studies were conducted after 2004. Information on the German translation is not available.

7. Family Burden Interview Schedule

This 100-item structured personal interview was developed in the USA. It takes about 60 minutes to administer in person and can also be used as a briefer telephone interview, as has been done in two follow-up assessments. Interviewers do not need a special background, and a manual is available describing the modular structure of the instrument. Psychometric information is available (Tessler & Gamache, 1994).

Despite the length of the instrument and the time required to complete it, the interview is regularly used throughout the world. Most of the 19 references found since 2000 originate from outside the USA: Spain, China,

Brasil, Nepal, India and Australia. The Spanish, Chinese and Brazilian versions have been validated (Chien & Norman, 2004; Siu & Yeung, 2005; Bandeira et al, 2005; Vilaplana et al, 2007). Translation into Arabic is mentioned, but no further information is available.

Scales suitable for both clinical and research use

2. Family Burden Scale

This instrument, developed in Greece, is a structured personal interview that requires 30 minutes to administer. It is designed for use with the first-degree relatives of patients with schizophrenia. Interviewers require a clinical background but no special training. The validation of the Greek version was conducted in 2004 (Madianos et al, 2004). Since 2000, eight studies with this instrument were found. The studies were conducted in Australia, China, Brazil, India and Puerto Rico. The Brazilian version has been validated (Bandeira et al, 2005, 2007). Information on other translations (Spanish, Chinese) is not available.

4. Significant Other Scale

This personal interview with family members whose relative is a patient with schizophrenia takes 15 minutes to administer. It is comprehensive and designed to generate separate scores for subjective and objective burden. The instrument has been used in a randomised trial comparing intermittent and maintenance medication. In 1999 the only psychometric information pertained to interrater reliability.

Since 2000 six studies have been reported, three of them on postpartum psychosis. A Chinese version has been validated (Tsang et al, 2000).

5. Family Problems Questionnaire (FPQ)

This instrument was developed in Italy for use in routine clinical practice. Its first version (Questionnaire for Family Problems; Morosini et al, 1991), a comprehensive self-administered questionnaire, was administered to a variety of relatives of recently admitted psychiatric patients at two points in time. An international version of the questionnaire, the FPQ, was developed and validated in five European languages (English, German, Greek, Italian and Portuguese). It was used in a BIOMED study on family burden and coping in schizophrenia (Magliano et al, 1998, 1999). It contains 29 items grouped in five factors. Three of these have to do with burden: objective burden, subjective burden and criticism. The other two factors concern support and positive attitudes to the patient. The psychometric properties are well established.

Since 2000, seven studies have been reported, five of them by the author of the instrument. One study in the Netherlands and one in the UK were found. No information on more translations is available.

6. Involvement Evaluation Questionnaire (IEQ)

This instrument was initially developed in the Netherlands to compare the family impact of day hospitalisation against in-patient hospitalisation (Schene, 1987). It was subsequently revised to render it suitable for a survey of a large organisation of relatives of patients with psychotic disorders (Schene *et al*, 1998). In the mid-1990s the IEQ was adapted for use in studies concerning carers of patients suffering from mood disorders, to allow comparisons to be made of the impact of schizophrenia and depression on carers (van Wijngaarden *et al*, 2009).

The core IEQ is a 31-item questionnaire and may be used as a self-administered or mail questionnaire. It is extended with six extra modules, containing the 12-item General Health Questionnaire, socio-demographic variables, and items on extra financial expenses, carer's use of professional help, and consequences for the patient's children. The whole 77-item instrument takes about 30 minutes to administer. Factor analysis identified four factors, which can be added into a total score (see Table 7.4).

The IEQ is available in 15 languages. The English, Danish, Italian and Spanish translations have been developed, validated and used in the BIOMED-financed Epsilon study of schizophrenia in five European countries (van Wijngaarden *et al*, 2000). Validation data on the Malawi, Swedish, Chinese, German, Polish and Portuguese version are available (Bernert *et al*, 2001; Magne-Ingvar & Öjehagen, 2005; Sefasi *et al*, 2008; Tang *et al*, 2008; Hadrys *et al*, 2010; Portuguese data available from the author). Also, the original Dutch version has been further validated (van Wijngaarden *et al*, 2001, 2003; van Wijngaarden, 2003). The Finnish, French, Greek and Arabic versions have not yet been validated.

The IEQ has been widely used. In total 33 international publications since 2000 were found of studies in Malawi, Italy, Australia, Sweden, the Netherlands, Finland, Hong Kong, Germany, France, the UK and Austria.

8. Burden Assessment Scale

This instrument, developed in the USA, can be administered as a personal interview, a telephone interview and as a self-administered questionnaire. The 19 questions can be answered in 5 minutes. A 6-month time frame is recommended, which contrasts with the 4 weeks used in most other instruments. The instrument is appropriate for use with a variety of family members of people with a severe mental illness, including (but not limited to) the primary carer. Psychometric information is available. Factor analysis identified five factors (see Table 7.4).

Since 2000 the Burden Assessment Scale has been used in 15 reported studies throughout the world: Australia, Sweden, Canada, the USA, Israel and Sri Lanka. Translations into Spanish, Swedish and Singhalese are mentioned but only the Swedish version has been validated (Ivarsson *et al*, 2004).

9. Experience of Caregiving Inventory (ECI)

This questionnaire was developed in the UK by collecting items from in-depth interviews and focus groups with 120 carers. It takes about 15 minutes to complete and has two main sections. The first section contains 52 statements and carers are asked how often during the last month they have thought about the issue outlined in the statement. The second section contains 14 questions about symptoms, in the format 'During the past month how often have you thought about her being ... [symptom]'. The questionnaire has been used in descriptive, epidemiological and programme-evaluation studies, as well as in randomised clinical trials. The psychometric properties are well established (Szmukler et al, 1996a,b).

Since 2008, 24 studies using the ECI have been reported. Most studies (16) were conducted in the UK, the rest in Hong Kong, Norway, Australia and Canada. In 2000 the original version of the ECI was further validated (Joyce et al, 2000). The Chinese version also has been validated (Lau & Pang, 2007). Information on other translations was not found.

10. Perceived Family Burden Scale

This 24-item questionnaire was developed in Canada for the measurement of burden experienced by relatives of patients with schizophrenia. Items were generated from a literature review and consultation with relatives' groups. Psychometrics were tested in a small sample ($n = 52$) and further replication in a larger sample was needed, according to the authors (Levene et al, 1996). Until 1999, the scale had been used only in descriptive studies.

No additional information on the psychometric properties of the original version of this instrument were found. However, the Chinese translation has been validated (Tsang, 2005; Tsang et al, 2005). In total five studies were found, conducted in Hong Kong, Canada and Norway.

11. Interview Schedule for Families and Relatives of Severely Mentally Ill Persons

This instrument was found in the present literature review. In fact it is not a new instrument but the latest version of an instrument initially developed in 1985. The 95-item interview covers several dimensions of burden, most subjective. Also relatives' experiences and attitudes concerning participation in care and psychiatric services are assessed. The instrument contains no subscales nor a total score. Psychometric testing was limited to test–retest reliability, feasibility, acceptability and content validity. The interview can be used in longitudinal research (Östman & Hansson, 2000). The 2000 validation study was the only reference since 2000.

Popularity and dispersion

In the previous section the use and spread of the 11 instruments were mentioned. Table 7.5 summarises these results. As can be seen, during

Table 7.5 Popularity and dispersion of instrument

Instrument	No. references since 2000	No. studies in other countries	No. other countries	No. validated translations
1	10	9	6	1
2	8	6	5	1
3	4	4	2	
4	6	6	4	1
5	7	2	2	4
6	33	23	10	9
7	19	15	6	3
8	15	10	5	1
9	24	8	4	1
10	5	5	3	1
11	1			

the last decade some of the instruments have become more popular and widespread than the others. This is true especially for the Involvement Evaluation Questionnaire, the Experience of Caregiving Inventory and the Family Burden Interview Schedule. Remarkably, most new studies were conducted in countries other than the country of origin. Apparently these instruments have been noticed, adapted and applied abroad. There are two exceptions: the Family Problems Questionnaire, which has mainly been used in Italy by the author herself, and the Experience of Caregiving Inventory, which in most cases has been used in the UK.

When instruments are adopted throughout the world, it is important that their translations are validated. The Involvement Evaluation Questionnaire has the most validated versions, and more validations are on their way. Four validated versions resulted from the BIOMED II study; the others were published in the last decade. The Family Problems Questionnaire was validated in four languages in the BIOMED I study, but since then no new validated language versions have been reported. The Familly Burden Interview Schedule has been validated in three languages.

As reported above, ten instruments from the review in the second edition of this book have not been mentioned again in the international literature since 2000. Some of these were specialised instruments. Apparently there seems to be only limited interest in these kind of instruments in research studies. The literature overview shows that the instruments that have been adopted in other countries are all multidimensional instruments, covering a broad range of burden domains (see Table 7.2). Also, researchers apparently tend to seek well-developed instruments. In fact, the four most used instruments since 2000 all have subscale scores based on factor analysis (see Table 7.4).

In summary, while in 1999 it was still unclear which instruments had the potential to become standard measures, by 2009 an 'elite' group seemed to have formed. However, which instrument to pick will depend on the purposes of the research. If the purpose is to conduct a theoretical study linking burden with other constructs, then instruments 1, 3 and 7 may be relevant. If the purpose is to study the family burden associated with caring for a person with depression, then instruments 1, 3, 6 and 9 should be considered. For those whose research interest is relatives of persons with schizophrenia, instruments 1, 2, 4, 5, 6, 9 and 10 are appropriate. For more general use with heterogeneous patient populations, researchers may find instruments 1, 6, 7, 8 and 9 useful. For measuring change in longitudinal studies, instruments 5, 6, 7, 9 and 11 should be considered, as they have previously been used for this purpose. However, one has to check whether sensitivity to change has been studied.

The section on individual instruments and Table 7.3 may also be useful in helping researchers to select an instrument that meets other specific requirements, such as time to administer, interviewer background and method of administration. For example, if one knows in advance that a brief, self-administered questionnaire is to be used, then this narrows down the range of options. However, we recommend that researchers do not make final choices based on this review alone, but contact the authors of the instruments directly and obtain copies of their instruments before making a final choice.

Conclusion

In the last decade there seems to have formed a consensus among researchers on which carer burden instruments are most useful. The general tendency is towards instruments that cover a wide range of burden dimensions and have good psychometric properties. Surprisingly, the length of the instrument does not seem to matter (e.g. the Family Burden Interview Schedule). Five instruments stand out, in popularity and/or in dispersion throughout the world. Those researchers looking for an instrument that covers many domains, that are well validated, and/or that can be used in multi-country studies are likely to use the Involvement Evaluation Questionnaire, the Family Problems Questionnaire, the Family Burden Interview Schedule, the Experience of Caregiving Inventory or the Burden Assessment Scale. Researchers looking for instruments closer to specific research goals can have a pick from the other instruments, with the exception of the added Swedish instrument (no. 11), which needs more psychometric testing.

References

Bandeira, M., Calzavara, M. G. P. & Varella, A. A. B. (2005) Escala de sobrecarga dos familiars de pacientes psiquiátricos: adaptação transcultural para o Brasil (FBIS–BR). [Family burden scale for caregivers of psychiatric patients: transcultural adaptation to Brazil (FBIS–BR).] Jornal Brasileiro de Psiquiatria, 54, 206–214.

Bandeira, M., Calzavara, M. G. P., Freitas, L. C., *et al* (2007) Family Burden Interview Scale for relatives of psychiatric patients (FBIS–BR): reliability study of the Brazilian version. *Revista Brasileira de Psiquiatria*, **29**, 47–50.

Bernert, S., Kilian R., Matschinger, H., *et al* (2001) Die Erfassung der Belastung der Angehörigen psychisch erkrankter Menschen – Die deutsche Version des Involvement Evaluation Questionnaires (IEQ–EU). [The assessment of burden on relatives of mentally ill people: the German version of the Involvement Evaluation Questionnaire (IEQ–EU).] *Psychiatrische Praxis*, **28** (suppl. 2), s97–s101.

Biegel, D. E., Song, L. Y. & Chakravarthy, V. (1994) Predictors of caregiver burden among support group members of persons with chronic mental illness. In *Family Caregiving Across the Lifespan* (eds E. Kahana, D. E. Biegel & M. L. Wykle), pp. 178–215. Family Caregiver Applications Series No. 4. Sage.

Birchwood, M. & Smith, J. (1992) Specific and non-specific effects of educational intervention for families living with schizophrenia. *British Journal of Psychiatry*, **160**, 645–652.

Chien, W.-T. & Norman, I. (2004) The validity and reliability of a Chinese version of the Family Burden Interview Schedule. *Nursing Research*, **53**, 314–322.

Clark, R. E. & Drake, R. E. (1994) Expenditures of time and money by families of people with severe mental illness and substance use disorders. *Community Mental Health Journal*, **30**, 145–163.

Cook, J. A. & Pickett, S. A. (1987) Feelings of burden and criticalness among parents residing with chronically mentally ill offspring. *Journal of Applied Social Sciences*, **12**, 79–107.

Fadden, G. B. (1984) *The Relatives of Patients with Depressive Disorders: A Typology of Burden and Strategies of Coping*. MPhil thesis, Institute of Psychiatry, University of London.

Fadden, G. B., Bebbington, P. & Kuipers, L. (1987*a*) The burden of care: the impact of functional psychiatric illness on the patient's family. *British Journal of Psychiatry*, **150**, 285–292.

Fadden, G. B., Bebbington, P. & Kuipers, L. (1987*b*) Caring and its burdens: a study of the spouses of depressed patients. *British Journal of Psychiatry*, **151**, 660–667.

Fisher, G. A., Benson, P. R. & Tessler, R. C. (1990) Family response to mental illness: developments since deinstitutionalization. *Research in Community and Mental Health*, **6**, 203–236.

Gallop, R., McKeever, P., Mohide, E. A., *et al* (1991) *Family Care and Chronic Illness: The Caregiving Experience. A Review of the Literature*. Faculty of Nursing, University of Toronto.

Gopinath, P. S. & Chaturvedi, S. K. (1986) Measurement of distressful psychotic symptoms perceived by the family: preliminary findings. *Indian Journal of Psychiatry*, **28**, 343–345.

Gopinath, P. S. & Chaturvedi, S. K. (1992) Distressing behaviour of schizophrenics at home. *Acta Psychiatrica Scandinavica*, **86**, 185–188.

Greenberg, J. S., Greenley, J. R., McKee, D., *et al* (1993) Mothers caring for an adult child with schizophrenia: the effects of subjective burden on maternal health. *Family Relations*, **442**, 205–211.

Gubman, G. D. & Tessler, R. C. (1987) The impact of mental illness on families. *Journal of Family Issues*, **8**, 226–245.

Gubman, G. D., Tessler, R. C. & Willis, G. (1987) Living with the mentally ill: factors affecting household complaints. *Schizophrenia Bulletin*, **13**, 727–736.

Hadrys, T., Adamowski, T. & Kiejna, A. (2010) Mental disorder in Polish families: is diagnosis a predictor of caregiver's burden? *Social Psychiatry and Psychiatric Epidemiology*, March 23, Epub ahead of print.

Herz, M. I., Glazer, W. & Mostert, M. (1991) Intermittent vs maintenance medication in schizophrenia. *Archives of General Psychiatry*, **48**, 333–339.

Ivarsson, A. B., Sidenvall, B. & Carlsson, M., *et al* (2004) The factor structure of the Burden Assessment Scale and the perceived burden of caregivers for individuals with severe mental disorders. *Scandinavian Journal of Caring Sciences*, **18**, 396–401.

Jacob, M., Frank, E., Kupfer, D. J., *et al* (1987) Recurrent depression: an assessment of family burden and family attitudes. *Journal of Clinical Psychiatry*, **48**, 395–400.

Joyce, J., Leese, M. & Szmukler G. (2000) The Experience of Caregiving Inventory: further evidence. *Social Psychiatry and Psychiatric Epidemiology*, **35**, 185–189.

Lau, D. Y. K. & Pang, A. H. T. (2007) Validation of the Chinese version of Experience of Caregiving Inventory in caregivers of persons suffering from severe mental illness. *Hong Kong Journal of Psychiatry*, **17**, 24–31.

Levene, J. E., Lancee, W. J. & Seeman, M. V. (1996) The Perceived Family Burden Scale: measurement and validation. *Schizophrenia Research*, **22**, 151–157.

Madianos, M. & Madianou, D. (1992) The effects of long-term community care on relapse and adjustment of persons with chronic schizophrenia. *International Journal of Mental Health*, **21**, 37–49.

Madianos, M., Gournas, G., Tomaras, V., *et al* (1987) Family atmosphere on the course of chronic schizophrenia treated in a community mental health center: a prospective longitudinal study. In *Schizophrenia: Recent Biosocial Developments* (eds C. Stefanis & A. Rabavilas), pp. 246–256. Human Sciences Press.

Madianos, M., Economou, M., Dafni, O., *et al* (2004) Family disruption, economic hardship and psychological distress in schizophrenia: can they be measured? *European Psychiatry*, **19**, 408–414.

Magliano, L., Fadden, G., Madianos, M., *et al* (1998) Burden on the families of patients with schizophrenia: results of the BIOMED I study. *Social Psychiatry and Psychiatric Epidemiology*, **33**, 405–412.

Magliano, L., Fadden, G., Fiorillo, A., *et al* (1999) Family burden and coping strategies in schizophrenia: are key relatives really different to other relatives? *Acta Psychiatrica Scandinavica*, **99**, 10–15.

Magne-Ingvar, U. & Öjehagen, A. (2005) Significant others of persons with mental health problems: the testing of a questionnaire on the burden of significant others. *Nordic Journal of Psychiatry*, **59**, 441–447.

Miller, F., Dworkin, J., Ward, M., *et al* (1990) A preliminary study of unresolved grief in families of seriously mentally ill patients. *Hospital and Community Psychiatry*, **41**, 1321–1325.

Morosini, P., Roncone, R., Veltro, F., *et al* (1991) Routine assessment tool in psychiatry: a case of questionnaire of family attitudes and burden. *Italian Journal of Psychiatry and Behavioural Sciences*, **1**, 95–101.

Östman, M. & Hansson, L. (2000) Family burden and care participation. A test–retest reliability study of an interview instrument concerning families with a severely mental ill family member. *Nordic Journal of Psychiatry*, **54**, 327–342.

Pai, S. & Kapur, R. L. (1981) The burden on the family of a psychiatric patient: development of an interview schedule. *British Journal of Psychiatry*, **138**, 332–335.

Pai, S. & Kapur, R. L. (1982) Impact of treatment intervention on the relationship between dimensions of clinical psychopathology, social dysfunction and burden on the family. *Psychological Medicine*, **12**, 651–658.

Platt, S. (1985) Measuring the burden of psychiatric illness on the family: an evaluation of some rating scales. *Psychological Medicine*, **15**, 383–393.

Platt, S., Weyman, A., Hirsch, S., *et al* (1980) The Social Behaviour Assessment Schedule (SBAS): rationale, contents, scoring and reliability of a new interview schedule. *Social Psychiatry*, **15**, 43–55.

Platt, S., Weyman, A. & Hirsch, S. (1983) *Social Behaviour Assessment Schedule* (3rd edition). NFER-Nelson.

Reinares, M., Vieta, E., Colom, F., *et al* (2004) Evaluación de la carga familiar: una propuesta de escala autoaplicada derivada de la escala de desempeño psicosocial. [An assessment of family burden: a proposal for a self-administered scale derived from the Spanish version of the Social Behaviour Assessment Schedule.] *Revista de Psiquiatría de la Facultad de Medicina de Barcelona*, **31**, 7–13.

Reinhard, S. C, Gubman, G. D., Hortwitz, A. V., *et al* (1994) Burden Assessment Scale for families of the seriously mentally ill. *Evaluation and Program Planning*, **17**, 261–269.

Schene, A. H. (1987) *The Burden on the Family Scale*. Department of Ambulatory and Social Psychiatry, University of Utrecht.

Schene, A. H. (1990) Objective and subjective dimensions of family burden. Toward an integrative framework for research. *Social Psychiatry and Psychiatric Epidemiology*, **25**, 289–297.

Schene, A. H. & van Wijngaarden, B. (1992) *The Involvement Evaluation Questionnaire*. Department of Psychiatry, University of Amsterdam.

Schene, A. H., Tessler, R. C. & Gamache, G. M. (1994) Instruments measuring family or caregiver burden in severe mental illness. *Social Psychiatry and Psychiatric Epidemiology*, **29**, 228–240.

Schene, A. H., Tessler, R. C. & Gamache, G. M. (1996) Caregiving in severe mental illness: conceptualization and measurement. In *Mental Health Service Evaluation* (eds H. C. Knudsen & G. Thornicroft), pp. 296–316. Cambridge University Press.

Schene, A. H., van Wijngaarden, B. & Koeter, M. W. J. (1998) Family caregiving in schizophrenia: domains and distress. *Schizophrenia Bulletin*, **24**, 609–618.

Schene, A. H., Tessler, R. C. & Gamache, G. M., *et al* (2001) Measuring family or care-giver burden in severe mental illness: the instruments. In *Mental Health Outcome Measures* (eds M. Tansella & G Thornicroft) (2nd edition), pp. 48–71. Gaskell.

Schofield, H., Murphy, B., Herrman, H., *et al* (1997) Family caregiving: measurement of emotional well being and various aspects of the caregiving role. *Psychological Medicine*, **27**, 647–657.

Sefasi, A., Crumlish, N., Samalani, P., *et al* (2008) A little knowledge: caregiver burden in schizophrenia in Malawi. *Social Psychiatry and Psychiatric Epidemiology*, **43**, 160–164.

Siu, B. W. M. & Yeung, T. M. H. (2005) Validation of the Cantonese version of Family Burden Interview Schedule on caregivers of patients with obsessive–compulsive disorder. *Hong Kong Journal of Psychiatry*, **15**, 109–117.

Szmukler, G. I., Burgess, P., Herrman, H., *et al* (1996a) Caring for relatives with serious mental illness: the development of the Experience of Caregiving Inventory. *Social Psychiatry and Psychiatric Epidemiology*, **31**, 137–148.

Szmukler, G. I., Herrman, H., Colusa, S., *et al* (1996b) A controlled trial of a counselling intervention for caregivers of relatives with schizophrenia. *Social Psychiatry and Psychiatric Epidemiology*, **31**, 149–155.

Tang, V. W. K., Leung, S. K. & Lam, L. C. W. (2008) Validation of the Chinese version of the Involvement Evaluation Questionnaire. *Hong Kong Journal of Psychiatry*, **18**, 6–14.

Tessler, R. C. & Gamache, G. (1994) Continuity of care, residence, and family burden in Ohio. *Milbank Memorial Fund Quarterly*, **72**, 149–169.

Tessler, R. C., Fisher, G. & Gamache, G. (1992) *The Family Burden Interview Schedule Manual*. Social and Demographic Research Institute, University of Massachusetts.

Tsang, H. (2005) The Chinese version of the Perceived Family Burden Scale for individuals suffering from schizophrenia. *Transcultural Psychiatry*, **38**, 533–536.

Tsang, H., Lam, P. & Yee-chiu, I. (2000) A simplified Chinese version of the Significant Others Scale as a measure of social support for people with mental illness. *Psychiatric Rehabilitation Skills*, **4**, 367–375.

Tsang, H., Chan, A. S., Chung, A. W., *et al* (2005) Reliability of the Chinese version of the Perceived Family Burden Scale. *International Journal of Rehabilitation Research*, **28**, 289–291.

van Wijngaarden, B. (2003) *Consequences for Caregivers of Patients with Severe Mental Illness: The Development of the Involvement Evaluation Questionnaire*. Dissertation, University of Amsterdam.

van Wijngaarden, B., Schene, A. H., Koeter, M., *et al* (2000) Caregiving in schizophrenia: development, internal consistency and reliability of the Involvement Evaluation Questionnaire – European version. *British Journal of Psychiatry*, **177** (suppl. 39), s21–s27.

van Wijngaarden, B., Schene, A. H. & Koeter, M. (2001) Caregiving consequences in the Netherlands and other European countries: the development and use of the Involvement Evaluation Questionnaire (IEQ). In *Family Interventions in Mental Illness: International Perspectives* (eds H. P. Lefley & D. B. Johnson), pp. 145–169. Praeger.

van Wijngaarden, B., Schene, A. H., Koeter, M., *et al* (2003) People with schizophrenia in five countries: conceptual similarities and intercultural differences in family caregiving. *Schizophrenia Bulletin*, **29**, 573–586.

van Wijngaarden, B., Koeter, M. W. J., Knapp, M., *et al* (2009) Caring for people with depression or with schizophrenia: are the consequences different? *Psychiatry Research*, **169**, 62–69.

Vilaplana, M., Ochoa, S., Martínez, A., *et al* (2007) Validation in Spanish population of the Family Objective and Subjective Interview (ECFOS–II) for relatives of patients with schizophrenia. *Actas Españolas de Psichitría*, **35**, 372–381.

Weissman, M. M. (1975) The assessment of social adjustment. A review of techniques. *Archives of General Psychiatry*, **32**, 357–365.

Weissman, M. M. (1981) The assessment of social adjustment. An update. *Archives of General Psychiatry*, **38**, 1250–1258.

Zarit, S. H., Reever, K. E. & Bach-Peterson, J. (1980) Relatives of the impaired elderly: correlates of feelings of burden. *Gerontologist*, **20**, 649–655.

CHAPTER 8

Measures of quality of life for persons with severe mental disorders

Anthony F. Lehman and Antonio Lasalvia

This chapter provides clinicians, researchers, programme evaluators and administrators with current information on the assessment of quality-of-life (QOL) outcomes for persons with severe mental illnesses. Measures are summarised according to purpose, content, psychometric properties, patient subgroups with whom used and key references. A series of QOL measures are summarised and reflect considerable variability on the parameters examined. Comprehensive, reliable, and valid measures of QOL are available, although further development of QOL assessment methods is needed. More importantly, we must strive for a better understanding of how to interpret and use QOL outcome information.

The broad impact that severe mental illnesses have on people's lives and the resulting complexity of the needs generated by such illnesses pose a particular challenge in the assessment of the outcomes of services for these persons (Lehman *et al*, 1982; Ruggeri & Tansella, 1995). Relevant outcome domains include psychiatric symptoms, functional status, access to resources and opportunities, subjective well-being, family burden and community safety. Because of this broad array of relevant outcomes and because of a prevailing concern that outcome assessments should include the patient's perspective (Lasalvia & Ruggeri, 2007), there has been increased attention paid over the past decade to the development of measures of patients' QOL.

This chapter summarises the measures of QOL that have been developed specifically for persons with severe mental illnesses. We do not consider generic health-related QOL measures, such as the WHOQOL–100 (WHOQOL Group, 1998a) or its abbreviated version, the WHOQOL–BREF (WHOQOL Group, 1998b), the Medical Outcome Study (MOS) 36-Item Short-Form Health Survey (SF–36) (Ware & Sherbourne, 1992) or the EQ–5D (Kind, 1996). Although these measures have been widely used for assessing QOL in studies conducted on psychiatric populations, they have been designed to asses it in a wide spectrum of physical disorders and in a variety of situations and population groups (e.g. cancer patients, refugees, the elderly and those with certain diseases, such as HIV/AIDS). 'Quality of life' is a broad term and conceptually could cover all outcome measures, including measures of clinical symptoms and functional status (Katschnig, 2000). However, many of these measures are reviewed elsewhere in this volume or have been reviewed previously. Therefore, they are not included in this review. Also excluded here are measures of client satisfaction with services and 'family burden', which are considered in detail in Chapters 6 and 7, respectively.

The measures reviewed here are those that emphasise the patient's QOL, that is, measures covering patients' perspectives on what they have (access to resources and opportunities), how they are doing (functional status) and how they feel about their life circumstances. At a minimum, QOL covers a sense of well-being and in order to be selected for this review a measure had to assess at least this domain; as will be seen, most measures also cover the broad areas of functioning and resources.

Specific measures

The vast majority of QOL measures identified were designed for mixed diagnostic groups of persons with mental illnesses, primarily schizophrenia but also including affective disorders and a variety of other chronic Axis I disorders. This section is organised according to the mental illnesses targeted by the various measures: first, severe and persistent mental illnesses; then schizophrenia; and last depression and anxiety disorders. Each measure is summarised in terms of its name, key reference(s), original purpose, types of patients studied, type of instrument, number of items, length of administration, content and psychometric properties.

Severe and persistent mental illnesses

The main characteristics of QOL measures designed for severe and persistent mental illnesses are summarised in Table 8.1.

Community Adjustment Form (CAF)

This semi-structured self-report interview (Stein & Test, 1980; Hoult & Reynolds, 1984) was developed to assess life satisfaction and other QOL outcomes in a randomised study of an experimental system of community-based care for people with severe mental illness versus standard care in Dane County, Wisconsin. It consists of 140 items and requires approximately 45 minutes to complete. The areas assessed include: leisure activities; quality of living situation; employment history and status; income sources and amounts; free lodging and/or meals; contact with friends; family contact; legal problems; life satisfaction (21 items); self-esteem; medical care; and agency utilisation. No psychometric properties have been reported. The original patient sample studied included 130 people seeking admission to a state hospital. Over half were men (55%) and their mean age was 31 years. Half had a diagnosis of schizophrenia. They were treated both in the state hospital and in a community-based assertive community treatment programme. The results of the original Wisconsin study were replicated in Australia using the same measures (Hoult & Reynolds, 1984). This instrument was also used in a study examining the relationship between psychosocial functioning and subjective experience in individuals diagnosed with schizophrenia (Brekke *et al*, 1993); more recently its use was described in a series of papers produced by the same research group (Brekke *et al*, 2001, 2002). The CAF has never been used outside the USA, and no validated versions in languages other than English are available.

Quality of Life Checklist (QOLC)

This checklist (Malm *et al*, 1981) was developed to provide information about which aspects of QOL are particularly important to patients and clinician raters to assist in therapeutic planning. This 93-item rating scale is completed by a trained interviewer after conducting a 1-hour semi-structured interview. Scoring for all areas assessed is dichotomised as 'satisfactory' or 'unsatisfactory'. The areas assessed include: leisure activities, work, vocational rehabilitation, economic dependency, social relationships, knowledge and education, psychological dependency, inner experience, housing standard, medical care (psychiatric and general), religion. No psychometric properties are reported. Data analyses report simple frequencies of 'satisfactory' and 'unsatisfactory', by item. The patients studied included 40 persons with chronic schizophrenia in a Swedish out-patient clinic. They ranged in age from 18 to 50 and 27 (68%) were men. The QOLC has not been used by other research groups and, as far as we know, validated versions in languages other than English and Swedish are not available.

Satisfaction with Life Domains Scale (SLDS)

The SLDS was developed to evaluate the impact of the US National Institute of Mental Health (NIMH) Community Support Program (CSP) in New York State on the QOL of patients with a chronic mental illness (Baker & Intagliata, 1982; Johnson, 1991). It is a self-rated scale administered by a trained interviewer, consists of 15 items and requires approximately 10 minutes. Its individual items cover: satisfaction with housing, neighbourhood, food, clothing, health, people lived with, friends, family, relations with other people, work/day programming, spare time, fun, services and facilities in area, economic situation, place lived in now compared with state hospital. These can be summed into a total life satisfaction score. This total score correlates at $r = 0.64$ with the Bradburn Affect Balance Scale (Bradburn, 1969) and at $r = 0.29$ with the Global Assessment Scale (Endicott *et al*, 1976). No other psychometric data are provided. The frequencies and means on these items can be compared with item scores in a national QOL survey of the general population (Andrews & Withey, 1976). The patients studied included 118 out-patients with a chronic mental illness, aged 18–86 (mean 53.3) years, in two community support programmes; 61% were women and 84% lived in supervised residential settings. Diagnoses included 56%

Table 8.1 Quality-of-life measures designed for severe and persistent mental illnesses

Instrument	Acronym	Reference	No. of items	No. of domains	Mode of administration	Completion time (min)	Test-retest reliability	Internal consistency
Community Adjustment Form	CAF	Stein & Test (1980)	140	12	Clinician	45	na	na
Quality of Life Checklist	QOLC	Malm et al (1981)	93	11	Clinician	60	na	na
Satisfaction with Life Domains Scale	SLDS	Baker & Intagliata (1982)	15	15	Self-rated	10	na	na
Lehman Quality of Life Interview	QOLI	Lehman (1983a)	143	8	Clinician	45	0.41–0.95 (subjective QOL); 0.29–0.98 (objective QOL)	0.79–0.88 (subjective QOL); 0.44–0.82 (objective QOL)
Client Quality of Life Interview	CQLI	Mulkern et al (1986)	46	8	Self-rated (+19 items clinician)	30	na	na
California Well-Being Project Client Interview	CWBPCI	Campbell et al (1989)	151 patient; 76 family; 77 staff	60	Clinician; self-rated	na	na	na
Oregon Quality of Life Questionnaire	OQLQ	Bigelow et al (1991a,b)	146; 263	14	Trained interviewer; self-rated	45; 60	0.37–0.64	0.05–0.98
Lancashire Quality of Life Profile	LQOLP	Oliver (1991)	105	9	Clinician	55	0.49–0.78	0.84–0.86

Lancashire Quality of Life Profile – European Version	LQLP-EU	Gaite et al (2000)	105	9	Clinician	55	0.61–0.75	0.30–0.88
Wisconsin Quality of Life Index	W-QLI	Becker et al (1993)	113	8	Self-rated	20–30 patients; 10–20 staff	0.82–0.87	na
Quality of Life Interview Scale	QOLIS	Holcomb et al (1993)	87	8	Clinician	35	na	0.72–0.93
Quality of Life Self-Assessment Inventory	QLS–100	Skantze & Malm (1994)	100	14	Self-rated (+clinician)	10 (+40–50 min interview)	0.88 (overall score)	0.48–0.87
Lehman Quality of Life Interview – brief version	QOLI – BV	Lehman (1995)	78	8	Clinician	15	10	0.70–0.87 (life satisfaction); 0.56–0.82 (objective QOL)
Manchester Short Assessment of Quality of Life	MANSA	Priebe et al (1999)	16	9	Clinician	5	na	0.74

na not available.

139

schizophrenia, 14% affective disorders, 5% substance use disorders and 3% organic mental syndromes.

The SLDS has been translated and used worldwide in different settings and on various clinical populations (Caron *et al*, 1998; Prince & Prince, 2001; Carpiniello *et al*, 2002; Barbato *et al*, 2004). More recently, the instrument, translated into the respective national languages, has been used within the framework of the European Research Group On Schizophrenia (ERGOS) to assess the QOL of patients with schizophrenia from seven different sites across four European countries (France, Ireland, Portugal and Spain) (Kovess-Masféty *et al*, 2006).

Lehman Quality of Life Interview (QOLI)

The QOLI (Lehman *et al*, 1982; Lehman, 1983*a*, 1988) assesses the life circumstances of persons with severe mental illnesses in terms of both what they actually do and experience ('objective' QOL) and their feelings about these experiences ('subjective' QOL). It provides a broad-based assessment of the recent and current life experiences of the respondent in a wide variety of life areas of potential interest, including living situation, family relations, social relations, leisure activities, finances, safety and legal problems, work and school, and health (as well as religion and neighbourhood in some versions).

The QOLI is a structured self-report interview administered by trained interviewers. Its original, core version consists of 143 items and requires approximately 45 minutes to administer. It has since undergone a variety of revisions, primarily to improve its psychometric properties and to shorten it. The core version contains a global measure of life satisfaction as well as measures of objective and subjective QOL in eight life domains: living situation, daily activities and functioning, family relations, social relations, finances, work and school, legal and safety issues, and health. The sections on each life domain are organised such that information first is obtained about objective QOL and then about life satisfaction in that life area. This pairing of objective and subjective QOL indicators by domain is essential to the assessment model (Lehman, 1988).

All of the life satisfaction items in the interview utilise a fixed interval scale, which originally was developed in a national survey of the quality of American life (Andrews & Withey, 1976). The types of objective QOL indicators utilised vary considerably across the domains. In general they can be viewed as being of two types: measures of functioning (e.g. frequency of social contacts or daily activities) and measures of access to resources and opportunities (e.g. income support or housing type). The QOL indicators include both individual items (e.g. monthly income support) and scales (e.g. frequency of social contacts).

The variables generated by the QOLI include:

- *objective QOL indicators* – residential stability, homelessness, daily activities, frequency of family contacts, frequency of social contacts,

total monthly spending money, adequacy of financial supports, current employment status, number of arrests during the past year, victim of violent crime during past year, victim of non-violent crime during the past year, general health status
- *subjective QOL indicators* – satisfaction with living situation, leisure activities, family relations, social relations, finances, work and school, legal and safety, and health.

The psychometric properties of the QOLI have been extensively assessed. Internal consistency reliabilities range from 0.79 to 0.88 (median 0.85) for the life satisfaction scales, and from 0.44 to 0.82 (median 0.68) for the objective QOL scales. These reliabilities have been replicated in two separate studies of persons with severe mental illnesses. Test–retest reliabilities (1 week) have also been assessed for the QOLI: life satisfaction scales score 0.41–0.95 (median 0.72); objective QOL scales 0.29–0.98 (median 0.65). Construct and predictive validity have been assessed as good by confirmatory factor analyses and multivariate predictive models. The QOLI also differentiates between patients living in hospitals and supervised community residential programmes in the USA and the UK (Lehman *et al*, 1986; Simpson *et al*, 1989). Individual life satisfaction items clearly discriminate between persons with severe mental illness and the general population (Lehman *et al*, 1982). Further construct validation has been assessed in studies of the predictors of QOL among day treatment patients in the UK (Levitt *et al*, 1990) and the relationship between QOL and feelings of empowerment among persons with severe mental illnesses in the USA (Rosenfield & Nesse-Todd, 1993). A variety of methodological papers have explored other issues, such as the relationship between QOL: and clinical symptoms (Lehman, 1983*b*); gender, race and age (Lehman *et al*, 1992, 1995); and housing type (Lehman *et al*, 1991; Slaughter & Lehman, 1991).

The QOLI has been used almost exclusively with persons with severe mental disorders. The samples in published studies have included approximately equal numbers of men and women, about 75% Caucasian, ranging in age from 18 to 65 years. The predominant diagnosis in these studies has been schizophrenia (the diagnosis for 57–76% of patients). General population norms for individual life satisfaction items are available (Andrews & Withey, 1976).

A brief version of the QOLI is also available (QOLI–BV; Lehman, 1995). As with the core version, this brief version provides a broad-based QOL assessment and consists of 78 questions from the full version. It too is a self-report interview administered by trained interviewers. It requires on average 15 minutes and measures the same life domains as the core version, including the global measure of life satisfaction as well as measures of objective and subjective QOL in the eight life domains. This brief QOLI has been tested on a sample of 50 individuals with severe mental illness from a local psychosocial rehabilitation programme in a pilot study. Internal consistency reliabilities for the brief QOLI life satisfaction are comparable to those for the full version, ranging from 0.70 to 0.87 (median 0.83). Internal consistency reliabilities for the objective brief QOLI scales range from 0.56 to 0.82 (median 0.65). The QOLI–BV has displayed good reliability and validity for both patients with chronic severe mental disorders (Postrado & Lehman, 1995) and acute psychiatric in-patients (Russo et al, 1997); it has been shown to differentiate between patients with different severity of illness and functional status (Russo et al, 1997), and with patients with depression (Corrigan & Buican, 1995). It has been translated into several languages, including French (Lancon et al, 2000), Spanish (Duno et al, 2001), Indian (Lobana et al, 2001), Japanese (Horiuchi et al, 2006) and Norwegian (Nørholm & Bech, 2007), and shown to have good cross-cultural properties. The QOLI–BV has been used in a study on patients with first-episode psychosis (Melle et al, 2005), which found that the psychometric properties of the instrument do not significantly change when it is used with first-episode samples, thus providing further evidence that the QOL construct is substantially similar in this group of patients and in both clinical and non-clinical populations.

Client Quality of Life Interview (CQLI)

The CQLI (Goldstrom & Manderscheid, 1986; Mulkern et al, 1986) was developed as part of a battery of instruments to assess outcomes among persons with severe mental disorders who were served by the NIMH CSP. These instruments include the Uniform Client Data Instrument (UCDI), the UCDI Short Form, the CSP Participant Follow-up Form and the CQLI. The content of these instruments overlap to a considerable degree. All but the CQLI are completed by case managers or other professionals serving the clients and generally focus on functioning, services and clinical outcomes. Only the CQLI asks clients directly about the quality of their lives and therefore only it is reviewed here. The conceptual model underlying the CQLI assumes that certain life essentials are necessary precursors to a high quality of life. One major purpose of the CSP was to provide these essentials and thus to enhance QOL.

The CQLI is a structured self-report interview administered by a trained interviewer. It consists of 46 items rated by the respondent as well as 19 interviewer ratings. Ratings are done on fixed, ordinal scales. The content areas covered include: essentials of life (food, clothing, shelter, health and hygiene, money and safety), job training and education, daily activities and recreation, privacy, social supports, social time, self-reliance, and peace of mind. In each area questions generally cover both the quantity of resources or activities as well as the respondent's subjective feelings about these resources and activities. Many of the item sets lend themselves readily to composite scales, although the development or scoring of these scales is not available for the CQLI. Some of the scales parallel the UCDI (see above), for which scale computation guidelines as well as psychometric properties are available.

No formal psychometric analyses of the CQLI are available. Correlations of CQLI items rated by the clients with comparable items from the UCDI rated by the case manager were quite low. The CQLI ratings remained stable over a 14-month follow-up. The subsample in the CSP study who completed the CQLI were 109 severely mentally ill clients from six exemplary CSP programmes. They included 51% men; 82% Caucasian, 11% Black, 6% Hispanic, and 1% other; and had a mean age of 41.5 years. No diagnoses are indicated, but all were severely mentally ill.

California Well-Being Project Client Interview (CWBPCI)

The California Well-Being Project (Campbell *et al*, 1989) was a 3-year initiative funded by the California Department of Mental Health to develop a better understanding of the health and well-being concerns of persons who have been treated for mental illness, the so-called 'psychiatrically labelled'. This initiative was designed and conducted entirely by mental healthcare consumers. The Project consisted of three components:

1   research and analysis of well-being factors for individuals, assessed through a structured survey of consumers, family members and professionals
2   production of educational materials based upon this survey
3   dissemination of these educational materials to consumers, family members and mental health providers.

Three versions of the survey questionnaire on well-being were developed: one for consumers (151 items), one for family members (76 items) and another for mental health professionals (77 items). Time required for administration is not indicated. The questionnaires consist predominantly of Likert scaled questions, but with some open-ended questions interspersed. The questionnaires are designed to be administered either in face-to-face interviews (conducted by trained consumers), self-administered by mail, or group self-administration with an interviewer available to answer questions. The instrument is thus designed for flexibility in administration to provide the multiple perspectives of consumers, family members and professionals.

In the California survey the CWBPCI was administered to 331 persons who were 'psychiatrically labelled' and living in various settings, including psychiatric hospitals (non-state), skilled nursing facilities, board-and-care homes, satellite houses, single-occupancy hotels, community residential treatment centres, drop-in centres, client self-help groups, organisations serving people identified as 'homeless mentally ill' and on the streets. The final sample consisted of 61 randomly selected members of the California Network of Mental Health Consumers (surveyed by mail), 249 volunteer respondents from various facilities in California (face-to-face interviews, not randomly selected) and 21 randomly selected Project Return clients. The sample was 52% men, 67.5% Caucasian, 14.7% Black and 4.6% Hispanic.

They were predominantly young, with 41% below the age of 35 and 75% below 45, and the authors describe them as predominantly chronically mentally ill, but no further clinical details are given.

No information is provided on the instrument's psychometric properties, and for the most part data from individual items are reported as frequencies (or percentages) in a narrative section that discusses the many concerns of the respondents. Topics covered in this narrative include: adequate resources, age, alternatives to psychiatric hospitalisation, aspirations, benefit agencies, board and care residents, boredom, causes of psychological and emotional problems, children, client/consumer, conservatorship, control of emotional problems, creativity, stereotype of dangerousness, discrimination, electroconvulsive therapy, empowerment, ethnic/cultural group, family relationships, freedom, friends, gender, general population, hallucinations and/or voices, happiness, health, homelessness, hospitalisation, income, informed consent, internalised stigma, involuntary treatment/hospitalisation, labelling, loneliness/isolation, mass media, meaningful work and achievement/activity, medications, misdiagnosis, neighbourhood resistance, 'normal' people, patients' rights, personhood, poverty, privacy, pro-choice, professional–client relationship, public policy, quality of life, seclusion and restraint, self-esteem, self-help, sexual life, side-effects, social life, spiritual life, stigma, stress, tolerance, stereotype of unpredictability, validation, vocational rehabilitation, warmth and intimacy, well-being, and young adult chronic mentally ill.

A key measure derived from the interview is the Well-Being Quotient. This is derived from two questions providing information about the relative importance assigned to various factors that may affect well-being and whether the respondent currently lacks these factors. The questions read:

1   'Below is a list of things that some people have said are essential for their well-being. Please mark all of those things that you believe are *essential* for your well-being.'

2   'Of the things that people have mentioned that are essential for well-being, which of the following, if any, do you lack in your everyday life?'

The response factors include happiness, health, adequate income, meaningful work or achievement, comfort, satisfying social life, satisfying spiritual life, adequate resources, good food and a decent place to live, satisfying sexual life, creativity, basic human freedoms, warmth and intimacy, safety, and other. Besides simply rank ordering these factors according to the percentages of respondents who identify each factor in these questions, four well-being profiles are computed:

1   for each factor, the proportion of respondents who indicate that they lack a well-being factor that they consider essential

2   the proportion of respondents who do not lack a factor they consider essential

3   the proportion of clients who consider a factor essential regardless of whether they have it

4   the proportion of respondents who lack a given factor regardless of its essentialness.

The fact that it is consumer generated enhances its face validity even though no formal psychometric analyses were conducted. No published data on the performance of the CWBPCI have been made available in the international literature.

Oregon Quality of Life Questionnaire (OQLQ)

The OQLQ (Bigelow *et al*, 1982a,b) was based upon the Denver Community Mental Health Scale and has undergone a series of developments since. The original purpose of the OQLQ was to assess QOL outcomes among clients served by community mental health programmes, especially those developed under the NIMH CSP initiative. Bigelow *et al* (1991a,b) provide more recent psychometric data, alternative versions and further programme applications of the updated OQLQ.

The OQLQ exists in two versions: a structured self-report interview (263 items) and a semi-structured interviewer-rated interview (146 items). Both are administered by a trained (not necessarily clinical) interviewer. The theory underlying the OQLQ states that QOL derives from the social contract between an individual and society. Individuals' needs are met to the extent that persons fulfil the demands placed upon them by society. Most of the items use fixed, ordinal response categories, and the interview requires approximately 45 minutes to administer. The OQLQ yields 14 scale scores: psychological distress, psychological well-being, tolerance of stress, total basic need satisfaction, independence, interpersonal interactions, spouse role, social support, work at home, employability, work on the job, meaningful use of time, negative consequences of alcohol use, negative consequences of drug use.

The psychometric properties of the OQLQ have been evaluated extensively. Cronbach's alpha for the 14 scales on the self-report interview range from 0.05 to 0.98, with a median of 0.84. Eight of the scales have excellent reliability (alpha > 0.8), two have intermediate reliability (alpha 0.4–0.8) and four have poor reliability (alpha < 0.4). Test–retest reliabilities (interval not specified) ranged from 0.37 to 0.64, with a median of 0.50. The interrater reliability for the interviewer-rated version has been assessed in a small sample study ($n = 6$) and produced interrater agreement levels between 58% and 100% on the interviewer judgements. More than half the items showed greater than 90% agreement, and Cronbach alpha ranged from 0.32 to over 0.80 (more than half over 0.80). The predictive validity of the OQLQ has been evaluated by comparing: clients in different types of community mental health programmes (CSP, drug, alcohol and general psychiatric clinics); general community respondents from economically distressed and non-distressed communities; and changes in community mental health clients

145

over time. Results of these analyses support the overall predictive validity of the OQLQ.

The OQLQ has been applied to out-patients of mental health programmes as well as to samples of the general population. The out-patient samples included patients at intake to community mental health programmes in Oregon (which served people with chronic mental illness or drug and alcohol misuse, and general psychiatric patients). Their mean age was 33.8 (range 18–85) years and included 60% men and 96% 'non-Hispanics'. The community sample had 43% men (mean age 36.8 years) and was 92% non-Hispanic.

Lancashire Quality of Life Profile (LQOLP)

The LQOLP (Oliver, 1991; Oliver & Mohamad, 1992) was developed in the UK during the late 1980s by Oliver and colleagues in response to a requirement by the British government that all community care programmes serving persons with severe mental disorders assess the impact of their services on patients' QOL. The LQOLP is based upon the Lehman QOLI, but modified to reflect cultural variations and the broader survey intent of the government mandate for service-based evaluation of QOL. The theory underlying the LQOLP is essentially the same as that described under the Lehman QOLI above.

The LQOLP is a structured self-report patient interview designed for administration by clinical staff in community settings. It consists of 105 items and requires approximately 1 hour to complete. It assesses objective QOL and life satisfaction in nine life domains: work/education, leisure/participation, religion, finances, living situation, legal and safety, family relations, social relations, and health. The subjective components of these domains are evaluated on a seven-point Life Satisfaction Scale (LSS). In addition the instrument allows the assessment of the following additional areas: positive and negative affect (with the Bradburn Affect-Balance Scale), self-concept, global well-being (Cantril's Ladder and Happiness Scale), perceived QOL and the QOL of the patient independently of the patient's own opinion (with the Quality of Life Uniscale). Objective QOL information is collected by means of categorical or continuous measures, depending upon the content area. Life satisfaction ratings are on a seven-point Likert scale.

Psychometric properties of the life satisfaction have been evaluated in a series of pilot studies (Oliver, 1991; Oliver et al, 1997). Test–retest reliabilities for life satisfaction scores range from 0.49 to 0.78, depending upon the patient sample. Internal consistency reliabilities (Cronbach's alpha) of these scales range from 0.84 to 0.86. Content, construct and criterion validities were also assessed using a variety of techniques and judged to be adequate.

A European version of the instrument, the LQOLP–EU (Gaite et al, 2000), is also available. It was developed within the framework of the multisite EPSILON study of schizophrenia (Becker et al, 1999). In this context, the original English LQOLP was translated into Danish, Dutch, Italian and Spanish and tested for cross-cultural applicability and psychometric properties on a sample of over 400 patients with schizophrenia from five European sites. The internal consistency (Cronbach's alpha) of the total Life Satisfaction Scale (LSS) was 0.87. Of the nine subjective QOL domains, work and leisure showed the lowest internal consistency (0.30 and 0.56, respectively), the values of the remaining subscales ranging between 0.62 and 0.88. Test–retest intraclass correlation was good for the total LSS score (pooled estimate 0.82), ranging in the nine subjective domains from 0.61 (legal and safety) to 0.75 (living situation).

The LQLP has also been translated into and validated in other languages, such as German (Kaiser *et al*, 1996), Scandinavian languages (Hansson *et al*, 1998, 1999), French (Salomè *et al*, 2000) and Brazilian (de Souza & Coutinho, 2006). Both the original LQOLP and the LQOLP–EU have been used extensively in studies on QOL of people with serious mental illness: specifically, they have been used in comparison and multinational studies (Oliver *et al*, 1997; Hansson *et al*, 1999; Gaite *et al*, 2002), as a means of exploring unmet care needs (Lasalvia *et al*, 2005) and the impact of psychopathology (Lasalvia *et al*, 2002), with long-term patient populations (Ruggeri *et al*, 2005) and with patients experiencing their first episode of psychosis (Priebe *et al*, 2000).

Wisconsin Quality of Life Index (W–QLI)

The W–QLI (Becker *et al*, 1993; Becker, 1998; Diamond & Becker, 1999), initially called the name Quality of Life Index for Mental Health (QLI–MH), provides a patient-focused assessment of QOL that is intended to be responsive to the needs and constraints of clinical practice and research, and that incorporates the multiple perspectives of patients, families and clinicians. It is designed as a self-administered questionnaire, with which assistance may be given to patients with more severe impairments. Versions exist for patients, families and clinicians. It consists of 113 items; the patient version takes about 20–30 minutes and the provider version about 10–20 minutes. It has been field tested with a convenience sample of 40 out-patients meeting DSM–III–R criteria for schizophrenia.

The W–QLI produces eight scaled scores in the following domains: life satisfaction (using 15 items from Andrews & Withey, 1976); occupational activities; psychological well-being (using the Bradburn Affect Balance Scale; Bradburn, 1969); physical health; activities of daily living (using the Life Skills Profile; Rosen *et al*, 1989) and the QL Index (Spitzer *et al*, 1981); social relationships (using items from the International Pilot Study of Schizophrenia; Strauss & Carpenter, 1974); economics (adequacy and satisfaction with finances); and symptoms (using the Brief Psychiatric Rating Scale; Overall & Gorham, 1962). The W–QLI also includes some open-ended questions to generate individual goals for improvement with treatment. Finally, the instrument includes ratings of the importance of each domain to assess the salience of the scales to patients' overall QOL.

147

Test–retest reliabilities have been assessed on a subsample of 10 patients with schizophrenia over 3–10 days. The 'percentage match' for the various domains ranged from 0.82 to 0.87. Content validity is supported by the use of some previously developed scales and a scale development process that used key informants, including patients, family members and providers. Criterion validity has been assessed through correlations between patient W–QLI scores and provider ratings on the Uniscale and the Spitzer QL–Index (0.68 and 0.58, respectively).

The W–QLI is available in a French version (Diaz et al, 1999; Caron et al, 2003), which has been used on a sample of patients with first-episode psychosis engaged in a phase-specific community-focused treatment programme in Ontario, Canada (Malla et al, 2001, 2004).

Quality of Life Interview Scale (QOLIS)

The QOLIS (Holcomb et al, 1993) is designed as a QOL measure for assessing people with severe mental illness. It is a semi-structured interview administered by trained clinical interviewers and consists of 87 items. Length of time to administer is not reported.

The QOLIS was used with 201 patients with severe mental illness, including 100 long-term in-patients and 101 patients in surrounding community residences. Diagnoses included 45% schizophrenia, 16% organic mental disorders, 11% major affective disorders, 16% other. QOLIS items are rated on a Likert scale from 'strongly agree' to 'strongly disagree' and generate eight factors: autonomy, self-esteem, social support, physical health, anger/hostility, somatisation/anxiety, activity/mobility and accessibility to medical services. Factor analysis of an initial pool of 148 items yielded the proposed eight factors with 87 items. Alpha coefficients for these factors range from 0.72 to 0.93 (median 0.77). Step-wise multiple regression analyses were used to predict self-reported life satisfaction using the SLDS (Baker & Intagliata, 1982 – see above) and Global Assessment of Functioning Scale (GAF; Endicott et al, 1976) ($P < 0.0001$ for both analyses). All the QOLIS scales significantly discriminated between the in-patient and community-based samples. Canonical analysis of the QOLIS scales and the scales from the Quality of Life Scale (Heinrichs et al, 1984) showed substantial redundancy.

Quality of Life Self-Assessment Inventory (QLS–100)

The QLS–100 (Skantze et al, 1992; Skantze, 1998) provides information about which aspects of QOL are particularly important to patients and care providers to assist in therapeutic planning. It is an updated version of the QOL Checklist (Malm et al, 1981) and has been used with out-patients with chronic schizophrenia ($n = 66$). The QLS–100 is a 100-item self-report inventory completed by the patient, followed by a semi-structured interview with a clinician to confirm the patient's ratings of satisfaction and dissatisfaction and to discuss implications for treatment planning. It requires approximately 10 minutes for the patient to complete the self-rated inventory, plus 40–50 minutes for the semi-structured clinical interview.

The domains assessed include physical health, finances, household and self-care, contacts, dependence, work and leisure, knowledge and education, inner experiences, mental health, housing, housing environment, community services, and religion. For all areas, ratings are 'satisfactory' or 'unsatisfactory'. The test–retest (7–10 day) correlation for the overall scale is 0.88. Comparative data are available from healthy university students.

The psychometric properties of the QLS–100 have been assessed in two different cultures. In separate studies of 30 patients, the test–retest reliability (1–2 weeks) for the overall score was 0.88 in a Swedish sample (Skantze *et al*, 1992) and 0.91 in an Italian sample (Carpiniello *et al*, 1997). This indicates an acceptable level of stability of the questionnaire. The internal consistencies of the domains (Cronbach's alpha) ranged from 0.48 to 0.87 in the Swedish 1984 study, and from 0.87 to 0.90 in the Italian 1996 study. From these results, it would appear that items constituting the various subscales of the questionnaire tend to evaluate the same underlying dimension. The face validity of the QLS–100 may be regarded as good, since the items and domains were derived from many years of clinical experience and interviews with patients and family members familiar with the lifestyle of patients with schizophrenia. The measure also discriminated between different samples, namely out-patients with schizophrenia ($n = 61$) and university students ($n = 60$) in Sweden (Skantze *et al*, 1990), in-patients ($n = 14$) and out-patients ($n = 14$) with schizophrenia in Norway (Gråwe & Løvaas, 1994), and out-patients with schizophrenia ($n = 25$) and with major depression ($n = 20$) in Italy (Carpiniello *et al*, 1997).

Manchester Short Assessment of Quality of Life (MANSA)

The MANSA (Priebe *et al*, 1999) represents a briefer version of the LQOLP. The instrument is administered as a structured interview and comprises 4 objective questions and 12 subjective questions. The subjective items assess satisfaction with life as a whole, job, financial situation, number and quality of friendships, leisure activities, accommodation, personal safety, people with whom the individual lives (or living alone), sex life, relationship with family, physical health and mental health. The ratings are made on a seven-point scale and the mean ratings from the different domains form an overall QOL score. Administration of the MANSA takes 3–5 minutes. Good agreement has been shown between the MANSA and the LQOLP (all Pearson's coefficient correlations were above 0.82). Cronbach's alpha for satisfaction ratings resulted in a coefficient of 0.74, indicating good internal consistency.

The instrument has been translated into Dutch, German (Kaiser *et al*, 1999) and Swedish (Björkman & Svensson, 2005). According to its authors (Priebe *et al*, 1999), MANSA represents a viable and valid instrument to obtain condensed and accurate QOL data, and it is brief enough to be included in a minimum data-set. However, since test–retest reliability data are still not available, further testing of the measure's psychometric properties is needed.

Measures specifically designed for schizophrenia

Although all of the QOL measures reviewed above have been used with patient samples with a predominance of schizophrenia, none was specifically developed as a disease-specific QOL measure. The main characteristics of measures specifically designed for assessing QOL in schizophrenia are summarised in Table 8.2.

Quality of Life Scale (QLS)

The QLS (Heinrichs *et al*, 1984) was developed to assess the deficit syndrome in patients with schizophrenia. It is a semi-structured interview rated by trained clinicians. Its 21 items are rated on fixed interval scales based upon the interviewer's judgement of the patient's functioning in each of the 21 areas. The interview requires approximately 45 minutes. The 21 items of the QLS cover: commonplace activities, occupational role, work functioning, work level, possession of commonplace objects, interpersonal relations (household, friends, acquaintances, social activity, social network, social initiative, social withdrawal, sociosexual functioning), sense of purpose, motivation, curiosity, anhedonia, aimless inactivity, empathy, emotional interaction, and work satisfaction. These items reduce to four scales: intrapsychic foundations, interpersonal relations, instrumental role, and common objects and activities. A total score can be also computed. The interrater reliabilities on conjointly conducted interviews range from 0.84 to 0.97 on summary scales. Individual item intraclass correlations range from 0.5 to 0.9. Confirmatory factor analysis has been conducted.

This scale is widely used in the evaluation of psychopharmacological treatments for schizophrenia, predominantly with out-patients (Bobes & Garcia-Portilla, 2005).

Efforts aimed at identifying a core subset of QLS items that maintain the validity and psychometric property of the complete version have been undertaken in order to facilitate evaluation of treatment outcomes in schizophrenia in both routine care and clinical trials.

A brief QLS version containing seven items (the QLS7) was produced by Bilker *et al* (2003). Their abbreviated QLS included items representing all four interdependent theoretical constructs of the original 21-item QLS. For intrapsychic foundations, three of the seven items were retained (motivation, anhedonia and capacity for empathy); for interpersonal relations, two of eight items were retained (active acquaintances and social initiative); for instrumental role, only one item, occupational role functioning, of four was retained; for common objects and activities, one of the two items was retained (possession of objects reflecting participation in living). This study demonstrated that using only seven QLS items as predictors, the correlation was 0.98 between the predicted and true QLS totals. However, the patient sample used in this study included 31.3% drug-naive and 32.3% first-episode patients, a sample not representative of the distribution of patients with schizophrenia in the general population; moreover, the relationship

Table 8.2 Quality-of-life measures specifically designed for schizophrenia

Instrument	Acronym	Reference	No. of items	No. of domains	Mode of administration	Completion time (min)	Test-retest reliability	Internal consistency
Quality of Life Scale	QLS	Heinrichs et al (1984)	21	21	Clinician	40–45	0.5–0.9; 0.84–0.97 (interrater)	na
Subjective Well-being under Neuroleptics Scale	SWN	Naber (1995)	38	5	Self-rated	15–20	0.75–0.89	0.73–0.88
Schizophrenia Quality of Life Scale	SQLS	Wilkinson et al (2000)	30	3	Self-rated	5–10	na	0.78–0.93
Schizophrenia Quality of Life Scale – Revision 4	SQLS–R4	Martin & Allan (2007)	33	2	Self-rated	na	na	na
Quality of Life Questionnaire in Schizophrenia	S–QOL	Auquier et al (2003)	41	8	Self-rated	15	0.64–0.79	0.72–0.92
Subjective Quality of Life Analysis	S.QUA. L.A.	Nadalet et al (2005)	22	22	Self-rated	na	na	0.87–0.88

na not available.

of the QLS7 to severity of symptoms, side-effects, emotional distress and perceived QOL was not addressed.

Ritsner *et al* (2005*b*), using only five QLS items (social initiatives, adequacy, acquaintances, motivation, and time utilisation) as predictors, found a correlation of 0.98 between the predicted and true QLS totals. Additional analyses indicated that this five-item version exhibited similar performance to the original QLS regarding construct validity, test–retest reliability and responsiveness to change over time. Though the sample size and age at onset of illness were similar with respect to the study reported by Bilker *et al* (2003), all patients in this study were medicated, and their mean duration of illness was considerably longer, and better reflected the distribution of patients with schizophrenia in the general population. Moreover, in this study construct validity was assessed by investigating the correlation of the QLS items with severity of symptoms, side-effects, emotional distress and perceived QOL (all Pearson's *r* ranging from 0.46 to 0.55).

Subjective Well-being under Neuroleptics Scale (SWN)

The SWN (Naber, 1995, 1998) was specifically designed to measure the subjective experience of patients with schizophrenia while they are taking antipsychotic medication. The assumption at the basis of the instrument is that the aim of any successful antipsychotic treatment should not merely be to reduce psychotic symptoms but also to help patients to live and enjoy their lives. The benefit of drugs in the treatment of schizophrenia is beyond any doubt. However, most patients taking them experience a series of adverse effects, not restricted to motor symptoms but also affecting cognition and emotion. They are often too subtle to be detected by objective examination, but they are reported by patients, who complain of a reduced QOL, with restrictions of emotionality, straight thinking and spontaneity. This syndrome, similar to the negative symptoms of schizophrenia, has been named 'pharmacogenic depression' or 'neuroleptic-induced deficit syndrome'. To investigate this issue of major clinical relevance, a self-rating scale was developed to measure subjective well-being under neuroleptic treatment (SWN), to be used in clinical routine as well as in clinical trials.

The SNW is a 38-item self-rating scale that uses six-point Likert-type responses. It refers to the subjective experience in the past 7 days, with items such as 'I am full of energy and life' and 'I feel very comfortable in my body'. Naber (1998) found a five-factor solution of the scale, which was interpreted as: emotional regulation, self-control, mental functioning, social integration and physical functioning. Analyses of the SWN results from 216 patients with schizophrenia showed good practicability, internal consistency (Chronbach's alpha = 0.95 for total score and 0.73–0.88 for the five subfactors), test–retest reliability ($r = 0.75$–0.89) and sensitivity. In addition, it was found that only 4% of the patients were inconsistent in their ratings, that all 37 patients on stable medication were consistent in rating their subjective experience and that the 16 patients whose medication was changed in the study period also significantly changed on their SWN factor scores (Naber 1995, 1998).

A short form of the SWN has been developed based on reliability analyses (Naber *et al*, 2001). Items with a low item–test correlation were dropped. The SWN – short form is a 20-item Likert scale (10 positive and 10 negative items) with five subscores. The internal consistency of both the short and long version was comparable, and the versions were found to be highly correlated. The SWN – short form has been translated into 15 languages. Its psychometric properties have been replicated by Dutch and Italian authors (de Haan *et al*, 2002; Balestrieri *et al*, 2006). Several trials have shown that the SWN rating is strongly related to compliance (Naber, 1995; Karow *et al*, 2007) and that the scale is sensitive to the effects of antipsychotic treatment.

Schizophrenia Quality of Life Scale (SQLS)

The SQLS (Wilkinson *et al*, 2000) is a self-reported 30-item questionnaire for measuring QOL specific to patients with schizophrenia. It was developed as a measure for use in clinical trials and other research studies, rather than for the assessment of community programmes. The SQLS is composed of three scales: psychosocial, motivation/energy and symptoms/side-effects. Lower scores indicate higher levels of subjective QOL.

The validity and reliability of the scale have been tested. Content validity has been addressed by developing items on the basis of in-depth interviews with patients, rather than relying on the literature or clinical scales in this field. The content of the questionnaire addresses experiences of importance to individuals with the disorder. The scale development involved a sample of over 200 people with schizophrenia in contact with secondary services in the Liverpool area. Construct validity was explored by correlation of the scales of the SQLS with established measures of health status (the SF–36; Ware & Sherbourne, 1992) and psychological outcome the General Health Questionnaire (GHQ; Goldberg, 1979) and the Hospital Anxiety and Depression Scale (HADS; Zigmond & Snaith, 1983). All three scales (psychosocial, motivation/energy and symptoms/side-effects) showed good internal consistency (Cronbach's alpha 0.93, 0.78 and 0.80, respectively). Wilkinson *et al* (2000) did not consider it necessary to examine the instrument's test–retest reliability, as the alpha statistic indicated that responses were non-random and consequently reflective of an underlying phenomenon.

The SQLS has been translated into several languages, including Japanese (Kaneda *et al*, 2002) and Chinese (Luo *et al*, 2008).

The SQLS has gone through various revisions to improve its psychometric properties. The Schizophrenia Quality of Life Scale – Revision 4 (SQLS–R4) contains 33 items in two domains, psychosocial feelings (20 items) and vitality/cognition (13 items). The SQLS–R4 has been translated into 52 languages through standardised procedures (i.e. forward translation, reconciliation, and back-translation) (Oxford Outcomes, 2004).

The administration of the SQLS–R4 in a patient group in the UK provided preliminary evidence supporting its factor structure and internal validity

(Martin & Allan, 2007). Confirmatory factor analysis was conducted on the SQLS–R4 to determine its psychometric properties in 100 patients with a primary ICD–10 diagnosis of schizophrenia. Internal reliability of both SQLS–R4 vitality/cognition and psychosocial feelings subscales was found to be good.

Quality of Life Questionnaire in Schizophrenia (S–QOL)

The S–QOL (Auquier *et al*, 2003) is a self-administered instrument developed for assessing health-related QOL among people with schizophrenia. The questionnaire was based on Calman's approach to the patient's point of view; health-related QOL was defined as the discrepancies perceived by patients between their expectations and their current life experiences (Calman, 1984). Its primary use is intended to be in clinical trials. The questionnaire consists of 41 items grouped in eight subscales: psychological well-being, self-esteem, family relationships, relationship with friends, resilience, physical well-being, autonomy, and sentimental life. Each item is rated on a five-point Likert scale, ranging from 1 = 'less than expected' to 5 = 'more than expected', with the highest score indicating the most favourable quality of life, and the lowest the least favourable. The questionnaire takes approximately 15 minutes. It provides a global QOL index and scores in the eight subscales. In-depth interviews with 207 patients with chronic schizophrenia determined the pertinent issues for item development. Construct validity was confirmed using established clinical and health-related QOL measures: S–QOL dimension scores had medium to high correlations ($r > 0.5$) with dimension scores of the SF–36, the QOLI (Lehman, 1983*a,b*) and the EuroQol (EuroQol Group, 1990) scores. All domains achieved a Cronbach's alpha of at least 0.7 (ranging from 0.72 to 0.92). However, further work is needed to test its strengths and weaknesses in different contexts.

Subjective Quality of Life Analysis (S.QUA.L.A.)

The S.QUA.L.A. (Nadalet *et al*, 2005) is a self-administered questionnaire designed to measure subjective QOL in patients with schizophrenia. The instrument is based on Calman's (1984) phenomenological approach. It comprises 22 domains of life, such as perceived health, mental well-being, physical autonomy, environment, family and social relations, safety, and general conceptions like justice, freedom, truth, beauty and art, and politics. All domains are rated in terms of importance (from 'absolutely necessary' to 'without importance') and satisfaction (from 'very satisfied' to 'very disappointed'). Importance and satisfaction scores, for each domain, are multiplied to obtain another specific and integrative measure of partial QOL (called here 'profile').

The psychometric properties of the instrument were assessed in a sample of patients with chronic schizophrenia and a sample of healthy students. Construct and convergent validity of the questionnaire were tested using the subjective part of the QOLI. Results showed that the satisfaction areas of the S.QUA.L.A. are clearly related to those of the QOLI, suggesting the same construct. Cronbach's alpha for all profiles were in the range 0.87–0.88 for patients, and internal consistency was 0.81–0.83 for students. No test–retest data were provided by the authors.

Measures specifically designed for affective and anxiety disorders

The main characteristics of measures specifically designed for assessing QOL in patients with affective and anxiety disorders are summarised in Table 8.3.

Quality of Life Enjoyment and Satisfaction Questionnaire (Q–LES–Q)

The intent of the Q–LES–Q (Endicott et al, 1993) is to provide an easy-to-use assessment of patients' enjoyment and satisfaction with their lives. It is a self-administered 93-item questionnaire. The length of time to complete it is 40–45 minutes. The Q–LES–Q has been used with 95 out-patients meeting DSM–III–R criteria for major depression. It yields eight summary scale scores. Five of these are relevant to all subjects: physical health, subjective feelings, leisure time activities, social relationships, and general activities. The other three can be scored for appropriate subgroups: work, household duties, and school/course work. Items are posed as questions and respondents rate their degree of enjoyment or satisfaction on a five-point scale. The Q–LES–Q also includes single items assessing satisfaction with medication and overall life satisfaction.

Test–retest reliabilities (interval not specified) were assessed on 54 stable out-patients; these intraclass correlations ranged from 0.63 to 0.89 (median 0.74) on the various scales. Internal consistency reliabilities all exceeded 0.90 (median 0.92). Validity has been assessed with correlations of the Q–LES–Q scales with measures of illness severity and depression. The correlations of the Q–LES–Q scales ranged from –0.34 to –0.68 (median –0.54) with the Clinical Global Impressions Scale (CGI; National Institute of Mental Health, 1985) and showed comparable correlations with the Hamilton Rating Scale for Depression (HRSD; Hamilton, 1960), the Beck Depression Inventory (BDI; Beck & Beamesderfer, 1974) and the Symptom Checklist–90 (Derogatis et al, 1973). Changes in the Q–LES–Q correlated with changes in the CGI and the HRSD (correlations of change scores ranged from –0.30 to –0.54, median –0.46).

Research groups have found the Q–LES–Q to be a useful instrument for assessing the treatment of bipolar disorder (Revicki et al, 2003), depression (Seidman & Rabkin, 1998) and premenstrual dysphoric disorder (Pearlstein et al, 2000), and for evaluating QOL in chronic depression (Russell et al, 2001), bipolar disorder (Ozer et al, 2002) and post-traumatic stress disorder (Rapaport et al, 2002). However, the Q–LES–Q is a lengthy questionnaire: it takes 40–45 minutes to complete. Therefore, efforts have been made to identify a core subset of Q–LES–Q items that maintains the validity and psychometric properties of the full version. In this context, Ritsner et al (2005a) proposed an 18-item version of the instrument that predicted

Table 8.3 Quality-of-life measures specifically designed for affective and anxiety disorders

Instrument	Acronym	Reference	No. of items	No. of domains	Mode of administration	Completion time (min)	Test–retest reliability	Internal consistency
Quality of Life Enjoyment and Satisfaction Questionnaire	Q–LES–Q	Endicott et al (1993)	93	8	Self-rated	40–45	0.63–0.89	0.90
SmithKline Beecham Quality of Life Scale	SBQOL	Stoker et al (1992)	28	10	Self-rated	45	0.66–0.83	0.85–0.95
Quality of Life in Depression Scale	QLDS	Hunt & McKenna (1992a,b)	34	6	Self-rated	10–15	0.81	0.93
Quality of Life Inventory	QOLI	Frisch et al (1992)	16	16	Self-rated	na	0.80–0.91	0.77–0.89

na not available.

basic Q–LES–Q domains (physical health, subjective feelings, leisure time activities, social relationships) and general index scores with high accuracy. Q–LES–Q–18 showed high reliability (Cronbach's alpha ranging from 0.74 to 0.97), validity (correlation coefficients with QLS and LQOLP scores ranging from 0.55 to 0.64) and stability of test–retest ratings (intraclass correlation coefficients ranging from 0.71 to 0.83).

SmithKline Beecham Quality of Life Scale (SBQOL)

The SBQOL (Stoker et al, 1992) was specifically designed to provide a method for assessing QOL in patients with affective disorders. It is a 28-item self-report questionnaire (45 minutes). It was developed with 129 out-patients presenting in general practice and meeting criteria for either DSM–III–R major depression or generalised anxiety disorder. The items in the SBQOL are rated on a ten-point scale anchored by positive and negative extremes of the various constructs. Domains covered include psychic well-being, physical well-being, social relationships, activities/interests/hobbies, mood, locus of control, sexual function, work/employment, religion and finances. To provide an idiographic component, respondents are asked to rate themselves on these constructs from three perspectives: self now, ideal self and sick self. A summary score is then generated across the domains for the differences between self now and either ideal self or sick self.

Changes in the self now/sick self and self now/ideal self paralleled improvements in clinical depression (measured by the HRSD) over a 12-week therapeutic period. The self now/sick self and self now/ideal self 'distances' correlated with scores on the Sickness Impact Profile (Bergner et al, 1981) and the GHQ, two generic health-related QOL measures. One-day test–retest reliabilities for the self now, sick self, ideal self, self now/sick self and self now/ideal self scores ranged from 0.66 to 0.83 (median 0.70). Internal consistency reliabilities for these scores ranged from 0.85 to 0.95 (median 0.90).

Quality of Life in Depression Scale (QLDS)

The QLDS (Hunt & McKenna, 1992a,b) was designed to assess the impact of depression on the QOL of patients. It is a 34-item self-report questionnaire (10–15 minutes). It has been used in a study of 74 patients with depression in the UK. The QLDS generates a summary score encompassing six dimensions: domestic activities, interpersonal relationships, social life, cognition, personal hygiene, and leisure activities and relaxation. The 2-week test–retest reliability coefficient was 0.81 and the internal consistency reliability was 0.93. The QLDS score had a correlation of 0.79 with the General Well-Being Index (DuPuy, 1984). These results have been replicated on samples of non-elderly and elderly Dutch patients with major depression (Gregoire et al, 1994). Over the years, the QLDS has become a widespread measure for use in clinical trials to assess the QOL of patients with depression. The instrument has been produced in several languages, including French, Danish, German, Italian, Arabic and Spanish (McKenna et al, 2001).

Quality of Life Inventory (QOLI)

The QOLI (Frisch *et al*, 1992; Frisch, 1994) is a self-rated questionnaire specifically developed for use with people suffering from depressive and anxiety disorders. It measures life satisfaction in 16 domains: self-esteem, goals/values, health, learning, work, creativity, play, helping, friends, neighbourhood, community, home, children, love, money and relatives. Individuals are asked to judge both the importance of and their satisfaction with each domain on scales ranging from not at all important (0) to extremely important (2) and very dissatisfied (–3) to very satisfied (3). Overall life satisfaction is calculated by averaging the weighted satisfaction ratings with non-zero importance ratings.

The reliability and validity of the QOLI have been examined in samples of undergraduates, undergraduate counselling centre patients, psychiatric in-patients and criminal offenders (Frisch *et al*, 1992). Test–retest coefficients for the QOLI ranged from 0.80 to 0.91, and internal consistency coefficients ranged from 0.77 to 0.89 across three clinical and three non-clinical samples. Across all samples, QOLI item–total correlations were found to be adequate, and the QOLI had significantly positive correlations with seven related measures of subjective well-being, including a peer rating and a clinical interview measure. The QOLI also correlated negatively with scores on the Symptom Checklist–90–R, the BDI and the depression, dysthymia and anxiety subscales of the Millon Clinical Multiaxial Inventory–II (Millon, 1983). Non-clinical respondents had significantly higher QOLI scores than clinical groups (Frisch *et al*, 1992). Thus, the QOLI possesses good psychometric properties and appears to be a valid and reliable self-report measure of life satisfaction.

Bourland *et al* (2000) investigated the validity of the QOLI with two samples of older adults: a group with generalised anxiety disorder (GAD) and a non-clinical group. The measure successfully discriminated between the two groups, and it was significantly and negatively correlated with three psychopathology measures, indicating good criterion-related and divergent validity. Furthermore, the sensitivity of the QOLI to treatment-related change was confirmed in three studies, examining the relationship between QOL and depression (Grant *et al*, 1995), social phobia (Safren *et al*, 1997) and GAD (Stanley *et al*, 2003). A further study provided evidence on the psychometric qualities of the QOLI in clinical populations of patients with anxiety and depression (McAlinden & Oei, 2006).

Discussion

Selecting a QOL measure

Given that none of these QOL measures has been widely used or accepted as a standard, the choice of measure must rest with the investigator's particular purpose and needs. Some general comments and caveats are warranted for the investigator or programme evaluator seeking a QOL measure for people who are severely mentally ill, whether one of those described above or some other. First, a major concern with using normative QOL measures in this population is that floor effects are frequently encountered, especially in role-functioning domains (e.g. spouse, parent, employment role). Therefore, special attention must be paid to the instrument's sensitivity. Such floor effects are typically not a problem in the domains of life satisfaction and resources. Second, significant numbers of these patients have problems with task perseverance and comprehension. Therefore, pencil-and-paper questionnaires are ill-advised. Note that nearly all of the instruments discussed here are interviews. Finally, psychopathology affects patients' ratings of their QOL. Therefore, QOL assessments of these patients should be accompanied by a concomitant assessment of psychopathological symptoms, to reduce the confounding effects of psychiatric syndromes on QOL assessments.

Interpreting QOL information

A gnawing issue in the assessment of QOL is whether persons with mental illness can provide truly valid assessments of their QOL. On a general level it can be argued that psychometric studies of the validity of QOL measures for persons with mental illness have produced positive results (Lehman, 1996). That is, these have tended to support the construct, predictive and criterion validity of QOL measures. It has been repeatedly demonstrated that the so-called objective and subjective aspects of QOL are not highly correlated (Skantze, 1998; Ruggeri et al, 2001). Patients with schizophrenia, though functionally more impaired, express somewhat greater life satisfaction than do patients with depression (Lehman, 1983b; Oliver, 1991; Atkinson et al, 1997). African-American patients report lower incomes and rates of employment but somewhat greater life satisfaction than do Caucasian patients (Lehman et al, 1995). The maxim 'You can't buy happiness' seems to hold.

Still, the issue of validity of patient self-report frequently arises when QOL findings do not coincide with clinical, research or societal expectations. We must assume that there is something to this concern. As mentioned above, we do know that disorders of mood substantially affect satisfaction with life. Mood may also affect self-assessments of functional status. For example, a patient with depression may report low life satisfaction and cognitively distort and underestimate work achievements. Conversely, psychosis on average is only modestly related to level of life satisfaction (Lehman, 1983b; Oliver, 1991; Atkinson et al, 1997), probably because the effects of psychosis on life satisfaction depend upon the nature of the psychosis. Grandiose delusions may raise life satisfaction, while persecutory delusions will lower it. By definition, psychosis may distort the reality of level of functioning.

To some extent the issue reduces to our willingness to accept in-consistencies between outcomes rated by patients versus others (clinicians, family members) and to incorporate such differences of perception into treatment planning and research. An example illustrates this point. In a randomised trial of clozapine for patients with treatment-refractory schizophrenia, Cramer *et al* (2000) found that clozapine was associated with a significant improvement in clinical symptoms and clinician ratings of patients' QOL using the QLS (described above), but there was no significant change in patients' self-rated QOL using Lehman's QOLI. They concluded that patient self-reports of QOL are not as sensitive as clinician ratings of QOL to the types of clinical changes observed in clinical trials. At the very least we are left with the ambiguous finding that clozapine was associated with improved clinical symptoms and a perception by clinicians that patients were doing better, but the perception by patients that things had not changed significantly in their lives. This can be taken either as a plausible set of circumstances to inform future efforts to improve care or as evidence that patients misperceive their circumstances. If we are to adhere to the philosophy underlying QOL assessment that the goal is to address the patient's well-being as judged by the patient, then dismissing patient self-report as invalid is not productive.

Rather than reflecting measurement limitations, such inconsistent QOL findings may offer valuable information for clinical interventions and service planning. Counterintuitive QOL results may reflect the idiosyncratic views and values of persons afflicted by severe mental illness and should affect the clinician's approach to service planning. Patients are unlikely to be motivated to change circumstances with which they are content even if the clinician and family feel otherwise. Conversely, failure to address an area of life with which a patient is dissatisfied, even though the clinician and family view the patient's circumstances as satisfactory, can adversely affect the treatment alliance with the patient. Such disagreements about QOL may signal the need for a period of negotiation regarding treatment and service goals.

Counterintuitive QOL findings may also represent patients' accommodation to adversity. Patients who have lived with social isolation, unemployment, poverty or adverse living circumstances for extended periods of time may report relative positive life satisfaction. Their satisfaction reflects an accommodation to adversity and does not necessarily mean that they would not desire an improvement in life circumstances if the hope and opportunity for such changes were offered. Conversely, interventions that promote positive change, such as vocational rehabilitation or a novel antipsychotic medication (e.g. clozapine), may produce transient decreases in life satisfaction because of patients' renewed awareness of how their lives could be better. Such possibilities form the basis for caution and more thoughtful consideration about how we expect interventions to affect QOL.

Research needs

Studies are needed to examine in more detail the relationships between QOL judgements and psychopathology. A variety of research questions can be raised. How do patients' ratings of their QOL vary when they are and are not experiencing major symptoms? That is, holding objective life circumstances constant, how does life satisfaction vary with symptoms? If it does vary, how should this affect the timing of collection of life satisfaction assessments? Holding symptoms constant, how does life satisfaction vary across time as changes occur in objective life circumstances? Does psychopathology override the effects of changes in the patient's life circumstances or the patient's satisfaction with life? Does depression dampen the effects of improvements in objective life circumstances? Does psychosis distort changes in life satisfaction related to changes in life circumstances? For example, do we see expected changes in housing satisfaction among homeless people with a psychosis when they are given decent housing? Many of these questions could be answered from re-analyses of existing data-sets or from longitudinal studies that concurrently assess psychopathology, life satisfaction and objective life changes. In this regard, Malla & Payne (2005), in a review on first-episode psychosis, found that poor QOL is related to residual psychopathology, long delays in treatment and poor premorbid adjustment. However, according to the authors, the potential effects of improved treatment and/or early intervention on functional outcome and QOL have not been adequately examined, nor have the interrelationships between predictors and the underlying processes involved in determining variations in outcome.

An additional issue that must be addressed in QOL research is whether perceptions of QOL are primarily state or trait. Lykken & Tellegen (1996) suggest that there may be a strong hereditary component to 'happiness'. They found intraclass correlations on a measure of subjective well-being in the range 0.44–0.52 among monozygotic twins, whether reared together or apart, contrasting with correlations of –0.02 to 0.08 among dizygotic twins. Hence we must ask whether quality of life is a state or a trait. In contrast to the question about the effects of current mental status (a state) on subjective well-being, this question asks whether life satisfaction is primarily a function of enduring personality characteristics. In essence, are people inherently optimistic or pessimistic and is this the main determinant of life satisfaction? Again, this question should be examined through longitudinal studies to determine whether and how life satisfaction changes as circumstances change. Do people have an internal set point for life satisfaction to which they tend to return despite changes in life circumstances? How should this be incorporated into ongoing QOL research? Some data suggest that such enduring temperament characteristics may affect measures of general life satisfaction more than measures of domain-specific life satisfaction, such as housing or job satisfaction (Lehman *et al*, 1991; Slaughter & Lehman, 1991; Drake *et al*, 1996; Ruggeri *et al*, 2003).

Finally, we need a better understanding of how QOL varies naturally over time in psychiatric populations, the predictive validity of QOL measures for subsequent illness course and outcome, and the sensitivity of QOL measures to treatment effects among these patients, who may at best experience very modest improvements. There is a need for basic conceptual work to develop

161

better models for integrating QOL data into a general model of outcome for persons with severe mental illnesses.

References

Andrews, F. M. & Withey, S. B. (1976) *Social Indicators of Well-Being.* Plenum Press.

Atkinson, M., Zibin, S. & Chuang, H. (1997) Characterizing quality of life among patients with chronic mental illness: a critical examination of the self-report methodology. *American Journal of Psychiatry,* **154,** 99–105.

Auquier, P., Simeoni, M. C., Sapin, C., *et al* (2003) Development and validation of a patient-based health-related quality of life questionnaire in schizophrenia: the S–QoL. *Schizophrenia Research,* **63,** 137–149.

Baker, F. & Intagliata, J. (1982) Quality of life in the evaluation of community support systems. *Evaluation and Program Planning,* **5,** 69–79.

Balestrieri, M., Giaroli, G., Mazzi, M., *et al* (2006) Performance of the Italian version of the Subjective Well-being under Neuroleptic (SWN) scale in schizophrenic outpatients. *Pharmacopsychiatry,* **39,** 81–84.

Barbato, A., Monzani, E. & Schiavi, T. (2004) Life satisfaction in a sample of outpatients with severe mental disorders: a survey in northern Italy. *Quality of Life Research,* **13,** 969–973.

Beck, A. T. & Beamesderfer, A. (1974) Assessment of depression: the depression inventory. In *Modern Problems in Pharmacopsychiatry* (ed. P. Pichot), pp. 151–169. S. Karger.

Becker, M. (1998) A US experience: consumer responsive quality of life measurement. *Canadian Journal of Community Mental Health,* **17** (suppl. 3), 41–52.

Becker, M., Diamond, R. & Sainfort, F. (1993) A new patient focused index for measuring quality of life in persons with severe and persistent mental illness. *Quality of Life Research,* **2,** 239–251.

Becker, T., Knapp, M., Knudsen, H. C., *et al* (1999) The EPSILON study of schizophrenia in five European countries. Design and methodology for standardising outcome measures and comparing patterns of care and service costs. *British Journal of Psychiatry,* **175,** 514–521.

Bergner, M., Bobbit, R. A., Canter, W. B., *et al* (1981) The Sickness Impact Profile: development and final revision of a health status measure. *Medical Care,* **19,** 787–805.

Bigelow, D. A. & Young, D. J. (1991) Effectiveness of a case management program. *Community Mental Health Journal,* **27,** 115–123.

Bigelow, D. A., Brodsky, G., Steward, L., *et al* (1982*a*) The concept and measurement of quality of life as a dependent variable in evaluation of mental health services. In *Innovative Approaches to Mental Health Evaluation* (eds G. Stahler & W. Tash), pp. 345–366. Academic Press.

Bigelow, D. A., Gareau, M. J. & Young, D. J. (1982*b*) A quality of life interview. *Psychosocial Rehabilitation Journal,* **14,** 94–98.

Bigelow, D. A., McFarland, B. H., Gareau, M. J., *et al* (1991*a*) Implementation and effectiveness of a bed reduction project. *Community Mental Health Journal,* **27,** 125–133.

Bigelow, D. A., McFarland, B. H. & Olson, M. M. (1991*b*) Quality of life of community mental health program clients: validating a measure. *Community Mental Health Journal,* **27,** 43–55.

Bilker, W. B., Brensinger, C., Kurtz, M. M., *et al* (2003) Development of an abbreviated schizophrenia quality of life scale using a new method. *Neuropsychopharmacology,* **28,** 773–777.

Björkman, T. & Svensson, B. (2005) Quality of life in people with severe mental illness. Reliability and validity of the Manchester Short Assessment of Quality of Life (MANSA). *Nordic Journal of Psychiatry,* **59,** 302–306.

Bobes, J. & Garcia-Portilla, M. P. (2005) Quality of life in schizophrenia. In *Quality of Life in Mental Disorders* (eds H. Katschnig, H. Freeman & N. Sartorius), pp. 153–168. Wiley.

Bourland, S. L., Stanley, M. A., Snyder, A. G., et al (2000) Quality of life in older adults with generalized anxiety disorder. *Aging and Mental Health*, **4**, 315–323.

Bradburn, N. M. (1969) *The Structure of Psychological Well-Being*. Aldine.

Brekke, J. S., Levin, S., Wolkon, G. H., et al (1993) Psychosocial functioning and subjective experience in schizophrenia. *Schizophrenia Bulletin*, **19**, 599–608.

Brekke, J. S., Prindle, C., Bae, S. W., et al (2001) Risks for individuals with schizophrenia who are living in the community. *Psychiatric Services*, **52**, 1358–1366.

Brekke, J. S., Long, J. D. & Kay, D. D. (2002) The structure and invariance of a model of social functioning in schizophrenia. *Journal of Nervous and Mental Disease*, **190**, 63–72.

Calman, K. C. (1984) Quality of life in cancer patients: a hypothesis. *Journal of Medical Ethics*, **18**, 124–127.

Campbell, J., Schraiber, R., Temkin, T., et al (1989) *The Well-Being Project: Mental Health Clients Speak for Themselves*. California Department of Mental Health.

Caron, J., Tempier, R., Mercier, C., et al (1998) Components of social support and quality of life in severely mentally ill, low income individuals and a general population group. *Community Mental Health Journal*, **34**, 459–475.

Caron, J., Corbière, M., Mercier, C., et al (2003) The construct validity of the Client Questionnaire of the Wisconsin Quality of Life Index – a cross-validation study. *International Journal of Methods in Psychiatric Research*, **12**, 128–138.

Carpiniello, B., Lai, G. L., Pariante, C. M., et al (1997) Symptoms, standards of living and subjective quality of life: a comparative study of schizophrenic and depressed out-patients. *Acta Psychiatrica Scandinavica*, **96**, 235–241.

Carpiniello, B., Baita, A., Carta, M. G., et al (2002) Clinical and psychosocial outcome of patients affected by panic disorder with or without agoraphobia: results from a naturalistic follow-up study. *European Psychiatry*, **17**, 394–398.

Corrigan, P. W. & Buican, B. (1995) The construct-validity of subjective quality of life for the severely mentally ill. *Journal of Nervous and Mental Disease*, **183**, 281–285.

Cramer, J. A., Rosenheck, R., Xu, W., et al (2000) Quality of life in schizophrenia: a comparison of instruments. *Schizophrenia Bulletin*, **26**, 659–666.

de Haan, L., Weisfelt, M., Dingemans, P. M., et al (2002) Psychometric properties of the Subjective Well-Being Under Neuroleptics scale and the Subjective Deficit Syndrome Scale. *Psychopharmacology*, **162**, 24–28.

Derogatis, D. A., Lipman, R. S. & Covi, L. (1973) SCL–90: an outpatient psychiatric rating scale: preliminary report. *Psychopharmacological Bulletin*, **9**, 13–28.

de Souza, L. A. & Coutinho, E. S. (2006) The quality of life of people with schizophrenia living in community in Rio de Janeiro, Brazil. *Social Psychiatry and Psychiatric Epidemiology*, **41**, 347–356.

Diamond, R. & Becker, M. (1999) The Wisconsin Quality of Life Index: a multidimensional model for measuring quality of life. *Journal of Clinical Psychiatry*, **60** (suppl. 3), 29–31.

Diaz, P., Mercier, C., Hachey, R., et al (1999) An evaluation of psychometric properties of the Client's Questionnaire of the Wisconsin Quality of Life Index – Canadian version (CaW–QLI). *Quality of Life Research*, **8**, 509–514.

Drake, R. E., McHugo, G. J., Becker, D. R., et al (1996) The New Hampshire study of supported employment for people with severe mental illness. *Journal of Consulting and Clinical Psychology*, **64**, 391–399.

Duno, R., Pousa, E., Domenech, C., et al (2001) Subjective quality of life in schizophrenic outpatients in a Catalan urban site. *Journal of Nervous and Mental Disease*, **189**, 685–690.

DuPuy, H. (1984) The Psychological General Well-Being Index. In *Assessment of Quality of Life in Clinical Trials of Cardiovascular Therapies* (N. Wenger), pp. 170–183. Le Jacq.

Endicott, J., Spitzer, R., Fleiss, J., et al (1976) The Global Assessment Scale: a procedure for measuring overall severity of psychiatric disturbance. *Archives of General Psychiatry*, **33**, 766–771.

Endicott, J., Nee, J., Harrison, W., et al (1993). Quality of life enjoyment and satisfaction questionnaire: a new measure. *Psychopharmacology Bulletin*, **29**, 321–326.

163

EuroQol Group (1990) EuroQol – a new facility for measurement of health-related quality of life. *Health Policy*, **16**, 199–208.

Frisch, M. B. (1994) *Manual and Treatment Guide for the Quality of Life Inventory.* National Computer Systems, Inc.

Frisch, M. B., Cornell, J., Villanueva, M., *et al* (1992) Clinical validation of the Quality of Life Inventory: a measure of life satisfaction for use in treatment planning and outcome assessment. *Psychological Assessment*, **4**, 92–101.

Gaite, L., Vázquez-Barquero, J. L., Arrizabalaga, A. A., *et al* (2000) Quality of life in schizophrenia: development, reliability and internal consistency of the Lancashire Quality of Life Profile – European Version. *British Journal of Psychiatry*, **177**, suppl. 39, 49–54.

Gaite, L., Vázquez-Barquero, J. L., Borra, C., *et al* (2002) Quality of Life in patients with schizophrenia in five European countries: the EPSILON Study. *Acta Psychiatrica Scandinavica*, **105**, 283–292.

Goldberg, D. (1979) *Manual of the General Health Questionnaire.* NFER Publishing.

Goldstrom, I. D. & Manderscheid, R. W. (1986) The chronically mentally ill: a descriptive analysis from the Uniform Client Data Instrument. *Community Support Services Journal*, **2**, 4–9.

Grant, G. M., Salcedo, V., Hynan, L. S., *et al* (1995) Effectiveness of quality of life therapy for depression. *Psychological Reports*, **76**, 1203–1208.

Gråwe, R. W. & Løvaas, A-L. (1994) Quality of life among schizophrenic in- and out-patients. *Nordic Journal of Psychiatry*, **48**, 147–151.

Gregoire, J., de Leval, N., Mesters, P., *et al* (1994) Validation of the Quality of Life in Depression Scale in a population of adult depressive patients aged 60 and above. *Quality of Life Research*, **3**, 13–19.

Hamilton, M. (1960). A rating scale for depression. *Journal of Neurology, Neurosurgery and Psychiatry*, **23**, 56–62.

Hansson, L., Svensson, B. & Björkman, T. (1998) Quality of life of the mentally ill. Reliability of the Swedish version of the Lancashire Quality of Life Profile. *European Psychiatry*, **13**, 231–234.

Hansson, L., Middelboe, T., Merinder, L., *et al* (1999) Predictors of subjective quality of life in schizophrenic patients living in the community. A Nordic multicentre study. *International Journal of Social Psychiatry*, **45**, 247–258.

Heinrichs, D. W., Hanlon, T. E. & Carpenter, W. T. (1984) The Quality of Life Scale: an instrument for rating the schizophrenic deficit syndrome. *Schizophrenia Bulletin*, **10**, 388–398.

Holcomb, W. R., Morgan, P., Adams, N. A., *et al* (1993) Development of a structured interview scale for measuring quality of life of the severely mentally ill. *Journal of Clinical Psychology*, **49**, 830–840.

Horiuchi, K., Nisihio, M., Oshima, I., *et al* (2006) The quality of life among persons with severe mental illness enrolled in an assertive community treatment program in Japan: 1-year follow-up and analyses. *Clinical Practice and Epidemiology in Mental Health*, **2**, 18.

Hoult, J. & Reynolds, J. (1984) Schizophrenia: a comparative trial of community oriented and hospital oriented psychiatric care. *Acta Psychiatrica Scandinavica*, **69**, 359–372.

Hunt, S. M. & McKenna, S. P. (1992*a*) A new measure of quality of life in depression: testing the reliability and construct validity of the QLDS. *Health Policy*, **22**, 321–330.

Hunt, S. M. & McKenna, S. P. (1992*b*) The QLDS: a scale for measurement of quality of life in depression. *Health Policy*, **22**, 307–319.

Johnson, P. J. (1991) Emphasis on quality of life of people with severe mental illness in community-based care in Sweden. *Psychosocial Rehabilitation Journal*, **14**, 23–37.

Kaiser, W., Priebe, S., Hoffmann, K., *et al* (1996) Subiektiv Lebensqualität bei Patienten mit chronischer Schizophrenie [Subjective quality of life of patients with chronic schizophrenia.] *Nervenarzt*, **67**, 572–582.

Kaiser, W., Isermann, M., Hoffmann, K., *et al* (1999) Zur Kurzerfassung subjektiver Lebensqualität. Ergebnisse der Erprobung einer Kurzform des Berliner

Lebensqualitätsprofils (BELP-KF). [Short assessment of subjective quality of life. Application and results of a short form of the Berliner Lebensqualitätprofil (BELP-KF).] *Fortschritte der Neurologie und Psychiatrie*, **67**, 413–425.

Kaneda, Y., Imakura, A., Fujii, A., *et al* (2002) Schizophrenia Quality of Life Scale: validation of the Japanese version. *Psychiatry Research*, **113**, 107–113.

Karow, A., Czekalla, J., Dittmann, R. W., *et al* (2007) Association of subjective well-being, symptoms, and side effects with compliance after 12 months of treatment in schizophrenia. *Journal of Clinical Psychiatry*, **68**, 75–80.

Katschnig, H. (2000) Schizophrenia and quality of life. *Acta Psychiatrica Scandinavica*, **102** (suppl. 407), 33–37.

Kind, P. (1996) The EuroQoL instrument: an index of HRQOL. In *Quality of Life and Pharmacoeconomics in Clinical Trials* (2nd edition) (ed. B. Spilker), pp. 191–201. Lippincott-Raven.

Kovess-Masféty, V., Xavier, M., Moreno Kustner, B., *et al* (2006) Schizophrenia and quality of life: a one-year follow-up in four EU countries. *BMC Psychiatry*, **6**, 39.

Lancon, C., Auquier, P., Launois, R., *et al* (2000) Evaluation de la qualité de vie des patients schizophrènes: validation de la version courte de la QOLI. [Evaluation of the quality of life of schizophrenic patients: validation of the brief version of the Quality of Life Interview.] *Encephale*, **26**, 11–16.

Lasalvia, A. & Ruggeri, M. (2007) Assessing the outcome of community-based psychiatric care: building a feed-back loop from 'real world' services research into clinical practice. *Acta Psychiatrica Scandinavica*, **116** (suppl. 437), 6–15.

Lasalvia, A., Ruggeri, M. & Santolini, N. (2002) Subjective quality of life: its relationship with clinician-rated and patient-rated psychopathology. The South-Verona Outcome Project 6. *Psychotherapy and Psychosomatics*, **71**, 275–284.

Lasalvia, A., Bonetto, C., Malchiodi, F., *et al* (2005) Listening to patients' needs to improve their subjective quality of life. *Psychological Medicine*, **35**, 1655–1665.

Lehman, A. F. (1983*a*) The effects of psychiatric symptoms on quality of life assessments among the chronic mentally ill. *Evaluation and Program Planning*, **6**, 143–151.

Lehman, A. F. (1983*b*) The well-being of chronic mental patients: assessing their quality of life. *Archives of General Psychiatry*, **40**, 369–373.

Lehman, A. F. (1988) A quality of life interview for the chronically mentally ill. *Evaluation and Program Planning*, **11**, 51–62.

Lehman, A. F. (1995) *Quality of Life Toolkit*. Health Services Research Institute.

Lehman. A.F. (1996) Measures of quality of life among persons with severe and persistent mental disorders. *Social Psychiatry and Psychiatric Epidemiology*, **31**, 78–88.

Lehman, A. F., Ward, N. & Linn, L. (1982) Chronic mental patients: the quality of life issue. *American Journal of Psychiatry*, **10**, 1271–1276.

Lehman, A. F., Possidente, S. & Hawker, F. (1986) The quality of life of chronic mental patients in a state hospital and community residences. *Hospital and Community Psychiatry*, **37**, 901–907.

Lehman, A. F., Slaughter, J. C. & Myers, C. P. (1991) The quality of life of chronically mentally ill persons in alternative residential settings. *Psychiatric Quarterly*, **62**, 35–49.

Lehman, A. F., Slaughter, J. C. & Myers, C. P. (1992) Quality of life of the chronically mentally ill: gender and decade of life effects. *Evaluation and Program Planning*, **15**, 7–12.

Lehman, A. F., Rachuba, L. T. & Postrado, L. T. (1995) Demographic influences on quality of life among persons with chronic mental illnesses. *Evaluation and Program Planning*, **18**, 155–164.

Levitt, A. J., Hogan, T. P. & Bucosky, C. M. (1990) Quality of life in chronically mentally ill patients in day treatment. *Psychological Medicine*, **20**, 703–710.

Lobana, A., Mattoo Surendra, K., Basu, D., *et al* (2001) Quality of life in schizophrenia in India: comparison of three approaches. *Acta Psychiatrica Scandinavica*, **104**, 51–55.

Luo, N., Seng, B. K., Xie, F., *et al* (2008) Psychometric evaluation of the Schizophrenia Quality of Life Scale (SQLS) in English- and Chinese-speaking Asians in Singapore. *Quality of Life Research*, **17**, 115–122.

Lykken, D. & Tellegen, A. (1996) Happiness is a stochastic phenomenon. *Psychological Science*, **7**, 186–189.

Malla, A. & Payne, J. (2005) First-episode psychosis: psychopathology, quality of life, and functional outcome. *Schizophrenia Bulletin*, **31**, 650–671.

Malla, A. K., Norman, R. M., McLean, T. S., *et al* (2001) Impact of phase-specific treatment of first episode of psychosis on Wisconsin Quality of Life Index (client version). *Acta Psychiatrica Scandinavica*, **103**, 355–361.

Malla, A. K., Norman, R. M., McLean, T. S., *et al* (2004) Determinants of quality of life in first-episode psychosis. *Acta Psychiatrica Scandinavica*, **109**, 46–54.

Malm, U., May, P. R. A. & Dencker, S. J. (1981) Evaluation of the quality of life of the schizophrenic outpatient: a checklist. *Schizophrenia Bulletin*, **7**, 477–487.

Martin, C. R. & Allan, R. (2007) Factor structure of the Schizophrenia Quality of Life Scale Revision 4 (SQLS–R4). *Psychology, Health and Medicine*, **12**, 126–134.

McAlinden, N. M. & Oei, T. P. (2006) Validation of the Quality of Life Inventory for patients with anxiety and depression. *Comprehensive Psychiatry*, **47**, 307–314.

McKenna, S. P., Doward, L. C., Kohlmann, T., *et al* (2001) International development of the Quality of Life in Depression Scale (QLDS). *Journal of Affective Disorders*, **63**, 189–199.

Melle, I., Friis, S., Haahr, U., *et al* (2005) Measuring quality of life in first-episode psychosis. *European Psychiatry*, **20**, 474–483.

Millon, T. (1983) *Millon Multiaxial Inventory Manual* (3rd edition). National Computer System.

Mulkern, V., Agosta, J. M., Ashbaugh, J. W., *et al* (1986) *Community Support Program Client Follow-Up Study*. National Institute of Mental Health.

Naber, D. (1995) A self-rating to measure subjective effects of neuroleptic drugs, relationships to objective psychopathology, quality of life, compliance and other clinical variables. *International Clinical Psychopharmacology*, **10**, 133–138.

Naber, D. (1998) Subjective experiences of schizophrenic patients treated with antipsychotic medication. *International Clinical Psychopharmacology*, **13** (suppl. 1), 41–45.

Naber, D., Moritz, S., Lambert, M., *et al* (2001) Improvement of schizophrenic patients' subjective well-being under atypical antipsychotic drugs. *Schizophrenia Research*, **50**, 79–88.

Nadalet, L., Kohl, F. S., Pringuey, D., *et al* (2005) Validation of a subjective quality of life questionnaire (S.QUA.LA) in schizophrenia. *Schizophrenia Research*, **76**, 73–81.

National Institute of Mental Health (1985) Special feature: rating scales and assessment instruments for use in pediatric psychopharmacology research. *Psychopharmacology Bulletin*, **21**, 839–843.

Nørholm, V. & Bech, P. (2007) Quality of life assessment in schizophrenia: applicability of the Lehman Quality of Life Questionnaire (TL–30). *Nordic Journal of Psychiatry*, **61**, 438–442.

Oliver, J. P. J. (1991) The social care directive: development of a quality of life profile for use in community services for the mentally ill. *Social Work and Social Sciences Review*, **3**, 5–45.

Oliver, J. P. J. & Mohamad, H. (1992) The quality of life of the chronically mentally ill: a comparison of public, private, and voluntary residential provisions. *British Journal of Social Work*, **22**, 391–404.

Oliver J. P. J., Huxley, P. J., Priebe, S., *et al* (1997) Measuring the quality of life of severely mentally ill people using the Lancashire Quality of Life Profile. *Social Psychiatry and Psychiatric Epidemiology*, **32**, 76–83.

Overall, J. E. & Gorham, D. R. (1962) The Brief Psychiatric Rating Scale. *Psychological Reports*, **10**, 799–812.

Oxford Outcomes (2004) *The Revised Schizophrenia Quality of Life Questionnaire (SQLS–R4): User Manual for the SQLS–R4*. Oxford Outcomes Ltd.

Ozer, S., Ulusahin, A., Batur, S., *et al* (2002) Outcome measures of interepisode bipolar patients in a Turkish sample. *Social Psychiatry and Psychiatric Epidemiology*, **37**, 31–37.

Pearlstein, T. B., Halbreich, U., Batzar, E. D., *et al* (2000) Psychosocial functioning in women with premenstrual dysphoric disorder before and after treatment with sertraline or placebo. *Journal of Clinical Psychiatry*, **61**, 101–109.

Postrado, L. T. & Lehman, A. F. (1995) Quality of life and clinical predictors of rehospital-ization of persons with severe mental illness. *Psychiatric Services*, **46**, 1161–1165.

Priebe, S., Huxley, P., Knight, S., *et al* (1999) Application and results of the Manchester Short Assessment of Quality of Life (MANSA). *International Journal of Social Psychiatry*, **45**, 7–12.

Priebe, S., Roder-Wanner, U. U., Kaiser, W., *et al* (2000) Quality of life in first admitted schizophrenia patients: follow-up study. *Psychological Medicine*, **30**, 225–230.

Prince, P. N. & Prince, C. R. (2001) Subjective quality of life in the evaluation of programs for people with serious and persistent mental illness. *Clinical Psychology Review*, **21**, 1005–1036.

Rapaport, M. H., Endicott, J. & Clary, C. M. (2002) Posttraumatic stress disorder and quality of life: results across 64 weeks of sertraline treatment. *Journal of Clinical Psychiatry*, **63**, 59–65.

Revicki, D. A., Paramore, L. C., Sommerville, K. W., *et al* (2003) Divalproex sodium versus olanzapine in the treatment of acute mania in bipolar disorder: health-related quality of life and medical cost outcomes. *Journal of Clinical Psychiatry*, **64**, 288–294.

Ritsner, M., Kurs, R., Gibel, A., *et al* (2005a) Validity of an abbreviated quality of life enjoyment and satisfaction questionnaire (Q–LES–Q–18) for schizophrenia, schizoaffective, and mood disorder patients. *Quality of Life Research*, **14**, 1693–1703.

Ritsner, M., Kurs, R., Ratner, Y., *et al* (2005b) Condensed version of the Quality of Life Scale for schizophrenia for use in outcome studies. *Psychiatry Research*, **135**, 65–75.

Rosen, A., Hadzi-Pavlovic, D. & Parker, G. (1989) The Life Skills Profile: a measure assessing function and disability in schizophrenia. *Schizophrenia Bulletin*, **15**, 325–337.

Rosenfield, S. & Neese-Todd, S. (1993) Elements of a psychosocial clubhouse program associated with a satisfying quality of life. *Hospital and Community Psychiatry*, **44**, 76–78.

Ruggeri, M. & Tansella, M. (1995) Evaluating outcome in mental health care. *Current Opinion in Psychiatry*, **8**, 116–121.

Ruggeri, M., Warner, R., Bisoffi, G., *et al* (2001) Subjective and objective dimensions of quality of life in psychiatric patients: a factor-analytic approach. *British Journal of Psychiatry*, **178**, 268–275.

Ruggeri, M., Pacati, P. & Goldberg, D. (2003) Neurotics are dissatisfied with life, but not with services. The South Verona Outcome Project 7. *General Hospital Psychiatry*, **25**, 338–344

Ruggeri, M., Nosè, M., Bonetto, C., *et al* (2005) Changes and predictors of change in objective and subjective quality of life. A multiwave follow-up study in community psychiatric patients. *British Journal of Psychiatry*, **187**, 121–130.

Russell, J. M., Koran, L. M., Rush, J., *et al* (2001) Effect of concurrent anxiety on response to sertraline and imipramine in patients with chronic depression. *Depression and Anxiety*, **13**, 18–27.

Russo, J., Roy-Byrne, P., Reeder, D., *et al* (1997) Longitudinal assessment of quality of life in acute psychiatric inpatients: reliability and validity. *Journal of Nervous and Mental Disease*, **185**, 166–175.

Safren, S. A., Heimberg, R. G., Brown, E. J., *et al* (1997) Quality of life in social phobia. *Depression and Anxiety*, **4**, 126–133,

Salomé, F., Petitjean, F., Germain, C., *et al* (2000) Validation of the French version of the Lancashire Quality of Life Profile (LQOLP), a scale evaluating the quality of life in schizophrenic patients. *Annales Médico-Psychologiques*, **158**, 329–334 [in French].

Seidman, S. N. & Rabkin, J. G. (1998) Testosterone replacement therapy for hypogonadal men with SSRI-refractory depression. *Journal of Affective Disorders*, **48**, 157–161.

Simpson, C. J., Hyde, C. E. & Faragher, E. B. (1989) The chronically mentally ill in community facilities: a study of quality of life. *British Journal of Psychiatry*, **154**, 77–82.

Skantze, K. (1998) Subjective quality of life and standard of living: a 10-year follow-up of out-patients with schizophrenia. *Acta Psychiatrica Scandinavica*, **98**, 390–399.

Skantze, K. & Malm, U. (1994) A new approach to facilitation of working alliances based on patients' quality-of-life goals. *Nordic Journal of Psychiatry*, **1**, 37–55.

Skantze, K., Malm, U., Dencker, S. J., *et al* (1990) Quality of life in schizophrenia. *Nordic Journal of Psychiatry*, **44**, 71–75.

Skantze, K., Malm, U., Dencker, S. J., *et al* (1992) Comparison of quality of life with standard of living in schizophrenic out-patients. *British Journal of Psychiatry*, **161**, 797–801.

Slaughter, J. C. & Lehman, A. F. (1991) Quality of life of severely mentally ill adults in residential care facilities. *Adult Residential Care Journal*, **5**, 97–111.

Spitzer, W. O., Dobson, A., Hall, J., *et al* (1981) Measuring the quality of life in cancer patients: a concise Q/L index for use by physicians. *Journal of Chronic Disorders*, **34**, 585–597.

Stanley, M. A., Beck, J. G., Novy, D. M., *et al* (2003) Cognitive–behavioral treatment of late-life generalized anxiety disorder. *Journal of Consulting and Clinical Psychology*, **71**, 309–319.

Stein, L. I. & Test, M. A. (1980) Alternative to mental hospital treatment: I. Conceptual model, treatment program and clinical evaluation. *Archives of General Psychiatry*, **37**, 392–397.

Stoker, M. J., Dunbar, G. C. & Beaumont, G. (1992) The SmithKline Beecham 'quality of life' scale: a validation and reliability study in patients with affective disorder. *Quality of Life Research*, **1**, 385–395.

Strauss, J. S. & Carpenter, W. T. (1974) The prediction of outcome in schizophrenia: II. Relationships between predictor and outcome variables: a report from the WHO International Pilot Study of Schizophrenia. *Archives of General Psychiatry*, **31**, 37–42.

Ware, J. E. & Sherbourne, C. D. (1992) The MOS 36-Item Short-Form Health Survey (SF–36): I. Conceptual framework and item selection. *Medical Care*, **30**, 473–483.

WHOQOL Group (1998a) The World Health Organization Quality of Life Assessment (WHOQOL): development and general psychometric properties. *Social Science and Medicine*, **46**, 1569–1585.

WHOQOL Group (1998b) Development of the World Health Organization WHOQOL–BREF Quality of Life Assessment. *Psychological Medicine*, **28**, 551–558.

Wilkinson, G., Hesdon, B., Wild, D., *et al* (2000) Self-report quality of life measure for people with schizophrenia: the SQLS. *British Journal of Psychiatry*, **177**, 42–46.

Zigmond, A. S. & Snaith, R. P. (1983) The Hospital Anxiety and Depression Scale. *Acta Psychiatrica Scandinavica*, **67**, 361–370.

CHAPTER 9

Measuring social disabilities in mental health and employment outcomes

Durk Wiersma and Thomas Becker

Mental disorders, particularly schizophrenia and the major affective disorders, are in general strongly associated with social dysfunction. For a long time social dysfunction was considered an epiphenomenon of the disease process. Diagnostic criteria of mental disorders were and still are often derived from the domains of work and social relationships. There are, though, at least two related reasons why social functioning deserves a closer look:

1   There is an increasing trend to treat patients in the community instead of in hospital: this emphasis on community care requires careful evaluation with respect to its consequences. To what extent is survival in the community possible and what is the quality of life like there? Are community programmes better than hospital treatment, and for whom? Therefore, an emphasis on social dysfunction is justified in evaluating the outcome, costs and benefits of community care.

2   There is growing evidence that the time course of symptoms and social dysfunction may vary relatively independently. The social disablement of a patient may be characterised much more by social disabilities than by persistent psychiatric symptoms; the former may call for types of (non-clinical) care that are not readily available. For example, psychosocial rehabilitation focuses on those cognitive and social abilities of the patient which are crucial for a more or less independent life. Therefore, separate measurement is justified for the sake of the right choice of treatment.

Classification of social dysfunction

The standard diagnostic systems, primarily the ICD of the World Health Organization and the DSM of the American Psychiatric Association, offer no adequate solution to the problem of the classification and assessment of the social dysfunction that results from mental disorder. We have to look for other classification systems, such as the *International Classification of*

Functioning, Disability and Health (World Health Organization, 2001), known as ICF, the overall aim of which is to provide a unified and standard language and framework for the description of health and health-related states.

The ICF is the successor of the *International Classification of Impairments, Disabilities and Handicaps* (ICIDH) of the World Health Organization (1980), which offered a conceptual model to study the long-term consequences of disease or disorder in terms of impairments, functional disabilities and social handicaps, and the effectiveness of healthcare in handling these kinds of problem. The ICIDH model was rather simple and linear, in that it assumed that 'I' (impairment, defined as any loss or abnormality of psychological, physiological or anatomical structure or function; exteriorisation) may cause 'D' (disability, defined as any restriction or lack of ability to perform an activity in the manner or in the range considered normal for a human being; objectification), which in their turn may give rise to 'H' (handicap, defined as disadvantages experienced by the individual as a result of the impairments and/or disabilities, and also reflecting the interaction with the social environment that limits or prevents the fulfilment of social roles; socialisation); sometimes 'I' may directly cause 'H' without the intermediate steps of 'D', for example in the case of social stigma.

Although the ICIDH has, to a certain extent, been recognised as a valuable tool for assessment and research, it has already been criticised in relation to the many problems with the distinctions between the concepts: there is a lack of internal coherence within the framework with respect to how concepts are defined and used, and how categories are drawn up; and there is also much overlap between classifications. This applies even more to its application to mental health and complex mental disorders, for instance with respect to role disability and handicap. The ICF represents a move away from 'a consequence of disease' classification, and is more a 'components of health' classification, which takes a neutral stand with regard to aetiology and risk factors.

The ICF encompasses all aspects of human health and some health-relevant components of well-being and describes them in terms of health-related domains; its application is universal and not restricted to people with disabilities. The ICF organises information in two parts: part 1 deals with functioning and disability, and part 2 deals with contextual factors. Each part has two components: functioning and disability comprise two components or classifications of (a) body functions and structure, and (b) activities and participation; while contextual factors have (a) environmental factors and (b) personal factors.

The components of part 1, functioning and disability, can be used to indicate problems (e.g. impairments, activity limitation, restricted participation), summarised under the umbrella term 'disability', or to indicate non-problematic aspects of health, summarised under the umbrella term 'functioning'. A person's functioning and disability are conceived as dynamic interactions between health conditions (diseases, disorders, traumatic injuries) and contextual factors. The basis of the environmental factors component is the construct facilitating or hindering impact or features of the physical, social and attitudinal world. This chapter focuses on the component of activity and participation, which has nine domains covering the full range of life areas: learning and applying knowledge, general tasks and demands, communication, mobility, self-care, domestic life, interpersonal interactions and relationships, and finally, community, social and civic life.

All these domains can be qualified by describing performance (what does the individual do?) and capacity (what can the individual do?). Activity is the execution of a task or action by an individual who may experience a limitation or difficulty in relation to it. Participation is involvement in a life situation in which an individual may experience restrictions or problems. Limitations or restrictions are assessed against a generally accepted population standard; that is, an individual's capacity and performance are compared with those of an individual without a similar health condition. The limitation or restriction records the discordance between observed and expected performance.

The expected performance is the population norm, which represents the experience of people without the specific health condition. It is difficult to distinguish between 'activities' and 'participation' on the basis of the domains in the activities and participation component; similarly, differentiating between 'individual' and 'societal' perspectives on the basis of the domains has not been possible, given international variation and professional or theoretical frameworks. The ICF provides a list that can be used to differentiate between activities and participation in their own operational way. As a classification, the ICF does not model the 'process' of functioning and disability, but describes it by providing the means to map the different constructs and domains, or building blocks for those who wish to create models and study different aspects of this process.

Fig. 9.1 may be helpful in suggesting that an individual's functioning in a specific domain can be conceived as an interaction or complex relationship between the health condition and contextual factors, environmental factors – such as family support, individual or societal attitudes, and services (of all kinds) – and personal factors – such as gender, race, age and lifestyle (not classified further in the ICF).

The ICF is based on an integration of the medical and the social model of disability and uses a 'bio-psychosocial' approach. The medical model views disability as a problem of the individual directly caused by the disease, which requires medical care and individual treatment by a professional, while the social model sees disability mainly as a socially created problem and as a matter of integration into society.

Thus, the ICF attempts to achieve a synthesis in order to provide a coherent view of different perspectives of health from a biological, individual and societal perspective. Its use could lie in health and disability reporting based on surveys conducted at national and international level (e.g. the

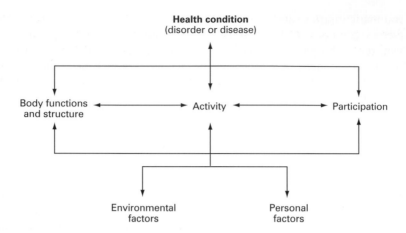

Fig 9.1 Interactions between the components of the *International Classification of Functioning, Disability and Health* (ICF).

World Health Survey, which measured the health status of the general population in 71 countries; www.who.int/healthinfo/surveys), in clinical and epidemiological use (in clinical settings for the assessment of functional status, for goal setting and treatment planning and monitoring, as well as for outcome measurement), in social policy (e.g. antidiscrimination law) and in intervention and implementation research.

In conclusion, the ICF, compared with the ICIDH, is a major improvement in terms of conceptual clarity, structure and meaning (e.g. distinction between structure and function, avoiding overlap, considering environmental factors). However, further detailed discussion of the ICF concept is beyond the scope of this chapter.

Social role theory

The categories of social disability and social role are of the utmost importance for psychiatry and mental healthcare. Functioning in social roles signifies the person's integration into the community. Sociologists, psychologists and anthropologists have used the concept of role to study both the individual and the social group within a single conceptual framework. Anthropologists such as Ralph Linton (1936) have traditionally treated role as a culturally derived blueprint for behaviour. In this sense it is an external constraint upon an individual and is a normative rather than a behavioural concept. Roles are always linked to a status or a position in a particular pattern or social structure, which consists of a network of social relations and communications. A role represents the dynamic aspect of a status. Linton and other anthropologists have made no distinction, however, between behavioural and normative aspects of role. Actual and ideal behaviours are used to describe the people studied. The assumption is that there exists a uniform mode of behaviour with regard to status. Empirical research has shown that these assumptions are not valid and that consensus concerning status and role behaviour is lacking.

Psychologists such as Newcombe (see Gordon, 1966) leaned heavily on interactional theory, and focused on the relationship of roles to the self and personality. They treated role and status as given and not as variables. Role is defined as the subjective perception of the direct interaction. This comes close to the symbolic interactionism which regards self-consciousness and the continuous interpretations of the actions of others as the motive for human action. The focus is on the individual response, based on the meaning attached to certain actions of other people. This interactionistic role concept, however, may not take properly into account the pathological changes in experiences and behaviour due to mental disorders.

In contrast, sociologists such as Parsons (1958), and many others known as structural functionalists, considered the reciprocal relationship or the socially preconditioned interaction of two or more persons as the core of the analysis. Parsons considered a role as the organised system of participation of an individual in a social system and defined it in terms of reciprocal orientations. Status and role are the building blocks or the means by which individuals are able to engage in a reciprocal relationship. One essential part of such a relationship is constituted by expectations, which, according to Dahrendorf (1965), could have the character of 'can', 'should' or 'must', implying the application of positive or negative sanctions in order to promote conformity with the prevailing norms and values. Other people are important here to define whether an individual is behaving 'normally' or 'deviantly' or is 'maladjusted'.

But there is, unfortunately, no consensus on how a social role is defined (see also Biddle, 1979). The following description, composed of common elements found in most of the definitions, may be sufficient:

A social role is a complex of expectations which people have as to the behaviour of a person who occupies a certain position in society.

A position is a location in a social structure which is associated with a set of social norms or expectations held in common by members of a social group. The group consists primarily of people with whom the individual frequently interacts, such as family members, friends, colleagues and so on. There are many positions in the social structure of a group, an association, a profession, a community or society as a whole, with a corresponding number of social roles. Role performance refers to the actual behaviour of the individual in the context of a particular role.

Therefore, a social disability or a role disability is a deficiency that leads to an inability to perform particular activities or to manifest particular behaviours, as these are expected in the context of a well defined social role.

173

It is important to understand that someone's behaviour should always be assessed against the background of how other people expect the individual to behave. This implies that such an assessment, above all, pertains to the individual's capacity for interpersonal functioning.

Social role theory does not produce a standard classification of roles that should be taken into account in order to give an adequate description of the individual's overall functioning or integration in the community. We therefore rely on what researchers put in their schedules.

Schedules assessing social functioning or social role performance

The numbers and contents of roles in existing schedules vary. There is an overwhelming number of schedules and instruments; many have been reviewed by Weissman (1975), Weissman *et al* (1981), Katschnig (1983) and Wing (1989), and more specifically by Hall (1980) with respect to ward behaviour, by Tyrer (1990) with respect to personality disorders, and by Wallace (1984) and Rosen *et al* (1989) with respect to schizophrenia.

There is substantial agreement on the adequacy of various instruments in assessing a number of roles. Several instruments are relevant in this respect (Hurry & Sturt, 1981):

- Groningen Social Disabilities Schedule (GSDS; Wiersma *et al*, 1988, 1990)
- Psychiatric Disability Assessment Schedule (DAS; World Health Organization, 1988, related to the ICIDH; and DAS–II, World Health Organization, 2001, related to the ICF)
- Role Activity Performance Scale (RAPS; Good-Ellis *et al*, 1987)
- Social Adjustment Scale (SAS; Weissman, 1975; Schooler *et al*, 1979)
- Social Behaviour Assessment Schedule (SBAS; Platt *et al*, 1980)
- Social Functioning Scale (SFS; Birchwood *et al*, 1990)
- Social Role Adjustment Instrument (SRAI; Cohler *et al*, 1968)
- Standardized Interview to Assess Social Maladjustment (Clare & Cairns, 1978)
- Structured and Scaled Interview to Assess Maladjustment (SSIAM; Gurland *et al*, 1972).

These are all well-known instruments, described in the literature, and data on reliability and validity are available.

It is striking that the instruments use different terms to describe role behaviours, half of them using terms with a negative connotation (maladjustment, disability) and half neutral terms (adjustment, performance). Nevertheless, their contents look much more the same, although there are large differences as to the precise wording, the description, the assessment, the anchor points and the scaling. Most also measure other concepts, such as social support, psychiatric symptoms, the burden of the illness on the family and satisfaction. There seems to be a consensus on the following areas of role behaviour:

- occupational role (work, education, household, regular activities)
- household role (participating and contributing to the household and its economic independence)
- marital role (emotional, sexual relationship with partner/spouse)
- parental role (relationship with children, caring)
- family or kinship role (relationship with parents and siblings, extended family)
- social role (relationship in the community – friends, acquaintances, neighbours)
- leisure activities and/or general interests
- self-care (personal grooming and appearance).

Each of these roles delineates an area of expected behaviour and, in their entirety, these role behaviours largely determine the level and quality or adequacy of an individual's functioning in the community. They describe general domains of roles and status which apply to everybody. Each area could be subdivided into smaller behavioural domains, such as instrumental tasks and affective or attitudinal aspects.

The description of expected behaviours could, of course, be different in various communities or cultures; for example, doing nothing is highly undesirable in Western countries but may be less so in Eastern countries. Taking part in the household (e.g. doing some cooking or household chores) may be quite different among men in various European countries. The applicability of the role concept is in principle not limited to time or place. It is very important to notice that the norms and values of the local community or of those with whom the person is interacting are decisive in the assessment. We should not assume general norms and values which apply to everybody. There is no general or objective standard of behaviour. Norms and values vary from community to community and the acceptability of particular behaviours will sometimes be the result of negotiations between those involved.

Thus, *ideal norms* with respect to what should be done are not relevant here. Empirical research has shown that they hardly apply in practice. Neither are *statistical norms* sufficient, because they do not do justice to the differences between social environments. We prefer the norms of the 'reference group', which comprises people who in social or other respects are of great importance to the individual (in this context, the concept of reference group is not used in the sociological sense that a person wants to be a member of a group he or she does not belong to). This pertains to people in the close environment, such as the partner and other members of the family and to all those with whom the individual comes into direct contact in performing his or her different roles: colleagues at work, friends and neighbours. The composition of the reference group will depend partly upon the role to be assessed.

Assessment and measurement of social or role disability

The following issues are crucial in the assessment of social or role disability and are based on the critical comments of several authors on existing schedules (see Platt, 1981; Katschnig, 1983; Link *et al*, 1990; Mueser & Tarrier, 1998) and on our own work (Wiersma, 1986; de Jong *et al*, 1994).

Independence of psychopathology

Considering the conceptual models of disability presented within the ICIDH, the ICF or others (e.g. Nagi, 1969, 1991) there should be a clear distinction between the signs and symptoms of psychopathology or psychological functioning, on the one hand, and social functioning, on the other; also, the concepts of impairment, functional limitation, disability and handicap should be considered conceptually distinct. Thus, hearing voices or feeling depressed does not automatically imply the presence of disability. Measurement of 'symptoms' and 'disability' should be kept distinct and should not be mixed, as is the case in the Global Assessment of Functioning (GAF) scale in DSM–III–R (American Psychiatric Association, 1987), which, however, can be split into a symptom assessment (GAF-s) and a disability assessment (GAF-d) to track rehabilitation progress independent of the severity of psychological symptoms. Moreover, proposals are made for separate axes for relational functioning (GARF) and occupational functioning (SOFAS) in DSM–IV (American Psychiatric Association, 1994: pp. 758–761). It ought also, however, to be kept well in mind that social or role disability should demonstrably or plausibly be caused by physical, psychological and/or psychopathological impairments or functional limitations. The assessment has to take place in the context of health experience or a health problem: if there is no health problem, there is no disability. That is, a person may not be working, not be married, have bad a relationship with their family or have financial problems for reasons other than a mental or personality disorder. The existence of such a difficulty does not in itself presuppose a mental health problem.

Actual role performance

The assessment of social or role disability should be based on the actual performance of activities, the actual manifestation of behaviours or the actual execution of tasks over a certain period (e.g. the last month). The focus is on observable phenomena and not on inferences from abstract concepts such as competence or abilities which are assumed to be present.

Criteria of assessment

Each community or society has more or less defined criteria of eligibility for sickness benefits, disability pensions, sheltered work or living and social assistance for entering or exiting social roles, such as the marital role, the work role (disability pension) or the parental role. These norms and regulations to a certain extent define the level and quality of functioning and are the first guideline for assessment. Further variables to be examined include the frequency of contacts, the number of tasks completed and the degree of conflict or depth of involvement or strength of motivation. Criteria of frequency and duration of deviation are important in assessing role disability, and so is the damage inflicted on the person him- or herself or on others, and the urge for help. This can mean that not fulfilling/occupying a social role implies a (severe or maximum) disability in role functioning, for example not having a job due to mental disorder and therefore being exempt from the obligation to look for work, or not fulfilling the parental role because of divesting of parental authority.

Restricted opportunities

The reduction in or the lack of performance should not result from personal or social circumstances that are beyond the control of the individual. An example is the hospitalised patient who cannot demonstrate certain behaviours because of the rules prevailing on the ward (e.g. visiting friends or family). Other examples of limited opportunities result from the inaccessibility of the labour market, the stigma attached to mental illness, and formal or informal rules precluding an (ex-)patient from normal role fulfilment (civil rights, driving licence). It is evident that these factors should not lead to a disability *per se*. The assessment of role performance has to take into account the influence of such circumstances.

Sources of information

There are three main sources on which the assessment can be based: the patient him- or herself; an informant (the partner or a parent or other family member, or even a friend); and an expert or mental health professional. Each source has its advantages and disadvantages, which influence the validity and reliability of the assessment. In role assessment there is consensus that several sources should be used rather than a single source. The patient should always be asked, although the severity of symptoms may negatively influence the report on his/her behaviour. Asking the patient is important in order to obtain information on his/

her perceptions, feelings and satisfaction with social situations and the performed activities.

The informant is of course also influenced to a certain extent by the patient's symptoms. But factual information on the patient's behaviour is of great value in order to see the agreement on the report of the same behaviours or other behaviours not reported by the patient, and the evaluation or judgement of the behaviours. It must be noted that an informant, as a rule, is familiar with behaviours concerning some specific roles only. It makes quite a difference whether the informant is the mother or a friend. It is important to find out the normative standards of the people with whom the patient interacts, although that may be difficult for certain groups, such as those who live alone.

The choice of an expert (a mental health professional, nurse or psychiatrist) may be obvious in case of the evaluation of a (hospital) treatment or of a long stay in hospital. In the latter case, staff are the persons who are most closely in touch with the patient. However, it should be noted that there are also disadvantages in using mental health staff as informants: differences in education, a lack of opportunities to observe the patient outside the treatment setting, and divergent expectations concerning normal and abnormal social behaviour.

Research on the GSDS showed that the influence of the informant on ratings is substantial: there is a 8–29% change in the ratings from ratings based on the patient's report only. It appeared that in most cases greater disability was rated as a result.

Method of measurement

There are various ways of measuring disabilities, each with specific advantages and disadvantages:

- *Self-report (paper-and-pencil test)*. This format is easy to administer, no training is required, there is no interview bias and the costs are low. However, it may be difficult for people who have problems with reading or who have a visual handicap. Problems may be underreported as a result of symptomatology; in the case of serious mental disorder there is often no completion or proper understanding of the questions. There is no allowance for the personal or social context, and by definition there is a lack of the opinion of others.
- *Personal interview*. This can be either a standardised respondent-based interview schedule or a semi-structured investigator-based interview. Both rely on an interview at least with the patient; the main differentiating characteristic is that in the latter case the interviewer or the investigator determines the rating or score. These methods require training, are time consuming, can suffer from an interviewer bias and are much more costly. The advantages are the direct observation of the patient's behaviour, the possibility of getting more precise

information, and the flexibility of taking into account the personal context of the person. For the assessment of social or role disabilities the semi-structured interview is preferred, because it is the most flexible method.

Conclusion

Some consensus is reached on the definition of social or role disability as:

- a restriction of the ability to perform activities (tasks) and to manifest behaviours as expected in the context of a social role
- violations of or deviations from norms and expectations within the relevant reference group caused by physical, psychological and/or psychopathological impairments
- not resulting from personal or social circumstances beyond the control of the individual.

Our research on social role disabilities (Wiersma *et al*, 1988, 1990; Kraaijkamp, 1992; Wiersma, 2005) has shown that agreement on the assessment of social disabilities is high and that these assessments can be performed reliably (interrater and test–retest reliability). Proper assessments take the patient's socio-demographic background adequately into account, differentiate between diagnostic and patient groups, have high internal and external validity and are sensitive to change. Social role functioning deserves its own place in a classification of the consequences of disease and in outcome research. It should not be mingled with other concepts, such as social support, adverse social circumstances or quality of life.

The new classification of the ICF offers a good solution to a number of conceptual problems. Important is the recognition of environmental (risk) factors that involve social expectations and opportunities in specific sociocultural environments, such as paternalism, stigma, access to care, or women's work participation, or physical circumstances, such as the design of public places or lead paint. These risk factors are important for identifying a mechanism for action or prevention. The model does not incorporate the concept of quality of life, which generally is not precisely defined but is rather often loosely described as total well-being with reference to the World Health Organization's definition of health as a state of complete physical, mental and social well-being, and not merely the absence of disease. Using this concept does not clarify much and might give rise to new conceptual difficulties.

Thirty years ago, social adjustment was said to be an umbrella concept encompassing skills, competence, integration, impairment, disability, inadequacy and so on. This has been replaced by the concept of quality of life, which is treated as a paradigm. Nowadays the words are 'social participation' and 'social inclusion', 'social recovery' and, thus, 'performance in social roles'. Recently, there has been increasing interest in considering social

179

functioning as an outcome measure, for example in schizophrenia studies (see Burns & Patrick, 2007; Juckel & Morosini, 2008). This is a challenge, not only for mental health practice to achieve good social functioning for patients, but also for researchers to define and measure it.

References

American Psychiatric Association (1987) *Diagnostic and Statistical Manual of Mental Disorders* (3rd edition, revised) (DSM–III–R). APA.

American Psychiatric Association (1994) *Diagnostic and Statistical Manual of Mental Disorders* (4th edn) (DSM–IV). APA.

Biddle, B. (1979) *Role Theory: Expectations, Identities and Behaviors*. Academic Press.

Birchwood, M., Smith, J., Cochrane, R., *et al* (1990) The Social Functioning Scale. The development and validation of a new scale of social adjustment for use in family intervention programmes with schizophrenic patients. *British Journal of Psychiatry*, **157**, 853–859.

Burns, T. & Patrick, D. (2007) Social functioning as an outcome measure in schizophrenia studies. *Acta Psychiatrica Scandinavica*, **116**, 403–418.

Clare, A. W. & Cairns, V. E. (1978) Design, development and use of a standardised interview to assess social maladjustment and dysfunction in community studies. *Psychological Medicine*, **21**, 589–604.

Cohler, B., Woolseau S., Cairns, V. E., *et al* (1968) Child rearing attitudes among mothers volunteering and revolunteering for a psychological study. *Psychological Reports*, **23**, 603–612.

Dahrendorf, R. (1965) *Homo Sociologicus. Ein Versuch zur Geschichte, Bedeutung und Kritik der Kategorie der sozialen Rolle* [Homo sociologicus: an attempt at the history, meaning and criticism of the social role category]. Westdeutscher Verlag.

De Jong, A. & Van der Lubbe, P. M. (1994) *Handleilting van de Groningse Vragenlijst over Sociaal Gedrag.* [*Manual of the Groningen Questionnaire About Social Behaviour.*] Department of Social Psychiatry, University of Groningen.

Good-Ellis, M. A., Fine, S. B., Spencer, J. H., *et al* (1987) Developing a role activity performance scale. *American Journal of Occupational Therapy*, **41**, 232–241.

Gordon, G. (1966) *Role Theory and Illness: A Sociological Perspective*. College and University Press.

Gurland, B. J., Yorkstone, N. J., Stone A. R., *et al* (1972) The Structured and Scaled Interview to Assess Maladjustment (SSIAM): description, rationale and development. *Archives of General Psychiatry*, **27**, 259–264.

Hall, N. J. (1980) Ward rating scales for longstay patients. A review. *Psychological Medicine*, **10**, 277–288.

Hurry, J. & Sturt, E. (1981) Social performance in a population sample: relation to psychiatric symptoms. In *What Is a Case?* (eds J. K. Wing, P. Bebbington & L. N. Robins), pp. 202–213. Grant McIntyre.

Juckel, G. & Morosini, P. L. (2008) The new approach: psychosocial functioning as a necessary outcome criterion for therapeutic success in schizophrenia. *Current Opinion in Psychiatry*, **21**, 630–639.

Katschnig, H. (1983) Methods for measuring social adjustment. In *Methodology in Evaluation of Psychiatric Treatment* (ed. T. Helgason), pp. 205–218. Cambridge University Press.

Kraaijkamp, H. J. M. (1992) *Moeilijke Rollen. Psychometrisch Onderzoek naar de Betrouwbaarheid en Validitcit van de Groningse Sociale Beperkingenschaal bij Psychiatrische Patinten.* [*Difficult Roles. A Study into the Reliability and Validity of the Groningen Social Disabilities Schedule in Psychiatric Patients.*] Thesis, University of Groningen.

Link, B. G., Mesagno, F. P., Lubner, M. E., *et al* (1990) Problems in measuring role strains and social functioning in relation to psychological symptoms. *Journal of Health and Social Behaviour*, **31**, 354–369.

Linton, R. (1936) *The Study of Man*. Appleton-Century.

Mueser, K. & Tarrier, N. (1998) *The Handbook of Social Functioning in Schizophrenia*. Allyn & Bacon.

Nagi, S. Z. (1969) *Disability and Rehabilitation*. Ohio State University Press.

Nagi, S. Z. (1991) Disability concepts revisited: implications for prevention. In *Disability in America. Toward a National Agenda for Prevention* (eds A. M. Pope & A. R. Tadov), appendix A, pp. 309–327. Institute of Medicine, National Academy Press.

Parsons, T. (1958) Definitions of health and illness in the light of American values and social structure. In *Patients, Physicians, Illnesses* (ed. E. G. Jaco), pp. 165–187. Free Press.

Platt, S. (1981) Social adjustment as a criterion of treatment success: just what are we measuring? *Psychiatry*, **44**, 95–112.

Platt, S., Weyman, A., Hirsch, S. R., *et al* (1980) The Social Behaviour Assessment Schedule (SBAS): rationale, contents, scoring and reliability of a new interview schedule. *Social Psychiatry and Psychiatric Epidemiology*, **15**, 43–55.

Rosen, A., Hadzi-Pavlovic, D. & Parker, G. (1989) The Life-Skills Profile: a measure assessing function and disability in schizophrenia. *Schizophrenia Bulletin*, **15**, 325–337.

Schooler, N., Hogerty, G. & Weissman, M. (1979) Social Adjustment Scale II. In *Resource Materials for Community Mental Health Program Evaluators* (eds W. A. Hargreaves, C. C. Atkinson & J. E. Sorenson), pp. 290–303. Departmentt of Health, Education and Welfare.

Tyrer, P. J. (1990) Personality disorder and social functioning. In *Measuring Human Problems: A Practical Guide* (eds D. F. Peck & C. M. Shapiro), pp. 119–142. Wiley.

Wallace, C. J. (1984) Community and interpersonal functioning in the course of schizophrenic disorders. *Schizophrenia Bulletin*, **10**, 233–257.

Weissman, M. M. (1975) The assessment of social adjustment. A review of techniques. *Archives of General Psychiatry*, **32**, 357–365.

Weissman, M. M., Shalomskas, D. & John, K. (1981) The assessment of social adjustment. An update. *Archives of General Psychiatry*, **38**, 1250–1258.

Wiersma, D. (1986) Psychological impairments and social disabilities: on the applicability of the ICIDH to psychiatry. *International Rehabilitation Medicine*, **8**, 3–7.

Wiersma, D. (2005) Role functioning as a component of quality of life in mental disorders. In *Quality of Life in Mental Disorders* (2nd edition) (eds H. Katschnig, H. Freeman & N. Sartorius), pp. 45–56. Wiley.

Wiersma, D., de Jong, A. & Ormel, J. (1988) The Groningen Social Disabilities Schedule: development, relationship with the ICIDH and psychometric properties. *International Journal of Rehabilitation Research*, **11**, 213–224.

Wiersma, D., de Jong, A., Kraaijkamp, H. I. M., *et al* (1990) *GSDS–II. The Groningen Social Disabilities Schedule, Second Version. Manual, Questionnaire and Rating Form*. Department of Social Psychiatry, University of Groningen.

Wing, J. K. (1989) The measurement of 'social disablement'. The MRC Social Behaviour and Social Role Performance Schedules. *Social Psychiatry and Psychiatric Epidemiology*, **24**, 173–178.

World Health Organization (1980) *The International Classification of Impairments, Disabilities and Handicaps*. WHO.

World Health Organization (1988) *Psychiatric Disability Assessment Schedule (DAS)*. WHO.

World Health Organization (2001) *The International Classification of Functioning, Disability and Health (WHO Disability Assessment Schedule II, WHO DAS II)*. WHO.

CHAPTER 10

Measuring the costs of mental healthcare

Paul McCrone and Scott Weich

The supply of resources in an economy is limited. However, the demand for resources is generally unlimited. This is particularly the case with healthcare; if the technology and expertise to treat people exist, then there will be a demand for such resources. If the technology and expertise do not exist, then there will be a demand for their provision. Scarcity of resources leads to competing alternatives. In the healthcare arena, policy-makers and clinicians are confronted with having to decide how healthcare resources should be allocated. What should guide decision-makers in this task of resource allocation? Obviously we would expect treatments and interventions to be looked at favourably if they are known to produce good outcomes. However, it is also necessary to know what the costs of achieving these outcomes are. This is particularly relevant given the high and increasing cost of healthcare. But economics should not be concerned with simply cutting costs. Costs are in effect proxies for units of production. More units of production could well result in improved outcomes. Therefore, the more expensive option might be the preferred one. If an evaluation does not include a cost component, then inefficient services may go undetected and resources will be used inappropriately. High-quality outcome and cost data are therefore required to advise policy-makers and clinicians as to the best use of their limited resources. This chapter examines the extent to which costs have been calculated in an appropriate way in mental healthcare evaluations.

Cost measurement has been undervalued in many studies. Sometimes costs have been omitted. In other cases, not all relevant costs have been collected. Costs are frequently measured incorrectly or not interpreted correctly. When costs have been measured, it has often been in an *ad hoc* fashion. Hardly any costing instruments have been published and described. One exception in the UK is the Client Service Receipt Inventory (Beecham, 1995; Beecham & Knapp, 2001). This is unfortunate, as costs are one of the few measures that have regularly exhibited variations among treatment interventions.

We need to be sure that the cost data being collected are appropriate. Although cost measurement has been performed imperfectly in many evaluations, a number of programmes and projects have sought to incorporate a cost–benefit or cost-effectiveness analysis in their evaluations. Without an adequate measurement of cost, the usefulness of such analyses will not be fully realised. Indeed, the very term 'cost-effective' has often been poorly understood and misused (Doubilet *et al*, 1986).

The aim of this chapter is to examine evaluations which have included an economic element. From these studies we can deduce what services were considered as relevant for the purposes of costing. Previous editions of this book reviewed economic studies across a wide range of areas up to 1998. Since then, the number of economic evaluations has risen substantially and it is beyond the scope of this review to include them all. As such, the focus of this chapter is on evaluations of three team approaches to delivering mental healthcare: assertive community treatment, home treatment/crisis intervention and early-intervention services. Studies were included if they were published between 1999 and July 2009 and were identified through searching Medline, Embase, Psychinfo and the NHS Economic Evaluation Database. (One paper the authors were aware of that was eventually published in 2010 was also included because of its relevance.)

Cost

Definition

It is important to have an understanding of the concept of cost prior to calculating it. Cost is often referred to as *opportunity cost*, which is the value of resources in their best alternative use. This is a definition used by economists in general. Health economists are no exception: 'The cost of a unit of a resource is the benefit that would be derived from using it in its best alternative use' (Drummond, 1980). Essentially, then, a cost occurs because with the existence of scarcity some opportunities have to be missed. For many products and services it is assumed that an appropriate proxy for opportunity cost is the market value of the product. However, for some products there is no market price and, therefore, an opportunity cost must be imputed.

How should cost be measured?

Cost can refer to an entire service, or to the cost of any one individual using the service. It would be advantageous to know what the cost is of one more person using the service, as decisions are often made about expanding or reducing services. If there is spare capacity (such as unused hospital beds) the extra cost might be small. Higher costs are incurred if a service is already operating at full capacity. Considering these *marginal costs* is intrinsically correct. They are, though, difficult to calculate. In the long run (the period in which the structure of a service can alter) *average costs* are assumed to approximate marginal costs. Most studies in mental healthcare focus upon policy-changing schemes and, therefore, examining average costs is appropriate.

The timescale over which costs are measured is crucial. It is important to choose a length of time that would be representative of service receipt. Six months to a year should be acceptable, although this does depend on the particular programme being evaluated. In addition, different service components require different costing procedures. For an outline of costing methods the reader is referred to Allen & Beecham (1993).

Components of cost packages

All relevant costs should be examined to assess the economic impact of a mental healthcare intervention (Glass & Goldberg, 1977; Drummond, 1980; Weisbrod, 1981; Rubin, 1982; Knapp & Beecham, 1990; Clark *et al*, 1993; Manning, 1999). It is rare that mental health service users will have contact with only one particular agency, and services often will have effects on each other via inter-agency cooperation, and substitution and complementary effects. The implementation of a mental health programme could, for example, decrease psychiatric service costs but increase those falling on social services departments or general practitioners. Indeed, overall costs may be higher than initially, but if only psychiatric service costs were calculated the results could show that the new programme was less costly. Thus it is important to capture the economic costs of the psychiatric service intervention *and* of the non-psychiatric service inputs. There may also be indirect effects of a mental healthcare intervention. A further category, non-measured costs, includes aspects of care that are either problematic to cost or where it would be inappropriate to cost them on the grounds of ethics.

A cost instrument should capture information that enables comprehensive costs to be calculated. It is realised, though, that there are limits on how comprehensive a cost evaluation should be. Collecting data on every possible cost may result in accuracy of measurement being sacrificed. It may sometimes be preferable to ensure that the major costs are measured with utmost accuracy, with perhaps less emphasis being placed upon minor services (Challis *et al*, 1993). Knapp & Beecham (1993) suggest that in mental healthcare evaluations it might be possible to cost a 'reduced list' of services, but they do urge caution in this in case important service inputs are neglected.

Mental health service costs

When contacts are made with specialist mental health providers, direct psychiatric service costs are incurred. Examples of these are indicated in Box 10.1. Many studies calculate only such costs. This may appear reasonable.

Box 10.1 Psychiatric service costs

Psychiatric hospital

- in-patient
- out-patient
- day-patient
- depot clinic
- emergency clinic
- psychologist
- occupational therapy

Community

- community psychiatric nurse
- psychiatrist home visit
- community mental health centre
- crisis house
- respite house
- drop-in/day centre

Patients in hospital will often not be using services that are provided by other agencies. In addition, staff conducting the research may be concerned only with the costs that fall to their service. These costs are relatively straightforward, and less time-consuming, to calculate than full costs. However, there will inevitably be other cost implications of mental health-care programmes, particularly when they are based in the community. To ignore these other costs reduces the impact and usefulness of an economic evaluation, and can make conclusions regarding cost-effectiveness invalid.

Non-psychiatric service costs

People with mental health problems often use services from a wide range of agencies. Box 10.2, though not an exhaustive list, reveals that the range of non-psychiatric services is extensive. We have disaggregated these costs into seven categories: family health services, employment, voluntary services, general hospital services, accommodation, law and order, and social services.

Indirect costs

Indirect costs are not readily observable, and it is unusual for payments to be made which are of equivalent value. Three main types are indirect cost are identified (Box 10.3). The burden on families is reflected by the cost of informal care. Time may need to be taken off work to care for a family member with a mental health problem, or leisure time may need to be given up. Many patients are also unemployed. There are clear costs associated with this lost employment. From the point of view of the user there is the absence of earnings. In addition, the whole of society suffers from reduced production. The degree of this depends on the workings of the labour market. It may be that lost employment opportunities are not included in

---

Box 10.2 Non-psychiatric service costs

Family health services
- general practitioner (GP)
- GP home visit
- optician
- chiropodist
- gynaecologist
- family planning clinic
- nurse
- domiciliary nurse
- dentist

Employment
- job centre
- job club
- disablement rehabilitation officer
- careers advice

Voluntary services
- counselling
- bereavement service
- Samaritans
- voluntary day centres
- churches

General hospital services
- in-patient
- out-patient
- day-patient
- accident and emergency
- physiotherapy

Accommodation
- supported residential care
- private accommodation
- dental services

Law and order
- police
- probation service
- court
- solicitor
- legal aid
- prison

Social services
- social worker
- social worker home visit
- home help
- meals on wheels
- social security officer
- counsellor

---

cost evaluations, as they will be the same whatever the intervention (i.e. clients will remain unemployed). However, the aim of many involved in mental healthcare is to help people to become rehabilitated, which should increase their employment prospects, and so the costs of lost employment are still relevant. The financial gains made from employment, in the form of earnings, are often included in cost–benefit analyses (where outcomes are monetised). Finally, the costs of time and travelling incurred when services are used should ideally be considered in a cost evaluation. The opportunity cost of this time is determined by what the patient would have been doing otherwise – and clearly this is difficult to value and is usually omitted.

Box 10.3 Indirect costs

Informal care
- lost employment of friends and relatives
- lost leisure time of friends and relatives

User time
- travelling
- waiting

Lost employment
- time off work due to mental health problem
- foregone potential employment
- lost production to economy

Welfare benefits

Costs arise because a productive activity has taken place, for example the provision of a particular service. Welfare benefits are not a means of production and therefore not a cost. They are a transfer payment from one group of economic agents (taxpayers) to another (recipients). The cost to taxpayers is offset by the gain to recipients and hence there is no residual cost (excluding the costs of administering the benefits system). However, to the individual service user welfare benefits are a definite gain, and to the rest of society they are a diversion of funds, even if this is deemed to be appropriate. The level of benefits may also be an indication of the cost of living (Knapp, 1991). It is useful for studies to record the receipt of welfare benefits, even if this is not essential for the costing process.

Areas in which costing has been undertaken

Many areas of mental healthcare have undergone economic evaluation, and costs have frequently been reported. Here we review studies of assertive community treatment, home treatment/crisis intervention and early-intervention services. It should be stressed that reporting costs alone is as dangerous as omitting them altogether – the cost element should be viewed in the context of a full evaluation.

Assertive community treatment

Services have been developed for patients who are hard to engage. These assertive community treatment or assertive outreach teams provide intensive support and tend to be characterised by low case numbers per worker and extended working hours. Frequently the aim is to reduce hospital care, but

187

of course by engaging patients more it may be that problems are more easily identified that may warrant admission.

In California, an assertive community treatment (ACT) service which included capitated payments was evaluated by Chandler *et al* (1999). Patients who had been staying in a long-term in-patient facility were randomised to the ACT intervention or to a comparison condition. Costs were measured but were confined to mental health services. Other healthcare costs and those due to contact with the criminal justice system were not included. ACT resulted in costs that were 72% of those in the comparison group (US$946 000 against US$1 234 000).

Ford *et al* (2001) compared three teams that originally provided intensive case management (ICM) with elements of ACT over 5 years. Only one of the teams continued to provide ACT as it did during the initial 18 months, one team merged with another and saw an increase in its case-load, while another team was disbanded. Costs were measured over the 5 years, and these included the ICM service itself plus other mental health services. Costs varied substantially between the three sites but outcomes were similar. This led the authors to suggest that intensive services were not required over this period of time in order to generate patient benefits.

An evaluation of ACT in north London, in comparison with standard care, measured costs of mental health services, other healthcare, justice services and informal care from family members (McCrone *et al*, 2009a). Interestingly, costs were higher for the ACT group over an 18-month follow-up (£34 572 versus £30 541), although this difference was not statistically significant.

Salkever *et al* (1999) compared ACT with usual care in 144 patients in South Carolina. They limited their analysis to the impact on the use of hospital admission over an 18-month follow-up and found that while ACT produced fewer admissions, the number of bed days did not differ significantly. It is therefore unclear what the overall cost impact of ACT had been.

ACT is often targeted at specific groups of patients. For example, Lehman *et al* (1999) compared it with usual care for 152 homeless patients in a randomised trial in Maryland. The authors took a relatively comprehensive approach to estimating costs for both groups over 12 months. Mental health services were included as well as substance misuse and general medical services. Out-patient costs were significantly higher for the ACT group but these were more than offset by significantly lower in-patient costs. Total mean costs for the ACT group were US$50 748, compared with US$66 480 for the usual-care group.

An evaluation of ICM compared with standard care measured costs over a 2-year follow-up (UK 700 Group, 2000). This study was the most comprehensive of those reviewed in terms of services included. In addition to specialist mental healthcare, costs were also calculated for primary care, general medical care, medication, accommodation, criminal justice services and social care. ICM not surprisingly resulted in higher costs for case managers, but overall costs were similar in the two groups (£24 553 for ICM and £22 704 for the standard service).

Home treatment/crisis intervention

Patients experiencing psychiatric emergencies or crises have frequently been admitted to in-patient units. However, owing to the high cost and the assumption that many patients would prefer to be cared for in other ways, a number of countries have developed home treatment (HT) or crisis intervention (CI) teams. These generally provide care just during the crisis and aim either to reduce rates of admission or the duration of in-patient stays.

A number of naturalistic before-and-after studies of crisis intervention services have been conducted. In Luxembourg, Damsa et al (2005) compared 6-month periods before and following the introduction HT/CI services. Costs were confined to out-patient and in-patient care. The costs of out-patient care increased over time (as we might expect) but the costs of in-patient care were substantially reduced. Costs per consultation were reduced by US$206 over time.

A well-conducted randomised controlled trial in Canada compared a residential crisis service with voluntary in-patient care for 119 patients presenting as a psychiatric emergency (Fenton et al, 2002). Outcomes included symptoms and days living in the community over 6-month follow-up. Costs were comprehensively measured during this period and included the index admission to hospital or the crisis house, other admissions, other mental healthcare, physical healthcare, medication and criminal justice services. Costs were significantly lower for the crisis house group ($19 941) than for the hospital group ($25 737). Outcomes were non-significantly worse for the crisis house group, which led to an interesting discussion as to whether these lower costs justified poorer outcomes.

Day hospitals have been seen as an alternative to admission for those presenting in psychiatric crisis. An interesting study in Manchester in the UK by Harrison et al (2003) compared day hospitalisation with a home treatment service. Patients receiving the former service had previously taken part in an earlier randomised comparison with in-patient care (Creed et al, 1997) and the home treatment sample were recruited subsequently. Costs were shown to be lowest for the day hospital group, followed by the home treatment group and the in-patient group. The non-randomised nature of the comparison makes interpretation challenging, as does the limited range of costs included (in-patient care, day hospital contacts and out-patient attendances). While these services were the key components of care for the day hospital and in-patient groups, the authors recognise that the home treatment intervention may have resulted in extra costs elsewhere in the system. In addition, the home treatment group were not all presenting as an emergency.

Also in the UK, two groups of patients experiencing a crisis that could lead to admission were compared before ($n = 65$) and after ($n = 116$) the introduction of a CI team (McCrone *et al*, 2009*b*). Service use was measured for the 6 months prior to and following the start of the crisis and included the intervention itself as well as other mental health and physical healthcare, social care and contacts with the criminal justice system. There was a reduction in the use of in-patient care following the introduction of the CI team and this led to average cost savings of £1681 per person. This was not statistically significant, but when patients who had contact with the CI team were compared with those who had not, the cost savings were £2189, which was significant.

The above study was followed by a randomised trial of CI compared with usual care in an adjacent area (McCrone *et al*, 2009*c*). Two hundred and sixty patients were included and service use was measured for the 6 months before baseline and 6-month follow-up. The range of services was similar to that in the previous study, covering all major health, social and criminal justice services. While the costs of non-in-patient care were significantly higher for the intervention group, total costs were significantly lower, owing to reduced in-patient care.

Crisis services have also been developed for children with mental health problems as an alternative to hospital admission. In a longitudinal study from the USA, Blumberg (2002) compared the use of in-patient care for children in the 3 years before and after such a team was introduced. In-patient bed use fell by 23%. These resulting cost savings offset the extra costs incurred in running the service. However, other community costs were not included in the analyses.

Early-intervention services

In most areas of healthcare it is considered appropriate to provide treatment as soon as an illness develops or even to provide interventions to prevent its occurrence. However, people who develop severe mental health problems frequently have a long period of untreated illness and preventive services are few. In recent years, though, early-intervention (EI) services and (to a lesser extent) early-detection services have been developed, and a growing number of economic evaluations of such services have been undertaken. As with HT/CI teams, one of the key aims of EI services is to reduce the need for hospital admission.

The EI services for young people with emerging psychosis in Melbourne, Australia, were among the first to be developed and assessed. An economic evaluation examined costs that were incurred in the 12 months following referral to the service for 51 patients and compared these with costs from an earlier period when there was no EI service for 51 matched controls (Mihalopoulos *et al*, 1999). Costs included the EI service itself, in-patient care, and other psychiatric and physical healthcare. Non-in-patient costs were substantially higher for the EI service (A$5666 compared with A$2688) but in-patient savings resulted in total costs for EI (A$16 694) being less than for the pre-EI service (A$24 074).

The above study was followed by a long-term follow-up (with around two-thirds of the sample included) in which costs and cost-effectiveness were assessed over a 7-year period for the control patients and a 6-year period for the EI patients (Mihalopoulos *et al*, 2009). Given the difference in the follow-up periods, the annual costs are most informative and these show a large saving for EI (A$3841 compared with A$10 627). Costs were limited to in-patient care, out-patient contacts and medication. However, it is unlikely that the inclusion of any other services would alter this result. Although this chapter is focusing on cost measurement, it is worth pointing out that outcomes were generally also better for the EI service.

A study from Canada has examined the impact on service use and costs of an EI service (Goldberg *et al*, 2006). Costs were compared over the 2 years before the introduction of the service and for the subsequent 2 years. Hospital bed costs and emergency room costs fell over time. Other services were not included and therefore it is not possible to tell whether the extra costs of the service were offset by reduced hospital costs.

A similar study from Sweden compared the costs of in-patient and out-patient care for patients treated while an EI service was in operation with the costs of a prospective control service (Cullberg *et al*, 2006). Costs were lower for the EI group during a 1-year follow-up, but costs were similar over a subsequent year, before the cost advantage for EI reappeared in the third year. Once again, though, the exclusion of other services from the costing was noticeable.

Only one randomised trial of EI services which has included an economic component has been identified (McCrone *et al*, 2010). The Lambeth EI service in London in the UK was compared with usual care and costs were measured for 126 patients over an 18-month follow-up. Costs included mental health services, physical healthcare, social care and criminal justice services. Non-in-patient costs were slightly higher for the EI service, but total mean costs (£11 685) were lower than for standard care (£14 062) owing to reduced use of in-patient services. This difference, however, was not statistically significant.

Conclusion

Cost information is vital for a complete and worthwhile evaluation of a mental healthcare intervention. However, cost estimations have, with some exceptions, often been poorly performed and many areas of service provision which are affected have been neglected. Clearly, there is a need for stringent methods of costing. Indeed, well-thought-out costing frameworks have been proposed (Weisbrod, 1981; Knapp & Beecham, 1990; Drummond *et al*, 1997). However, many of the recommendations mooted have not as yet been wholly accepted. Ignoring the importance of comprehensive costing can, at best, reduce the impact of wider evaluation and, at worse, provide wrong information to policy makers, which would be to the detriment of all.

References

Allen, C. & Beecham, J. (1993) Costing services: ideals and reality. In *Costing Community Care: Theory and Practice* (eds A. Netten & J. Beecham), pp. 25–42. Ashgate.

Beecham, J. (1995) Collecting and estimating costs. In *The Economic Evaluation of Mental Health Care* (ed. M. Knapp), pp. 61–82. Arena.

Beecham, J. & Knapp, M. (2001) Costing psychiatric interventions. In *Measuring Mental Health Needs* (2nd edition) (ed. G. Thornicroft), pp. 200–224. Gaskell.

Blumberg, S. H. (2002) Crisis intervention program: an alternative to inpatient psychiatric treatment for children. *Mental Health Services Research*, **4**, 1–6.

Challis, D., Chesterman, J. & Traske, K. (1993) Case management: costing the experiments. In *Costing Community Care: Theory and Practice* (eds A. Netten & J. Beecham), pp. 143–161. Ashgate.

Chandler, D., Spicer, G., Wagner, M., *et al* (1999) Cost-effectiveness of a capitated assertive community treatment program. *Psychiatric Rehabilitation Journal*, **22**, 327–336.

Clark, R. E., Drake, R. E. & Teague, G. B. (1993) The costs and benefits of case management. In *Case Management for Mentally Ill Patients* (eds M. Harris & H. C. Bergman), pp. 217–236. Harwood.

Creed, F., Mbaya, P., Lancashire, S., *et al* (1997) Cost effectiveness of day and inpatient psychiatric treatment: results of a randomised controlled trial. *BMJ*, **314**, 1381–1385.

Cullberg, J., Mattsson, M., Levander, S., *et al* (2006) Treatment costs and clinical outcome for first episode schizophrenia patients: a 3-year follow-up of the Swedish 'Parachute Project' and two comparison groups. *Acta Psychiatrica Scandinavica*, **114**, 274–281.

Damsa, C., Hummel, C., Sar, V., *et al* (2005) Economic impact of a crisis intervention in emergency psychiatry: a naturalistic study. *European Psychiatry*, **20**, 562–566.

Doubilet, P., Weinstein, M. C. & McNeil, B. J. (1986) Use and misuse of the term 'cost effective' in medicine. *New England Journal of Medicine*, **314**, 253–256.

Drummond, M. (1980) *Principles of Economic Appraisal in Health Care*. Oxford University Press.

Drummond, M. F., O'Brien, B., Stoddart, G. L., *et al* (1997) *Methods for the Economic Evaluation of Health Care Programmes*. Oxford University Press.

Fenton, W. S., Hoch, J. S., Herrell, J. M., *et al* (2002) Cost and cost-effectiveness of hospital vs residential crisis care for patients who have serious mental illness. *Archives of General Psychiatry*, **59**, 357–364.

Ford, R., Barnes, A., Davies, R., *et al* (2001) Maintaining contact with people with severe mental illness: 5-year follow-up of assertive outreach. *Social Psychiatry and Psychiatric Epidemiology*, **36**, 444–447.

Glass, N. J. & Goldberg, D. (1977) Cost–benefit analysis and the evaluation of psychiatric services. *Psychological Medicine*, **7**, 701–707.

Goldberg, K., Norman, R., Hoch, J., *et al* (2006) Impact of a specialized early intervention service for psychotic disorders on patient characteristics, service use , and hospital costs in a defined catchment area. *Canadian Journal of Psychiatry*, **51**, 895–903.

Harrison, J., Marshall, S., Marshall, J., *et al* (2003) Day hospital vs. home treatment. A comparison of illness severity and costs. *Social Psychiatry and Psychiatric Epidemiology*, **38**, 541–546.

Knapp, M. (1991) The direct costs of the community care of chronically mentally ill people. In *Evaluation of Comprehensive Care of the Mentally Ill* (eds H. Freeman & J. Henderson), pp. 142–175. Gaskell.

Knapp, M. & Beecham, J. (1990) Costing mental health services. *Psychological Medicine*, **20**, 893–908.

Knapp, M. & Beecham, J. (1993) Reduced list costings: examination of an informed short cut in mental health research. *Health Economics*, **2**, 313–322.

Lehman, A. F., Dixon, L., Hoch, J. S., *et al* (1999) Cost-effectiveness of assertive community treatment for homeless persons with severe mental illness. *British Journal of Psychiatry*, **174**, 346–352.

Manning, W. G. Jr. (1999) Panel on cost-effectiveness in health and medicine recommendations: identifying costs. *Journal of Clinical Psychiatry*, **60** (Suppl 3), 54–56.

McCrone, P., Killaspy, H., Bebbington, P., *et al* (2009a) The REACT study: cost-effectiveness analysis of assertive community treatment in north London. *Psychiatric Services*, **60**, 908–913.

McCrone, P., Johnson, S., Nolan, F., *et al* (2009b) Impact of a crisis resolution team on service costs in the UK. *Psychiatric Bulletin*, **33**, 17–19.

McCrone, P., Johnson, S., Nolan, F., *et al* (2009c) Economic evaluation of a crisis resolution service: a randomised controlled trial. *Epidemiologia e Psichiatria Sociale*, **18**, 54–58.

McCrone, P., Craig, T. K. J., Garety, P., *et al* (2010) Cost-effectiveness of an early intervention service for people with psychosis in south London: the LEO study. *British Journal of Psychiatry*, **96**, 377–382.

Mihalopoulos, C., McGorry, P. D. & Carter, R. C. (1999) Is phase-specific, community-orientated treatment of early psychosis an economically viable method of improving outcome? *Acta Psychiatrica Scandinavica*, **100**, 47–55.

Mihalopoulos, C., Harris, M., Henry, L., *et al* (2009) Is early intervention in psychosis cost-effective over the long term? *Schizophrenia Bulletin*, **35**, 909–918.

Rubin, J. (1982) Cost measurement and cost data in mental health settings. *Hospital and Community Psychiatry*, **33**, 750–754.

Salkever, D., Domino, M. E., Burns, B. J., *et al* (1999) Assertive community treatment for people with severe mental illness: the effect on hospital use and costs. *Health Services Research*, **34**, 577–601.

UK 700 Group (2000) Cost-effectiveness of intensive v. standard case management for severe psychotic illness. UK 700 case management trial. *British Journal of Psychiatry*, **176**, 537–543.

Weisbrod, B. A. (1981) A guide to benefit–cost analysis, as seen through a controlled experiment in treating the mentally ill. *Journal of Health Politics, Policy and Law*, **7**, 808–845.

CHAPTER 11

Assessing needs for mental healthcare

Mike Slade, Sonia Johnson, Michael Phelan
and Graham Thornicroft

A needs-led approach to mental healthcare

A *needs-led* approach to the provision of mental healthcare has been one of the most consistent themes to emerge within evolving community mental healthcare services. In England this was first expressed in the provisions of the National Health Service and Community Care Act 1990. The central tenet of a needs-led approach is that assessment of the needs of patients should be on the basis of their individual circumstances, problems and personal goals. Assessment should not be undertaken in terms of or on the basis of existing services, that is, assessment should not be *service based*. This means that assessment of need is a separate process from decisions about what care or treatment to provide.

Needs-led assessment should, for example, look at whether people have access to enough activities which are meaningful (to them) each day, rather than whether they need to attend a day centre. If the assessment indicates that there is a problem with daytime activities, one service response might be a place at a day centre. Another, however, might be support in undertaking voluntary work. Needs-led assessments have two advantages over service-based assessments: first, they point to the most appropriate form of service response (in terms of treatment or care) for the individual's difficulties; and second, they have the potential to indicate needs for which there is currently no service provision, which a service-based assessment by definition would not identify.

What is a need?

People with severe mental illness usually have a wide range of clinical and social needs. A variety of approaches to defining need have been proposed. The American psychologist Maslow (1954) established a hierarchy of need when attempting to formulate a theory of human motivation. In Maslow's model, fundamental physiological needs (such as the need for food) underpin the higher needs of safety, love, self-esteem and self-actualisation. He proposed that people are motivated by the requirement to meet these needs, and that higher needs could be met only after the lower and more fundamental needs were met. This approach can be illustrated by the example of a homeless man, who is not concerned about his lack of friends while he is cold and hungry. However, once these physiological needs have been met he may express more interest in having the company of other people.

Since the work of Maslow, other approaches have been developed to defining need with respect to healthcare. In the Medical Research Council's Needs for Care Assessment Schedule, a need is defined as being present when a person's level of functioning falls below, or threatens to fall below, some specified level and when there is some remediable, or potentially remediable, cause (Brewin *et al*, 1987). The sociologist Bradshaw (1972) proposed a taxonomy of four types of need: that which is 'felt' (but not expressed) by the patient; that which is 'expressed' by the patient; 'normative' need, which is assessed by an expert; and 'comparative' need, which arises from comparison with other groups or individuals. Such an approach underlines that need is a subjective concept, and that the judgement of whether a need is present or not will, in part, depend on whose viewpoint is being taken (Slade, 1994).

Stevens & Gabbay (1991) have distinguished between need (the ability to benefit in some way from healthcare), demand (wishes expressed by the service patient) and supply of services. These concepts can be illustrated by different components of mental health services. For instance, mental health services for homeless people who are mentally ill are rarely demanded by homeless people, but most professionals would agree that a need exists. In contrast, the demand for counselling services frequently outstrips supply. Clearly, the need, demand and supply of services will never be perfectly matched. If mismatch is to be minimised, then two principles need to underpin mental health service development: first, services must try to address the identified problems and difficulties of local patients (i.e. local services should be shaped by the specific needs of the population), rather than being provided in line with any national template or historical patterns; and second, a continued effort to demonstrate what is, and is not, effective with different groups is required, so that resources are provided for effective interventions, and not driven by demand or short-term political pressures.

There is no perfect individual needs assessment tool. The requirements of different people using mental health services will vary, and there is inevitable conflict between factors such as brevity and comprehensiveness. A number of measurement approaches have been developed, including the Needs for Care Assessment Schedule mentioned above, the Cardinal Needs Schedule (Marshall *et al*, 1995), the Bangor Assessment of Need Profile (Carter *et al*, 1996) and the Avon Mental Health Measure (Markovitz, 1996). However, an independent review (Evans *et al*, 2000) identified the most widely used needs assessment measure as the Camberwell Assessment of Need (CAN; Phelan *et al*, 1995; http://www.iop.kcl.ac.uk/prism/can), and the CAN is the main focus in the remainder of this chapter.

Camberwell Assessment of Need (CAN)

The Adult CAN is an individual needs assessment instrument for use with adults with severe mental illness. The original drive was to meet the requirements of the National Health Service and Community Care Act 1990. Four broad principles governed the development of the CAN:

1   Everyone has needs, and although people with mental health problems have some specific needs, the majority of their needs are similar to those of people who do not have a mental illness, such as having somewhere to live, something to do and enough money.
2   The majority of people with a severe mental illness have multiple needs, and it is vital that all of them are identified by those caring for them. Therefore a priority of the CAN is to identify, rather than describe in detail, serious needs. Specialist assessments can be conducted in specific areas if required, once the need is identified.
3   Needs assessment should be both an integral part of routine clinical practice and a component of service evaluation, so the CAN should be useable by a wide range of staff.
4   Need is a subjective concept and there will frequently be differing but equally valid perceptions regarding the presence or absence of a specific need. The CAN therefore records the views of staff and patients separately.

The specific criteria that were established for the CAN are that it:

*   has adequate psychometric properties
*   can be completed within 30 minutes
*   can be used by a wide range of professionals
*   is suitable for both routine clinical practice and research
*   can be used without formal training
*   incorporates the views of both patients and staff about needs
*   measures both met and unmet need
*   measures the level of help received from friends or relatives as well as from statutory services.

Four versions of the Adult CAN have been developed:

1   CAN–Research (CAN–R) – a long version intended for research use, to assess needs, formal and informal help received, and satisfaction with help, which can be completed by staff or service users or their carers (Phelan *et al*, 1995; Slade *et al*, 1999a; see also below)
2   CAN–Clinical (CAN–C) – a long version intended for clinical use, to assess needs, formal and informal help received, and to support care planning, which can be completed by staff or service users or their carers (Phelan *et al*, 1995; Slade *et al*, 1999a)

3   CAN Short Appraisal Schedule (CANSAS) – a brief assessment of needs which can be completed by staff or service users or their carers (Phelan *et al*, 1995; Slade *et al*, 1999*a*; Andresen *et al*, 2000)
4   CANSAS–Patient (CANSAS–P) – a brief self-completed assessment of needs intended for completion by the service user (Slade *et al*, 2006; Trauer *et al*, 2008).

All versions of the Adult CAN assess need in the same 22 domains of health and social needs:

1   accommodation
2   food
3   looking after the home
4   self-care
5   daytime activities
6   physical health
7   psychotic symptoms
8   information
9   psychological distress
10 safety to self
11 safety to others
12 alcohol
13 drugs
14 company
15 intimate relationships
16 sexual expression
17 child care
18 basic education
19 telephone
20 transport
21 money
22 benefits.

A *need rating* is made for each domain on the following scale:

0 = no serious problem   (no need)
1 = no/moderate problem due to help given   (met need)
2 = serious problem   (unmet need)
9 = not known

The need rating can be summed across all domains to give the total number of met needs and the total number of unmet needs, both ranging from 0 (no needs) to 22.

The adult CAN has been translated into many different languages, including: Afrikaans, Cantonese, Czech, Danish, Dutch, Finnish, French, German, Greek, Hindi, Hungarian, Icelandic, Italian, Lithuanian, Maltese, Mandarin Chinese, Norwegian, Polish, Portuguese, Portuguese (Brazil),

Spanish, Swedish and Turkish. Further information about translations is available at http://www.iop.kcl.ac.uk/prism/can.

Variants of the CAN

In addition to the four versions of the Adult CAN with its focus on assessing the needs of people with severe mental illness, variants for other patient groups have been developed.

The CAN–Forensic (CANFOR) assesses the needs of people with criminal justice and mental health issues (Thomas *et al*, 2003, 2008). CANFOR assesses need in 25 domains relevant to forensic mental health service users. It was developed for use in forensic mental health services, such as: high-security psychiatric services; medium-security psychiatric services; low-security psychiatric services; community forensic mental health services; probation services; and prison services.

The CAN–Elderly (CANE) is a comprehensive needs assessment tool for use by professionals working with the elderly (Reynolds *et al*, 2000; Orrell & Hancock, 2004). It was developed from the CAN to incorporate the special needs of elderly people. Twenty-four domains of individual need are assessed, as well as two questions to assess the needs of the person's carer.

The CAN–Developmental and Intellectual Disabilities (CANDID) is a needs assessment scale specifically designed for people with intellectual disabilities (learning disabilities, mental retardation) and mental health problems (Xenitidis *et al*, 2000, 2003). It assesses needs in 25 domains of life, and has both short and research versions.

The CAN–Mothers (CAN-M) is an assessment that highlights frequent problem areas for pregnant women and mothers with severe mental illness (Howard *et al*, 2007, 2008). It covers 26 domains of need.

A further CAN variant is under development for use in disaster situations internationally, which is called the Humanitarian and Emergency Settings Perceived Needs Scale (HESPER).

CAN–Research

Why is the CAN so widely used and developed? Perhaps the main reason is that it was one of the first measures internationally to have two key properties: psychometric robustness and separate assessments of the views of staff and service users. In the CAN, ratings for each domain of need can be made separately by staff and service users and informal carers (friends and family). This allows empirical research to be conducted into the differing perspectives of, in particular, staff and service users. The main research findings have been that:

- the ratings made by staff and service users consistently differ, and are not interchangeable or collapsible into a single summary rating (Lasalvia *et al*, 2000, 2007; Hansson *et al*, 2001; Fleury *et al*, 2006)

- one reason for this discordance is that patient ratings are statistically more reliable than staff ratings (Slade *et al*, 1999*b*; Ochoa *et al*, 2003)
- patient-rated unmet need has emerged as a key determinant of well-being, with an associative relationship shown with satisfaction (Leese *et al*, 1998; Wiersma & van Busschbach, 2001; Lasalvia *et al*, 2008) and a causal (i.e. not simply associative) relationship demonstrated with both quality of life (Hansson *et al*, 2003; Slade *et al*, 2004, 2005; Lasalvia *et al*, 2005) and therapeutic alliance (Junghan *et al*, 2007).

Three clinical principles emerge from this empirical foundation:

1   Unmet need is the most important CAN total score (Slade *et al*, 1999*a*; Killaspy *et al*, 2008) and converting unmet needs to met needs is a primary goal of mental health services (Drukker *et al*, 2008).
2   Agreement on needs predicts outcome (Fleury *et al*, 2006; Macpherson *et al*, 2007; Lasalvia *et al*, 2008) and agreement increases with longer-term staff–patient relationships (Macpherson *et al*, 2003; Najim & McCrone, 2005).
3   The service user's assessment of unmet needs should be given at least equal weight with the staff perspective when planning clinical action.

Implementing these three clinical principles will lead to evidence-based practice.

Other approaches to measuring needs in research

Before introduction of the CAN, the main available tool for individual needs assessment was the Medical Research Council's Needs for Care Assessment Schedule (Brewin *et al*, 1987), designed primarily as a research tool. Acceptance that needs may differ from different perspectives is inherent in the CAN procedures: the MRC Needs for Care Assessment Schedule, by contrast, aims for objective expert assessment of needs for specific items of care. Whether someone is deemed to have a need thus depends whether there is any item of care that might be expected to improve a symptom or deficit in functioning. The fact that this schedule is now used much less than the CAN is likely to reflect: the difficulty in attaining the goal of objectivity; loss of confidence in the idea that an independent expert stance is the best perspective for assessment; the relatively lengthy assessment; and the requirement for extensive training. Needs may be identified not only as met or unmet, as in the CAN, but also as unmeetable if the judgement is that there is no available intervention that might be expected to be effective.

A few published studies have reported needs assessments using this instrument with adults who were severely mentally ill. Some of the more interesting studies investigated whether their needs changed over time. For example, the rehabilitation service users investigated in the Camberwell High Contact Survey (Brewin *et al*, 1988) were followed up after 12 years (Reid *et al*, 2001) and found to have patterns and levels of problems and needs strikingly similar to those observed more than a decade earlier. Considerable stability (over 4 years) was also observed in a Dresden sample to whom this instrument was applied on several occasions (Kallert *et al*, 2004).

The Cardinal Assessment of Need is an adaptation of the Needs for Care Assessment Schedule, intended to be quicker and simpler to complete and to take explicit account of patient and carer views and of whether patients are willing to accept interventions (Marshall *et al*, 1995). It does not seem to have been widely used beyond the originating group, but has been applied in a cluster randomised trial testing the impact on outcomes of clinical care of feeding back to clinicians the results of needs assessments: the only effect was a positive one on patient satisfaction (Marshall *et al*, 2004).

Conclusion

The principal advances of the past decade in individual assessment of need have been a range of developments based on the CAN, very much the pre-eminent tool in this domain. Level of unmet needs, measured using this instrument and its variants, has emerged as the most favoured single indicator in this domain, used both for service evaluation purposes and in a very large range of research studies, especially in Europe. While a single measure dominates in this domain of outcome assessment more than in most, some questions do remain regarding its application: in particular, its sensitivity to change resulting from specific treatments has been questioned and this warrants further exploration (Wiersma *et al*, 2009).

We have concentrated on the assessment of need at the level of the individual service user, in keeping with the focus throughout this book. Beyond our scope is a second sense in which the term 'needs assessment' is used: of great importance to service planning is the assessment of the needs for healthcare of a population. It is obviously desirable that policy-making and service planning at this level be needs led, and a large body of work in public health, health economics, health policy and related disciplines addresses the question of how to extrapolate from sociodemographic, geographical, service user and clinical outcome data to the allocation of resources (see Knapp & McDaid, 2007). The emphasis on such assessment is intensified in current National Health Service policy by the requirement for commissioners of services to engage in the Joint Strategic Needs Assessment process, involving the collation and analysis of a range of population and health indicators (Department of Health, 2008).

References

Andresen, R., Caputi, P. & Oades, L. G. (2000) Interrater reliability of the Camberwell Assessment of Need Short Appraisal Schedule. *Australian and New Zealand Journal of Psychiatry*, **34**, 856–861.

Bradshaw, J. (1972) A taxonomy of social need. In *Problems and Progress in Medical Care: Essays on Current Research* (ed. J. McLachlan), pp. 69–82. Oxford University Press.

Brewin, C., Wing, J., Mangen, S., *et al* (1987) Principles and practice of measuring needs in the long-term mentally ill: the MRC Needs for Care Assessment. *Psychological Medicine*, **17**, 971–981.

Brewin, C., Wing, I., Mangen, S., *et al* (1988) Needs for care among the long-term mentally ill: a report from the Camberwell High Contact Survey. *Psychological Medicine*, **18**, 457–468.

Carter, M., Crosby, C., Geerthuis, S., *et al* (1996) Developing reliability in client-centred mental health needs assessment. *Journal of Mental Health*, **5**, 233–243.

Department of Health (2008) *Guidance on Joint Strategic Needs Assessment*. Department of Heallth. Available at http://www.dh.gov.uk/en/Publicationsandstatistics/Publications/PublicationsPolicyAndGuidance/DH_081097 (accessed 28 May 2009).

Drukker, M., van Dillen, K., Bak, M., *et al* (2008) The use of the Camberwell Assessment of Need in treatment: what unmet needs can be met? *Social Psychiatry and Psychiatric Epidemiology*, **43**, 410–417.

Evans, S., Greenhalgh, J. & Connelly, J. (2000) Selecting a mental health needs assessment scale: guidance on the critical appraisal of standardized measures. *Journal of Evaluation in Clinical Practice*, **6**, 379–393.

Fleury, M. J., Grenier, G. & Lesage, A. (2006) Agreement between staff and service users concerning the clientele's mental health needs: a Quebec study. *Canadian Journal of Psychiatry*, **51**, 281–286.

Hansson, L., Vinding, H. R., Mackeprang, T., *et al* (2001) Comparison of key worker and patient assessment of needs in schizophrenic patients living in the community: a Nordic multicentre study. *Acta Psychiatrica Scandinavica*, **103**, 45–51.

Hansson, L., Sandlund, M., Bengtsson-Tops, A., *et al* (2003) The relationship of needs and quality of life in persons with schizophrenia living in the community. A Nordic multi-center study. *Nordic Journal of Psychiatry*, **57**, 5–11.

Howard, L., Hunt, K., Slade, M., *et al* (2007) Assessing the needs of pregnant women and mothers with severe mental illness: the psychometric properties of the Camberwell Assessment of Need – Mothers (CAN–M). *International Journal of Methods in Psychiatric Research*, **16**, 177–185.

Howard, L., Slade, M., O'Keane, V., *et al* (2008) *The Camberwell Assessment of Need for Pregnant Women and Mothers with Severe Mental Illness*. Gaskell.

Junghan, U. M., Leese, M., Priebe, S., *et al* (2007) Staff and patient perspectives on unmet need and therapeutic alliance in community mental health services. *British Journal of Psychiatry*, **191**, 543–547.

Kallert, T. W., Leisse, M. & Winecke, P. (2004) Needs for care of chronic schizophrenic patients in long term community treatment. *Social Psychiatry and Psychiatric Epidemiology*, **39**, 386–396.

Killaspy, H., Rambarran, D. & Bledin, K. (2008) Mental health needs of clients of rehabilitation services: a survey in one trust. *Journal of Mental Health*, **17**, 207–218.

Knapp, M. & McDaid, D. (2007) Financing and funding mental health care services. In *Mental Health Policy and Practice Across Europe: The Future Direction of Mental Health Care* (eds M. Knapp, D. McDaid, E. Mossialos & G. Thornicroft), pp. 60–99. Open University Press.

Lasalvia, A., Ruggeri, M., Mazzi, M. A., *et al* (2000) The perception of needs for care in staff and patients in community-based mental health services. The South-Verona Outcome Project 3. *Acta Psychiatrica Scandinavica*, **102**, 366–375.

Lasalvia, A., Bonetto, C., Malchiodi, F., *et al* (2005) Listening to patients' needs to improve their subjective quality of life. *Psychological Medicine*, **35**, 1655–1665.

Lasalvia, A., Bonetto, C., Salvi, G., *et al* (2007) Predictors of changes in needs for care in patients receiving community psychiatric treatment: a 4-year follow-up study. *Acta Psychiatrica Scandinavica*, suppl. 437, 31–41.

Lasalvia, A., Bonetto, C., Tansella, M., *et al* (2008) Does staff–patient agreement on needs for care predict a better mental health outcome? A 4-year follow-up in a community service. *Psychological Medicine*, **38**, 123–133.

Leese, M., Johnson, S., Slade, M., *et al* (1998) User perspective on needs and satisfaction with mental health services. PRiSM Psychosis Study. 8. *British Journal of Psychiatry*, **173**, 409–415.

Macpherson, R., Varah, M., Summerfield, L., *et al* (2003) Staff and patient assessments of need in an epidemiologically representative sample of patients with psychosis – staff and patient assessments of need. *Social Psychiatry and Psychiatric Epidemiology*, **38**, 662–667.

Macpherson, R., Gregory, N., Slade, M., *et al* (2007) Factors associated with changing patient needs in an assertive outreach team. *International Journal of Social Psychiatry*, **53**, 389–396.

Markovitz, P. (1996) *The Avon Mental Health Measure*. Changing Minds.

Marshall, M., Hogg, L., Gath, D. H., *et al* (1995) The Cardinal Needs Schedule: a modified version of the MRC Needs for Care Schedule. *Psychological Medicine*, **25**, 605–617.

Marshall, M., Lockwood, A., Green, G., *et al* (2004) Systematic assessment of needs for care and care planning in severe mental illness: a cluster randomised controlled trial. *British Journal of Psychiatry*, **185**, 163–168.

Maslow, A. (1954) *Motivation and Personality*. Harper and Row.

Najim, H. & McCrone, P. (2005) The Camberwell Assessment of Need: comparison of assessments by staff and patients in an inner-city and a semi-rural community area. *Psychiatric Bulletin*, **28**, 13–17.

Ochoa, S., Haro, J. M., Autonell, J., *et al* (2003) Met and unmet needs of schizophrenia patients in a Spanish sample. *Schizophrenia Bulletin*, **29**, 201–210.

Orrell, M. & Hancock, G. (2004) *The Camberwell Assessment of Need for the Elderly (CANE)*. Gaskell.

Phelan, M., Slade, M., Thornicroft, G., *et al* (1995) The Camberwell Assessment of Need: the validity and reliability of an instrument to assess the needs of people with severe mental illness. *British Journal of Psychiatry*, **167**, 589–595.

Reid, Y., Johnson, S., Bebbington, P., *et al* (2001) The longer term outcomes of community care: a 12 year follow up of the Camberwell High Contact Study. *Psychological Medicine*, **31**, 351–359.

Reynolds, T., Thornicroft, G., Abas, M., *et al* (2000) Camberwell Assessment of Need for the Elderly (CANE): development, validity, and reliability. *British Journal of Psychiatry*, **176**, 444–452.

Slade, M. (1994) Needs assessment. Involvement of staff and users will help to meet needs. *British Journal of Psychiatry*, **165**, 293–296.

Slade, M., Loftus, L., Phelan, M., *et al* (1999a) *The Camberwell Assessment of Need*. Gaskell.

Slade, M., Leese, M., Taylor, R., *et al* (1999b) The association between needs and quality of life in an epidemiologically representative sample of people with psychosis. *Acta Psychiatrica Scandinavica*, **100**, 149–157.

Slade, M., Leese, M., Ruggeri, M., *et al* (2004) Does meeting needs improve quality of life? *Psychotherapy and Psychosomatics*, **73**, 183–189.

Slade, M., Leese, M., Cahill, S., *et al* (2005) Patient-rated mental health needs and quality of life improvement. *British Journal of Psychiatry*, **187**, 256–261.

Slade, M., McCrone, P., Kuipers, E., *et al* (2006) Use of standardised outcome measures in adult mental health services: randomised controlled trial. *British Journal of Psychiatry*, **189**, 330–336.

Stevens, A. & Gabbay, J. (1991) Needs assessment needs assessment. *Health Trends*, **23**, 20–23.

Thomas, S., Harty, M., Parrott, J., *et al* (2003) *The Forensic CAN: Camberwell Assessment of Need Forensic Version (CANFOR)*. Gaskell.

Thomas, S. D., Slade, M., McCrone, P., *et al* (2008) The reliability and validity of the Forensic Camberwell Assessment of Need (CANFOR): a needs assessment for forensic mental health service users. *International Journal of Methods in Psychiatric Research*, **17**, 111–120.

Trauer, T., Tobias, G. & Slade, M. (2008) Development and evaluation of a patient-rated version of the Camberwell Assessment of Need Short Appraisal Schedule (CANSAS–P). *Community Mental Health Journal*, **44**, 113–124.

Wiersma, D. & van Busschbach, J. (2001) Are needs and satisfaction of care associated with quality of life? An epidemiological survey among the severely mentally ill in the Netherlands. *European Archives of Psychiatry and Clinical Neuroscience*, **251**, 239–246.

Wiersma, D., Brink, R., Wolters, K., *et al* (2009) Individual unmet needs for care: are they sensitive as outcome criterion for the effectiveness of mental health services interventions? *Social Psychiatry and Psychiatric Epidemiology*, **44**, 317–324.

Xenitidis, K., Thornicroft, G., Leese, M., *et al* (2000) Reliability and validity of the CANDID – a needs assessment instrument for adults with learning disabilities and mental health problems. *British Journal of Psychiatry*, **176**, 473–478.

Xenitidis, K., Slade, M., Bouras, N., *et al* (2003) *CANDID: Camberwell Assessment of Need for Adults with Developmental and Intellectual Disabilities*. Gaskell.

CHAPTER 12

Measuring stigma and discrimination related to mental illness[1]

Elaine Brohan, Mike Slade, Sarah Clement
and Graham Thornicroft

There has been a substantial increase in research on the stigma related to mental illness over the past 10 years (Major & O'Brien, 2005; Weiss *et al*, 2006). This chapter clarifies current practice in one area: the survey measurement of stigma among those who have personal experience of mental illness. The definition and construct of stigma are first discussed, and then the method and results of a review of current measures of personal mental illness stigma are presented.

Defining stigma

The classic starting point for defining the stigma of mental illness is Goffman's 'an attribute that is deeply discrediting'. The recognition of this attribute leads the stigmatised person to be 'reduced ... from a whole and usual person to a tainted or discounted one' (Goffman, 1963, p. 3). This presents stigma as the relationship between attribute and stereotype. In Goffman's terms, attributes can be categorised in three main groups: abominations of the body (e.g. physical disability or visible deformity); blemishes of individual character (e.g. mental illness, criminal conviction); and 'tribal' stigmas (e.g. race, gender, age).

The work of Jones *et al* (1984) built on these categorisations with a focus on the study of 'marked relationships'. In this definition, stigma occurs when the mark links the identified person, via attributional processes, to undesirable characteristics, which discredit him or her. They propose six dimensions of stigma:

1   concealability – how obvious or detectable a characteristic is to others
2   course – whether the difference is lifelong or reversible over time
3   disruptiveness – the impact of the difference on interpersonal relationships

---

1 This chapter is based on Brohan, E., Slade, M., Clement, S., *et al* (2010) Experiences of mental illness stigma, prejudice and discrimination: a review of measures. *BMC Health Services Research*, **10**, 80.

4   aesthetics – whether the difference elicits a reaction of disgust or is perceived as unattractive

5   origin – the causes of the difference, particularly whether the individual is perceived as responsible for this difference

6   peril – the degree to which the difference induces feelings of threat or danger in others.

Elliott *et al* (1982) emphasised the social interaction in stigma. In their definition, stigma is a form of deviance that leads others to judge an individual as illegitimate for participation in a social interaction. This occurs because of a perception that that person lacks the skills or abilities to carry out such an interaction, and is also influenced by judgements about the dangerousness and unpredictability of the person. Once the individual is considered illegitimate, then he or she is beyond the rules of normal social behaviour and may be ignored or excluded by the group.

Link & Phelan (2001) note that the stigma concept has been criticised as being too vaguely defined and individually focused. In response to these criticisms, they define stigma as 'the co-occurrence of its components: labeling, stereotyping, separation, status loss, and discrimination' in a context in which power is exercised (Link & Phelan, 2001, p. 363). Others consider the core elements of stigma to involve the following process: labelling, separation, stereotype awareness, stereotype endorsement, prejudice and discrimination, with social, economic or political power being necessary to stigmatise (Rüsch *et al*, 2005).

Corrigan (2005) has proposed a framework in which stigma is categorised as either public stigma or self-stigma, and within these two domains stigma is broken down into three elements: stereotypes, prejudice and discrimination. This is revised in the definition of Thornicroft *et al* (2007), in which stigma includes three elements: problems of knowledge (ignorance or misinformation); problems of attitudes (prejudice); and problems of behaviour (discrimination).

Phelan *et al* (2008) investigated the possible intersection of conceptual models of stigma and prejudice, and concluded that the two sets of models have much in common, with most differences being a matter of focus and emphasis. They argue that stigma and prejudice have three functions: exploitation and domination (keeping people down); norm enforcement (keeping people in); and disease avoidance (keeping people away).

Research asking people with serious mental illness how they understand the concept of stigma found that this group conceptualised it as encompassing: ignorance, labels, prejudice, isolation, exclusion, being treated differently, being made to feel different and unfair treatment (Rethink, 2009).

For the purpose of this review, stigma is taken as an overarching term to include elements of stereotyping, prejudice and discrimination. This is in keeping with models in which the cognitive, affective and behavioural dimensions of stigma are respectively represented by stereotyping, prejudice and discrimination (Fiske, 1998; Corrigan & Watson, 2002; Thornicroft *et al*, 2007).

Measuring stigma

In this chapter, the personal stigma of mental illness is considered in three main ways: perceived stigma, experienced stigma and self-stigma. Measures of stigma intended for use with groups other than those with personal experience of mental illness are not included in this review.

Perceived stigma

Van Brakel *et al* (2006) provide a definition of research into perceived or felt stigma as that in which 'people with a (potentially) stigmatized health condition are interviewed about stigma and discrimination they fear or perceive to be present in the community or society'. In turn, they draw upon a definition of felt stigma from Scrambler & Hopkins (1986, p. 33), who state that it 'refers principally to the fear of enacted stigma, but also encompasses a feeling of shame associated with [the illness]'. Felt stigma may be thought of as encompassing elements of both perceived stigma and self-stigma. For the purposes of this review, perceived stigma is consistent with the definition of Van Brakel *et al*, and does not include feelings of shame, which are instead included under self-stigma.

LeBel (2008) highlights that perceived stigma can include both the following:

- what an individual thinks *most people* think or believe about the stigmatised group in general
- how the individual thinks *society views him or her personally* as a member of the stigmatised group.

For the purposes of this review, both of these elements are included as perceived stigma.

Experienced stigma

Experienced stigma is the 'experience of actual discrimination and/or participation restrictions on the part of the person affected' (Van Brakel *et al*, 2006). This is similar to Scrambler & Hopkins' (1986, p. 33) concept of enacted stigma or 'instances of discrimination ... on the grounds of their perceived unacceptability or inferiority'. The definition by Van Brakel *et al* is used in this review.

Self-stigma

Corrigan & Watson (2002) use the term 'public stigma' to describe the ways in which the general public stigmatise people with a mental illness. They describe self-stigma as the internalisation of this public stigma. An extended definition describes it as 'the product of internalisation of shame, blame, hopelessness, guilt and fear of discrimination associated with mental illness' (Corrigan, 1998). It has also been defined as a process, either conscious or unconscious, wherein the person with mental illness accepts diminished expectations both for and by himself or herself (Caltaux, 2003).

Van Brakel *et al* (2006) describe it as 'feelings of loss of self-esteem and dignity, fear, shame, guilt, etc.' In this way, it is contains elements of felt stigma, as described above (Scrambler & Hopkins, 1986).

If self-stigma is considered as a reaction to public stigma, then it may be appropriate also to consider measures of other reactions to public stigma under this section, such as energisation, righteous anger or no observable response (Corrigan & Watson, 2002). The coping literature overlaps with this to a large degree, particularly with behavioural aspects of self-stigma such as disclosure or social withdrawal – see Zeidner & Endler (1996) for a review of the coping literature and the Stigma Coping Orientation Scales (Link *et al*, 1989, 2001) for further information. For the purposes of this review, these additional measures of self-stigma were not considered. The focus was solely on instruments which were described as measuring the personal stigma associated with mental illness.

Method of the review

A literature review was conducted to examine the measurement of these three stigma constructs. The Medline, Psychinfo and British Nursing Index databases were searched for journal articles containing the MESH terms 'mental AND ill*' *or* 'mental AND distress' *and* 'stigma*' for the period 1990–2009. A total of 984 articles were located. Papers were included in the review if they included a survey measure of perceived, experienced or self-stigma which had been used with a sample of adults with a primary diagnosis of a mental illness. Only English-language papers were included in the review. Forty-eight papers met these inclusion criteria. The reference lists of these papers were checked and a personal database of stigma papers was also searched. One systematic review of stigma and mental health was located and the reference list was scanned (Mak *et al*, 2007). The reference lists of three review papers on stigma and mental illness were also checked (Link & Phelan, 2001; Link *et al*, 2004; Rüsch *et al*, 2005). This resulted in the identification of a further 27 papers.

Results of the review

From the 75 identified papers, 18 were excluded. The reasons for this are shown in Fig. 12.1. As seen in Fig. 12.1, 57 studies were included in the review. In these studies, 12 measures of mental illness stigma were used. All but one of the papers describing the development of these measures are included in the 57 identified papers. The paper not included was published

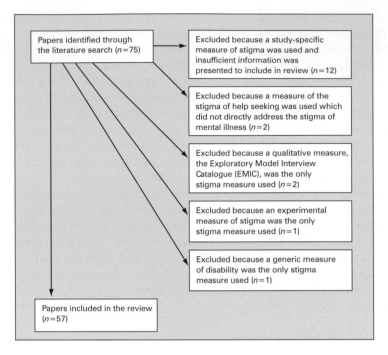

Fig. 12.1 Reasons for exclusion of papers from review.

in 1987, before the period for this review (Link, 1987). Tables 12.1–12.3 give a summary descriptions of the 14 scales identified in the review. In Table 12.1 and below, the subscales of each measure are categorised as measuring perceived, experienced or self-stigma. These categorisations are based on the definitions for these constructs given above. Efforts were made to categorise the subscales in a manner consistent with descriptions in the papers on scale development. In cases where a subscale contained items which fell under more than one construct, the subscale was placed under the construct which represented the most items. The studies are ordered in terms of frequency of studies identified which use the measures. Table 12.2 presents the psychometric properties. Table 12.3 lists the studies in the review that used the identified scales.

Measures of perceived stigma

Seven of the measures in Table 12.1 assess aspects of perceived stigma (the PDD, SSMIS, DSSS, ISE, SESQ, HSS and DISC). This is the most frequently addressed aspect of mental illness stigma, with 45 (79%) of the identified studies using one of these measures. The PDD scale is most commonly used, being applied in 82% of the studies (Link, 1987). This scale measures the individual's perception of how 'most other people' view individuals with a mental illness. Corrigan & Watson (2002) refer to this construct as 'stereotype awareness'. In their measure, the SSMIS, they adapt the PDD to create ten items for inclusion as their 'stereotype awareness' subscale (Corrigan *et al*, 2006). Similarly, the 'feelings of stigmatisation' subscale of the SESQ is an adapted eight-item version of the PDD (Hayward *et al*, 2002). This construct is also known as stigma consciousness (Pinel, 1999). The four-item 'public stigma' subscale of the DSSS also measures stereotype awareness (Kanter *et al*, 2008).

As mentioned above, stereotype awareness is only one aspect of perceived stigma. Several of the other identified scales instead focus on personal expectations or fears of encountering stigma, that is, a personally relevant version of stereotype awareness. This is addressed in the ISE, HSS and DISC. The HSS investigates perceptions of how people feel they have been personally viewed or treated by society (Harvey, 2001). The DISC contains four items which address anticipated discrimination, or the expectation of being stigmatised in various aspects of life (Thornicroft *et al*, 2009). In the two-item perceived stigma subscale of the ISE, one of the items addresses stereotype awareness, while the other addresses personal fear of encountering stigma (Stuart *et al*, 2005).

Measures of experienced stigma

Ten of the measures in Table 12.1 assess aspects of experienced stigma: the ISMI, CESQ, RES, DSSS, SRES, SS, ISE, MIDUS, DISC and EDS. Of the identified studies, 26 (46%) use one of these measures. In all scales, 'experienced stigma' refers to either experiencing stigma in general or a report of experiences of stigma in specific areas of life.

The 'discrimination experience' subscale of the ISMI contains five items which address both perceived and general experiences of discrimination (Ritsher *et al*, 2003). This subscale was included under the category of 'experienced discrimination' as more of the scale items address this construct. The CESQ 'discrimination' subscale asks about experiences of stigma in specific areas of life (Wahl, 1999). In Table 12.1, the CESQ 'stigma' subscale is also placed under the 'experienced stigma' construct. This decision was taken as the majority of items refer to general stigma experiences. The RES is based on 6 items from the SRES (Link *et al*, 1997) and 5 items from the CESQ (Wahl, 1999). The SRES was developed prior to the CESQ and the developers now recommend the use of the CESQ rather than the SRES (Link *et al*, 2004). The 12-item 'discrimination' subscale of the SS asks about general stigma experiences (e.g. 'Have you been talked down to?') and specific experiences (e.g. in education) (King *et al*, 2007). Several items also address feelings about stigma. The ISE asks two general questions about experiences of stigma (Stuart *et al*, 2005). The DSSS 'stigmatising experiences' subscale contains six items which relate to times at which the respondent may have felt stigmatised because of experiencing or disclosing depression (Kanter *et al*, 2008). The DISC contains 32 items

Table 12.1 Constructs of the scales assessing stigma and discrimination

Scale	Measures of perceived stigma	Measures of experienced stigma	Measures of self-stigma	Other
1. Perceived Devaluation and Discrimination Scale (PDD) (Link, 1987)	Perceived discrimination (6 items) Perceived devaluation (6 items)	No	No	No
2. Internalised Stigma of Mental Illness (ISMI) (Ritsher et al, 2003)	No	Discrimination experience (5 items)	Alienation (6 items) Stereotype endorsement (7 items) Social withdrawal (6 items)	Stigma resistance (5 items)
3. Self-stigma of Mental Illness Scale (SSMIS) (Corrigan et al, 2006)	Stereotype awareness (10 items)	No	Stereotype agreement (10 items) Stereotype self-concurrence (10 items) Self-esteem decrement (10 items)	No
4. Consumer Experiences of Stigma Questionnaire (CESQ) (Wahl, 1999)	No	Experiences of stigma (9 items) Experiences of discrimination (12 items)	No	No
5. Rejection Experiences Scale (RES) (Bjorkman et al, 2007)	No	Rejection experiences (11 items)	No	No
6. Depression Self-stigma Scale (DSSS) Kanter et al, 2008)	Public stigma (4 items)	Stigmatising experiences (6 items)	General self-stigma (9 items) Secrecy (9 items)	Treatment stigma (4 items)
7. Self-reported Rejection Experiences Scale (SRES) (Link et al, 1997)	No	Rejection experiences (12 items)	No	No
8. Stigma Scale (SS) King et al, 2007)	No	Discrimination (12 items)	Disclosure (11 items)	Positive aspects (5 items)
9. The Inventory of Stigmatising Experiences (ISE) (Stuart et al, 2005)	Perceived stigma (2 items)	Experienced stigma (2 items)	Social withdrawal (1 item)	Impact of stigma (5 items)

Scale	Measures of perceived stigma	Measures of experienced stigma	Measures of self-stigma	Other
10. Self-esteem and Stigma Questionnaire (SESQ) (Hayward et al, 2002)	Feelings of stigmatisation (8 items)	No	No	Self-esteem (6 items)
11. Stigmatisation Scale (HSS) (Harvey, 2001; Bagley & King, 2005)	Perceived stigma (15 items)	No	No	No
12. MacArthur Foundation Midlife Development in the United States (MIDUS) (Kessler et al, 1999)	No	Major discrimination (11 items) Day-to-day discrimination (11 items)	No	No
13. Discrimination and Stigma Scale (DISC) (Thornicroft et al, 2009)	Anticipated discrimination (4-items)	Experienced discrimination (32 items)	No	No
14. Experiences of Discrimination Scale (EDS) (Thompson et al, 2004)	No	Has discrimination occurred (1 item) Specific settings of discrimination (8 items)	No	Stressfulness of discrimination in specific settings (8 items)

which address experiences of stigma in various areas of life, including work, family and mental health service use (Thornicroft et al, 2009).

Two of the identified measures (the MIDUS and EDS) record experienced stigma as well as multiple reasons for this stigma. Both ask about the perceived reason for poor treatment, including areas such as mental illness, disability, gender, ethnicity/race, age, religion, physical appearance and socioeconomic status. The MIDUS contains 11 items which measure 'major discrimination' and 11 items which measure 'day to day' experiences of discrimination (Kessler et al, 1999). The EDS has eight items which address specific areas in which stigma has been experienced (Thompson et al, 2004).

Measures of self-stigma

Five of the measures assessed aspects of self-stigma: the ISMI, SSMIS, DSSS, SS and ISE. Of the studies identified, 19 (33%) used one of these measures. Self-stigma covers cognitive, affective and behavioural responses to perceived or experienced stigma. All three elements were reflected in the measures reviewed.

Table 12.2 Structure and psychometric properties of the scales assessing stigma and discrimination

Scale (see Table 12.1)	Scale structure and psychometric properties
1. Perceived Devaluation and Discrimination Scale (PDD) (Link, 1987)	12-item self-complete measure. Each item is rated on a six-point Likert scale anchored at 1 = strongly disagree and 6 = strongly agree. The internal consistency of the scale ranges from $\alpha = 0.86$ to $\alpha = 0.88$ (Link et al, 2001).
2. Internalised Stigma of Mental Illness (ISMI) (Ritsher et al, 2003)	29-item self-complete measure. Each item is rated on a four-point Likert scale anchored at 1 = strongly disagree and 4 = strongly agree. Internal consistency ($\alpha = 0.90$), test–retest reliability ($r = 0.92$).
3. Self-stigma of Mental Illness Scale (SSMIS) (Corrigan et al, 2006)	40-item self-complete measure. Each item is rated on a 9-point Likert scale anchored at 0 = strongly disagree and 9 = strongly agree). Internal consistency for subscales ranged from $\alpha = 0.72$ to $\alpha = 0.91$. Test–retest reliability for subscales ranged from 0.68 to 0.82. The stereotype awareness items were adapted from the PDD (Link, 1987).
4. Consumer Experiences of Stigma Questionnaire (CESQ) (Wahl, 1999)	21-item self-complete postal survey. Each item is rated on a five-point Likert scale anchored at 1 = never and 5 = very often. Has also been used as an interview. Psychometric properties not reported.
5. Rejection Experiences Scale (RES) (Bjorkman et al, 2007)	11-item self-complete scale, developed in Swedish. Each item rated on a five-point Likert scale anchored 1 = never and 5 = very often. Internal consistency $\alpha = 0.85$. The scale was developed based on the 6 items from the SRES (Link et al, 1991) and five items from the CESQ (Wahl, 1999).
6. Depression Self-stigma Scale (DSSS) Kanter et al, 2008)	32-item self-complete measure. Each item rated on a seven-point Likert scale anchored at 1 = completely agree and 7 = completely disagree. Internal consistency for subscales range $\alpha = 0.78$ to $\alpha = 0.95$ (Rusch et al, 2008).
7. Self-reported Rejection Experiences Scale (SRES) (Link et al, 1997)	12-item self-complete measure. Six items about experiences related to mental illness and 6 about experiences related to drug use. Each item is scored using a yes/no response. Internal consistency $\alpha = 0.80$. Link et al (2004) recommend the use of the CESQ rather than SRES.
8. Stigma Scale (SS) (King et al, 2007)	28-item self-complete measure. Each item is rated on a four-point Likert scale anchored at 0 = strongly disagree and 4 = strongly agree. Test–retest reliability (kappa range 0.49–0.71) and internal consistency $\alpha = 0.87$
9. The Inventory of Stigmatising Experiences (ISE) (Stuart et al, 2005)	10-item interview-based measure with qualitative components. Each item is scored on a five-point Likert scale anchored at 1 = never and 5 = always. The scale is intended as a measure of 'the extent and impact of stigma'. Stigma experiences scale KR-20 = 0.83, stigma impact scale $\alpha = 0.91$.

Scale (see Table 12.1)	Scale structure and psychometric properties
10. Self-esteem and Stigma Questionnaire (SESQ) (Hayward *et al*, 2002)	14-item self-complete measure. The feelings of stigmatisation items are adapted from the PDD (Link, 1987). It also contains five self-esteem items which address the respondent's confidence in their ability to complete various tasks. A sixth self-esteem item is taken from the Rosenberg (1977) self-esteem scale. All items are rated on a six-point Likert scale, anchored at 1 = strongly agree and 6 = strongly disagree. Internal consistency $\alpha = 0.80$. Item-total correlation $r = 0.4$ or greater for each item. Test–retest stigma scale = 0.63, self-esteem scale (0.71), $\alpha = 0.79$ to 0.71.
11. Stigmatisation Scale (HSS) (Harvey, 2001; Bagley & King, 2005)	15-item self-complete measure. Adapted from 18-item measure by Harvey (2001). Each item is rated on a five-point Likert scale anchored at 0 = never and 4 = always. Internal consistency $\alpha \geq 0.80$.
12. MacArthur Foundation Midlife Development in the United States (MIDUS) (Kessler *et al*, 1999)	22-item interview-based measure. Each item was rated on a five-point Likert scale anchored at 1 = all of the time and 5 = never. Assess discrimination for any reason, including disability, gender, ethnicity/race, age, religion, physical appearance, and SES. The disability category was further split into physical and mental disability. Dichotomous response for each question followed by a frequency scale anchored at 1 = often and 4 = never. Internal consistency $\alpha = 0.87$.
13. Discrimination and Stigma Scale (DISC) (Thornicroft *et al*, 2009)	36-item interview-based measure. All items are rated on a seven-point Likert scale anchored at –3 = strong disadvantage and 3 = strong advantage.
14. Experiences of Discrimination Scale (EDS) (Thompson *et al*, 2004)	Interview-based measure which assesses experienced discrimination resulting from mental illness and other stigmatised identities. It asks whether discrimination has occurred, what the basis for this discrimination was, whether discrimination occurred in eight specific settings and the level of stress associated with discrimination in each setting. Modified version of the Schedule of Racist Events Scale (Landrine & Klonoff, 1996).

Three subscales of the ISMI particularly addressed self-stigma: alienation, stereotype endorsement and social withdrawal (Ritsher *et al*, 2003). These can be considered affective, cognitive and behavioural dimensions respectively. The 'discrimination experience' subscale was excluded as it was considered to measure 'experienced stigma'. The 'stigma resistance' subscale was also excluded. Three subscales of the SSMIS also measure self-stigma: stereotype agreement, stereotype self-concurrence and self-esteem decrement (Corrigan *et al*, 2006). The SS contains a 'disclosure' subscale, which focuses on cognitive, affective and behavioural aspects of disclosure

Table 12.3 Studies using scales to assess stigma and discrimination[a]

Scale	Number of studies found in review using measure
PDD	35
	Link *et al*, 1991; Link *et al*, 1997; Rosenfield, 1997; Markowitz, 1998; Wright *et al*, 2000; Blankertz, 2001; Link *et al*, 2001; Markowitz, 2001; Perlick *et al*, 2001; Sirey *et al*, 2001; Yanos *et al*, 2001; Hayward *et al*, 2002; Link *et al*, 2002; Freidl *et al*, 2003; Ritsher *et al*, 2003; Roeloffs *et al*, 2003; Chung & Wong, 2004; Graf *et al*, 2004; Ritsher & Phelan, 2004; Bagley & King, 2005; Berge & Ranney, 2005; Hansson & Bjorkman, 2005; Kahng & Mowbray, 2005; Knight *et al*, 2006; Mueller *et al*, 2006; Rüsch *et al*, 2006*a,b*; Bjorkman *et al*, 2007; Freidl *et al*, 2007; Lundberg *et al*, 2007; Vauth *et al*, 2007; Freidl *et al*, 2008; Kleim *et al*, 2008; Link *et al*, 2008; Lundberg *et al*, 2008; Lysaker *et al*, 2008*a*; MacInnes & Lewis, 2008
ISMI	7
	Ritsher & Phelan, 2004; Lysaker *et al*, 2007*a,b*; Werner *et al*, 2007; Lysaker *et al*, 2008*a,b*; Yanos *et al*, 2008
SSMIS	5
	Rüsch *et al*, 2006*b*; Tsang *et al*, 2006; Fung *et al*, 2007; Watson *et al*, 2007; Fung *et al*, 2008
CESQ	3
	Dickerson *et al*, 2002; Bagley & King, 2005; Charles *et al*, 2007
RES	3
	Hansoon & Bjorkman, 2005; Lundberg *et al*, 2007; Lundberg *et al*, 2008
DSSS	1
	Rusch *et al*, 2008
SRES	1
	Wright *et al*, 2000

a. No studies were found for scales 8–14, the SS, ISE, SESQ, HSS, MIDUS, DISC and EDS.

(King *et al*, 2007). The ISE contains one item on social withdrawal (Stuart *et al*, 2005). Two subscales of the DSSS address self-stigma: general self-stigma, and secrecy (Kanter *et al*, 2008). General self-stigma includes aspects of personally relevant stereotype awareness (as discussed above). Secrecy addresses a similar construct to the disclosure subscale of the SS and the social withdrawal subscale of the ISMI.

Other subscales

Several other subscales were identified in the review, including 'stigma resistance' in the ISMI (Ritsher *et al*, 2003), 'positive aspects' in the SS (King *et al*, 2007), 'impact of stigma' in the ISE (Stuart *et al*, 2005), 'self-esteem' in the SESQ (Hayward *et al*, 2002), 'treatment stigma' in the DSSS (Kanter *et al*, 2008) and 'stressfulness of discrimination in specific settings' in the EDS (Thompson *et al*, 2004). These subscales did not clearly fit into one of the three stigma constructs. Stigma resistance, positive aspects and self-esteem would most closely fit with self-stigma. Treatment stigma is measuring a related construct, rather than mental illness stigma. Two other measures of help-seeking, the Stigma Scale for Receiving Psychological Help for depression (SSRPH; Komiya *et al*, 2000) and the Self-Stigma of Seeking Help (SSOSH; Vogel *et al*, 2006), were excluded from this review for this reason (see Fig. 12.1). Stressfulness is examining the magnitude of experienced discrimination, so would most clearly fit with this 'other' subscale.

Discussion

This chapter examined definitions of stigma, prejudice and discrimination, and presented a review of the survey measurement of mental illness stigma. Stigma was used as an over-arching term to incorporate stigma, prejudice and discrimination. Fourteen scales were identified that assessed aspects of perceived, experienced and self-stigma in 57 studies. Perceived stigma was most frequently assessed in 79% of studies, followed by experienced discrimination in 46% of studies and self-stigma in 33% of studies. This is in keeping with a previous review which considered the measurement of mental illness stigma among those with personal experience of mental illness ($n = 24$) (Link *et al*, 2004). It found that 50% ($n = 12$) of studies used a survey-based measure of status loss/discrimination (expectations), 33% ($n = 8$) used a survey-based measure of status loss/discrimination (experiences) and 13% ($n = 3$) measured emotional reactions. These categories broadly map onto the perceived, experienced and self-stigma categories used in this chapter. Although interesting to see that the ranking of areas of emphasis is the same, this should be interpreted with caution owing to the different categorisations used and, as the sample includes experimental and qualitative studies as well as those using survey measures, this underemphasises the proportions for survey-based measures alone.

Conclusions

This chapter has provided an overview of commonly used measures of personal mental illness stigma, as a resource to provide guidance on which measure may be most appropriate in future research. This contributes evidence to support the evaluation of outcomes as part of anti-stigma campaigns or social inclusion interventions, fitting with the Medical Research Council's guidance on developing and evaluating complex interventions (Craig *et al*, 2008). It builds on existing reviews by exploring this area of stigma measurement in detail and including recently developed measures.

This chapter has focused on survey measures. However, as mentioned in the discussion, alternative methods of considering this topic (e.g. qualitative and experimental investigations such as Dinos *et al*, 2004 and Teachman *et al*,

2006) provide valuable material and should be consulted by those wishing to use non-survey-based measures.

Throughout the chapter, stigma was categorised as perceived, experienced or self-stigma. These distinctions were useful for organising the chapter. However, many inter-connections exist between the concepts, and there was sometimes difficulty in judging which was the most appropriate to use in categorising a subscale. This points to the complex nature of stigma, as highlighted in the introduction, and reinforces the necessary interplay of cognitive, affective and behavioural aspects of perceived, experienced and self-stigma, in fully understanding the individual's position in relation to stigma.

References

Bagley, C. & King, M. (2005) Exploration of three stigma scales in 83 users of mental health services: implication for campaigns to reduce stigma. *Journal of Mental Health*, 14, 343–355.

Berge, M. & Ranney, M .(2005) Self-esteem and stigma among persons with schizophrenia: implications for mental health. *Care Management Journal*, 6, 139–144.

Bjorkman, T., Svensson, B. & Lundberg, B. (2007) Experiences of stigma among people with severe mental illness. Reliability, acceptability and construct validity of the Swedish versions of two stigma scales measuring devaluation/discrimination and rejection experiences. *Nordic Journal of Psychiatry*, 61, 332–338.

Blankertz, L. (2001) Cognitive components of self esteem for individuals with severe mental illness. *American Journal of Orthopsychiatry*, 71, 457–465.

Caltaux, D. (2003) Internalized stigma: a barrier to employment for people with mental illness. *International Journal of Therapy and Rehabilitation*, 10, 539–543.

Charles, H., Manoranjitham, S. D. & Jacob, K. S. (2007) Stigma and explanatory models among people with schizophrenia and their relatives in Vellore, South India. *International Journal of Social Psychiatry*, 53, 325–332.

Chung, K. F. & Wong, M. C. (2004) Experience of stigma among Chinese mental health patients in Hong Kong. *Psychiatric Bulletin*, 28, 451–454.

Corrigan, P. W. (1998) The impact of stigma on severe mental illness. *Cognitive and Behavioral Practice*, 5, 201–222.

Corrigan, P. W. (2005) *On the Stigma of Mental Illness*. American Psychological Association.

Corrigan, P. W. & Watson, A. C. (2002) The paradox of self-stigma and mental illness. *Clinical Psychology: Science and Practice*, 9, 35–53.

Corrigan, P. W., Watson, A. C. & Barr, L. (2006) The self-stigma of mental illness: implications for self-esteem and self-efficacy. *Journal of Social and Clinical Psychology*, 25, 875–884.

Craig, P., Dieppe, P., MacIntyre, S., *et al* (2008) Developing and evaluating complex interventions: the new Medical Research Council guidance. *BMJ*, 337, 979–983.

Dickerson, F. B., Sommerville, J., Origoni, A. E., *et al* (2002) Experiences of stigma among outpatients with schizophrenia. *Schizophrenia Bulletin*, 28, 143–156.

Dinos, S., Stevens, S., Serfaty, M., *et al* (2004) Stigma: the feelings and experiences of 46 people with mental illness. Qualitative study. *British Journal of Psychiatry*, 184, 176–181.

Elliott, G. C., Ziegler, H. L., Altman, B. M., *et al* (1982) Understanding stigma: dimensions of deviance and coping. *Deviant Behaviour*, 3, 275–300.

Fiske, S. (1998) Stereotyping, prejudice, and discrimination. In *The Handbook of Social Psychology* (eds D. T. Gilbert & S. T. Fiske), pp. 357–411. McGraw-Hill.

Freidl, M., Lang, T. & Scherer, M. (2003) How psychiatric patients perceive the public's stereotype of mental illness. *Social Psychiatry and Psychiatric Epidemiology*, **38**, 269–275.

Freidl, M., Spitzl, S. P., Prause, W., *et al* (2007) The stigma of mental illness: anticipation and attitudes among patients with epileptic, dissociative or somatoform pain disorder. *International Review of Psychiatry*, **19**, 123–129.

Freidl, M., Spitzl, S. P. & Aigner, M. (2008) How depressive symptoms correlate with stigma perception of mental illness. *International Review of Psychiatry*, **20**, 510–514.

Fung, K. M., Tsang, H. W., Corrigan, P. W., *et al* (2007) Measuring self-stigma of mental illness in China and its implications for recovery. *International Journal of Social Psychiatry*, **53**, 408–418.

Fung, K. M., Tsang, H. W. & Corrigan, P. W. (2008) Self-stigma of people with schizophrenia as predictor of their adherence to psychosocial treatment. *Psychiatric Rehabilitation Journal*, **32**, 95–104.

Goffman, I. (1963) *Stigma: Notes on the Management of Spoiled Identity.* Penguin Books.

Graf, J., Lauber, C., Nordt, C., *et al* (2004) Perceived stigmatization of mentally ill people and its consequences for the quality of life in a Swiss population. *Journal of Nervous and Mental Disease*, **192**, 542–547.

Hansson, L. & Bjorkman, T. (2005) Empowerment in people with a mental illness: reliability and validity of the Swedish version of an empowerment scale. *Scandinavian Journal of Caring Sciences*, **19**, 32–38.

Harvey, R. D. (2001) Individual differences in the phenomenological impact of social stigma. *Journal of Social Psychology*, **141**, 174–189.

Hayward, P., Wong, G., Bright, J. A., *et al* (2002) Stigma and self-esteem in manic depression: an exploratory study. *Journal of Affective Disorders*, **69**, 61–67.

Jones, E., Farina, A., Hastorf, A., *et al* (1984) *Social Stigma: The Psychology of Marked to Relationships.* W. H. Freeman.

Kahng, S. K. & Mowbray, C. T. (2005) What affects self-esteem of persons with psychiatric disabilities: the role of causal attributions of mental illnesses. *Psychiatric Rehabilitation Journal*, **28**, 354–361.

Kanter, J. W. P., Rusch, L. C. M. & Brondino, M. J. P. (2008) Depression Self-Stigma: a new measure and preliminary findings. *Journal of Nervous and Mental Disease*, **196**, 663–670.

Kessler, R. C., Mickelson, K. D. & Williams, D. R. (1999) The prevalence, distribution, and mental health correlates of perceived discrimination in the United States. *Journal of Health and Social Behavior*, **40**, 208–230.

King, M., Dinos, S., Shaw, J., *et al* (2007) The Stigma Scale: development of a standardised measure of the stigma of mental illness. *British Journal of Psychiatry*, **190**, 248–254.

Kleim, B., Vauth, R., Adam, G., *et al* (2008) Perceived stigma predicts low self-efficacy and poor coping in schizophrenia. *Journal of Mental Health*, **17**, 482–491.

Knight, M. T. D., Wykes, T. & Hayward, P. (2006) Group treatment of perceived stigma and self-esteem in schizophrenia: a waiting list trial of efficacy. *Behavioural and Cognitive Psychotherapy*, **34**, 305–318.

Komiya, N., Good, G. E. & Sherrod, N. B. (2000) Emotional openness as a predictor of college students' attitudes toward seeking psychological help. *Journal of Counseling Psychology*, **47**, 138–143.

Landrine, H. & Klonoff, E. A. (1996) The Schedule of Racist Events: a measure of racial discrimination and a study of its negative physical and mental health consequences. *Journal of Black Psychology*, **22**, 144–168.

LeBel, T. (2008) Perceptions of and responses to stigma. *Sociology Compass*, **2**, 409–432.

Link, B. G. (1987) Understanding labeling effects in the area of mental disorders: an assessment of the effect of expectations of rejection. *American Journal of Community Psychology*, **11**, 261–273.

Link, B. G. & Phelan, J. C. (2001) Conceptualizing stigma. *Annual Review of Sociology*, **27**, 363–385.

Link, B. G., Cullen, F. T., Struening, E., *et al* (1989) A modified labeling theory approach to mental disorders: an empirical assessment. *American Sociological Review*, **54**, 400–423.

Link, B. G., Mirotznik, J. & Cullen, F. T. (1991) The effectiveness of stigma coping orientations: can negative consequences of mental illness labeling be avoided? *Journal of Health and Social Behavior*, **32**, 302–320.

Link, B. G., Struening, E. L., Rahav, M., *et al* (1997) On stigma and its consequences: evidence from a longitudinal study of men with dual diagnosis of mental illness and substance abuse. *Journal of Health and Social Behavior*, **38**, 177–190.

Link, B. G., Struening, E. L., Neese-Todd, S., *et al* (2001) Stigma as a barrier to recovery: the consequences of stigma for the self-esteem of people with mental illness. *Psychiatric Services*, **52**, 1621–1626.

Link, B. G., Struening, E. L., Neese-Todd, S., *et al* (2002) On describing and seeking to change the experience of stigma. *Psychiatric Rehabilitation Skills*, **6**, 201–231.

Link, B. G., Yang, L. H., Phelan, J. C., *et al* (2004) Measuring mental illness stigma. *Schizophrenia Bulletin*, **30**, 511–541.

Link, B. G., Castille, D. M. & Stuber, J. (2008) Stigma and coercion in the context of outpatient treatment for people with mental illnesses. *Social Science and Medicine*, **67**, 409–419.

Lundberg, B., Hansson, L., Wentz, E., *et al* (2007) Sociodemographic and clinical factors related to devaluation/discrimination and rejection experiences among users of mental health services. *Social Psychiatry and Psychiatric Epidemiology*, **42**, 295–300.

Lundberg, B., Hansson, L., Wentz, E., *et al* (2008) Stigma, discrimination, empowerment and social networks: a preliminary investigation of their influence on subjective quality of life in a Swedish sample. *International Journal of Social Psychiatry*, **54**, 47–55.

Lysaker, P. H., Davis, L. W., Warman, D. M., *et al* (2007*a*) Stigma, social function and symptoms in schizophrenia and schizoaffective disorder: associations across 6 months. *Psychiatry Research*, **149**, 89–95.

Lysaker, P. H., Roe, D. & Yanos, P. T. (2007*b*) Toward understanding the insight paradox: internalized stigma moderates the association between insight and social functioning, hope, and self-esteem among people with schizophrenia spectrum disorders. *Schizophrenia Bulletin*, **33**, 192–199.

Lysaker, P. H., Tsai, J., Yanos, P., *et al* (2008*a*) Associations of multiple domains of self-esteem with four dimensions of stigma in schizophrenia. *Schizophrenia Research*, **98**, 194–200.

Lysaker, P. H., Buck, K. D., Taylor, A. C., *et al* (2008*b*) Associations of metacognition and internalized stigma with quantitative assessments of self-experience in narratives of schizophrenia. *Psychiatry Research*, **157**, 31–38.

MacInnes, D. L. & Lewis, M. (2008) The evaluation of a short group programme to reduce self-stigma in people with serious and enduring mental health problems. *Journal of Psychiatric and Mental Health Nursing*, **15**, 59–65.

Major, B. & O'Brien, L. T. (2005) The social psychology of stigma. *Annual Review of Psychology*, **56**, 393–421.

Mak, W. W. S., Poon, C. Y. M., Pun, L. Y. K., *et al* (2007) Meta-analysis of stigma and mental health. *Social Science and Medicine*, **65**, 245–261.

Markowitz, F. E. (1998) The effects of stigma on the psychological well-being and life satisfaction of persons with mental illness. *Journal of Health and Social Behavior*, **39**, 335–347.

Markowitz, F. E. (2001) Modeling processes in recovery from mental illness: relationships between symptoms, life satisfaction, and self-concept. *Journal of Health and Social Behavior*, **42**, 64–79.

Mueller, B., Nordt, C., Lauber, C., *et al* (2006) Social support modifies perceived stigmatization in the first years of mental illness: a longitudinal approach. *Social Science and Medicine*, **62**, 39–49.

Perlick, D. A., Rosenheck, R. A., Clarkin, J. F., *et al* (2001) Stigma as a barrier to recovery: adverse effects of perceived stigma on social adaptation of persons diagnosed with bipolar affective disorder. *Psychiatric Services*, **52**, 1627–1632.

Phelan, J. C., Link, B. G. & Dovidio, J. F. (2008) Stigma and prejudice: one animal or two? *Social Science and Medicine*, **67**, 358–367.

Pinel, E. C. (1999) Stigma consciousness: the psychological legacy of social stereotypes. *Journal of Personality and Social Psychology*, **76**, 114–128.

Rethink (2009) *How Can We Make Mental Health Education Work? Example of a Successful Programme Challenging Stigma and Discrimination*. Rethink.

Ritsher, J. B. & Phelan, J. C. (2004) Internalized stigma predicts erosion of morale among psychiatric outpatients. *Psychiatry Research*, **129**, 257–265.

Ritsher, J. B., Otilingam, P. G. & Grajales, M. (2003) Internalized stigma of mental illness: psychometric properties of a new measure. *Psychiatry Research*, **121**, 31–49.

Roeloffs, C., Sherbourne, C., Unutzer, J., *et al* (2003) Stigma and depression among primary care patients. *General Hospital Psychiatry*, **25**, 311–315.

Rosenberg, M. (1977) *Conceiving the Self*. Basic Books.

Rosenfield, S. (1997) Labeling mental illness: the effects of received services and perceived stigma on life satisfaction. *American Sociological Review*, **62**, 660–672.

Rusch, L. C. M., Kanter, J. W. P., Manos, R. C. M., *et al* (2008) Depression stigma in a predominantly low income African American Sample with elevated depressive symptoms. *Journal of Nervous and Mental Disease*, **196**, 919–922.

Rüsch, N., Angermeyer, M. C. & Corrigan, P. W. (2005) Mental illness stigma: concepts, consequences, and initiatives to reduce stigma. *European Psychiatry*, *20*(8), 529–539.

Rüsch, N., Holzer, A., Hermann, C., *et al* (2006*a*) Self-stigma in women with borderline personality disorder and women with social phobia. *Journal of Nervous and Mental Disease*, **194**, 766–773.

Rüsch, N., Lieb, K., Bohus, M., *et al* (2006*b*) Self-stigma, empowerment and perceived legitimacy of discrimination among women with mental illness. *Psychiatric Services*, **57**, 399–402.

Scrambler, G. & Hopkins, A. (1986) Being epileptic: coming to terms with stigma. *Sociology of Health and Illness*, **8**, 26–43.

Sirey, J. A., Bruce, M. L., Alexopoulos, G. S., *et al* (2001) Stigma as a barrier to recovery: perceived stigma and patient-rated severity of illness as predictors of antidepressant drug adherence. *Psychiatric Services*, **52**, 1615–1620.

Stuart, H., Milev, R. & Koller, M. (2005) The Inventory of Stigmatizing Experiences: its development and reliability. *World Psychiatry*, **4**, 33–37.

Teachman, B. A., Wilson, J. G. & Komarovskaya, I. (2006) Implicit and explicit stigma of mental illness in diagnosed and healthy samples. *Journal of Social and Clinical Psychology*, **25**, 75–95.

Thompson, V. L., Noel, J. G. & Campbell, J. (2004) Stigmatization, discrimination, and mental health: the impact of multiple identity status. *American Journal of Orthopsychiatry*, **74**, 529–544.

Thornicroft, G., Rose, D., Kassam, A., *et al* (2007) Stigma: ignorance, prejudice or discrimination? *British Journal of Psychiatry*, **190**, 192–193.

Thornicroft, G., Brohan, E., Rose, D., *et al* (2009) Global pattern of anticipated and experienced discrimination against people with schizophrenia. *Lancet*, **373**, 408–415.

Tsang, H. W. H., Fung, K. M. T. & Corrigan, P. W. (2006) Psychosocial treatment compliance scale for people with psychotic disorders. *Australian and New Zealand Journal of Psychiatry*, **40**, 561–569.

Van Brakel, W. H., Anderson, A. M., Mutatkar, R. K., *et al* (2006) The Participation Scale: measuring a key concept in public health. *Disability and Rehabilitation*, **28**, 193–203.

Vauth, R., Kleim, B., Wirtz, M., *et al* (2007) Self-efficacy and empowerment as outcomes of self-stigmatizing and coping in schizophrenia. *Psychiatry Research*, **150**, 71–80.

Vogel, D. L., Wade, N. G. & Haake, S. (2006) Measuring self-stigma associated with seeking psychological help. *Journal of Counseling Psychology*, **53**, 325–337.

Wahl, O. F. (1999) Mental health consumers experience of stigma. *Schizophrenia Bulletin*, **25**, 467–478.

Watson, A. C., Corrigan, P., Larson, J. E., *et al* (2007) Self-stigma in people with mental illness. *Schizophrenia Bulletin*, **33**, 1312–1318.

Weiss, M. G., Ramakrishna, J. & Somma, D. (2006) Health-related stigma: rethinking concepts and interventions. *Psychology, Health and Medicine*, **11**, 277–287.

Werner, P., Aviv, A. & Barak, Y. (2007) Self-stigma, self-esteem and age in persons with schizophrenia. *International Psychogeriatrics*, **20**, 174–187.

Wright, E. R., Gronfein, W. P. & Owens, T. J. (2000) Deinstitutionalization, social rejection, and the self-esteem of former mental patients. *Journal of Health and Social Behavior*, **41**, 68–90.

Yanos, P. T., Rosenfeld, S. & Horowitz, A. V. (2001) Negative and supportive social interactions and quality of life among persons diagnosed with severe mental illness. *Community Mental Health Journal*, **37**, 405–419.

Yanos, P. T., Roe, D., Markus, K., *et al* (2008) Pathways between internalized stigma and outcomes related to recovery in schizophrenia spectrum disorders. *Psychiatric Services*, **59,** 1437–1442.

Zeidner, M. & Endler, N. S. (1996) *Handbook of Coping: Theory, Research, Applications*. John Wiley & Sons.

Part III
Symptom severity outcome measures

CHAPTER 13

Top-down versus bottom-up measures of depression

David Goldberg

How a clinician decides the severity of a depression

In order to make the *diagnosis* of depressive episode, a clinician merely has to be satisfied that there are five or more depressive symptoms from a list of nine, present for at least 2 weeks. It should be remembered that the concept is atheoretical, and is derived from the collective clinical experience of international psychiatrists, who have decided to draw an arbitrary line between what will count as 'clinically significant' and what they will regarded as 'subclinical'.

In order to decide *how severe* such an episode is, other things must also be taken into account, including suicidal risk, the presence of a history or a family history of depression, and the degree of disability associated with the depressive symptoms. ICD–10 (World Health Organization, 1992) defines three degrees of severity:

- F32.0 Mild depressive episode. Depressed mood, loss of interest, increased fatiguability – at least two of these, plus two of the other seven symptoms. None of the symptoms should be present to an intense degree. The minimum episode length is 2 weeks. The individual is usually distressed by the symptoms and has some difficulty continuing with ordinary work and social activities, but does not cease to function completely.
- F32.1 Moderate depressive episode. At least two of the above three, plus either three or four other symptoms. Several symptoms are present in marked degree. An individual will usually have considerable difficulty continuing social, work and domestic activities.
- F32.2 Severe depressive episode. The sufferer usually shows considerable distress or agitation – unless retardation is a marked feature. Loss of self-esteem and feelings of uselessness or guilt are likely to be prominent and suicide is a distinct danger. A somatic syndrome is usually present. All three of the above three symptoms are present, plus at least four of the others, some of which are of severe intensity. If symptoms are widespread and severe, the diagnosis can be

made in less than 2 weeks. It very unlikely that a person with a severe depressive episode could continue social, domestic or work activities, except to a very limited extent.

This adds distress, intensity and impairment to the list of symptoms, but there are problems with each of these. There is no accepted definition of distress, but a simple enquiry about how much the symptoms just described upset the patient is probably sufficient, if only to distinguish between sub-clinical and mild depression. Intensity can probably be dealt with the reply to much the same question, since it follows that an 'intense' symptom will be distressing, so if many symptoms are present the clinician can re-phrase the same question, and ask 'Which of these symptoms are the most distressing?'

There are two problems with social impairment, the first being that some people allow themselves to be functionally disabled at very low symptom levels, while more phlegmatic people may continue with their usual activities despite experiencing many symptoms. The other is a more difficult problem, since impairment is a global concept affecting the entire individual – we can be socially impaired for many reasons other than depression, and it may be difficult to decide whether undoubted impairment is due to depression or some other factor, such as a physical illness. In the case of those who were not impaired at all before their depressive symptoms started but are now impaired, there is no problem – but if there was pre-existing impairment then the clinician must decide on the size of the incremental increase in impairment. This may not be at all easy to do.

Top-down measures of the severity of depression

Since the concept of depression is itself quite arbitrary, one approach is 'top down' and simply uses the list of symptoms in one of the international classifications. For example, the nine-item Patient Health Questionnaire (PHQ–9; Kroenke et al, 2001) simply uses the symptoms listed in DSM–IV (American Psychiatric Association, 1994), each of which is rated on a four-point frequency scale, ranging from 'not at all' to 'nearly every day'. This approach produces a very close fit with DSM diagnoses made by a clinician, since it is using almost identical criteria. The main difference between the DSM criteria and the PHQ–9 is that the wording has been modified – so, instead of asking about 'recurrent thoughts of death' it asks about 'thoughts that you would be better off dead or of hurting yourself in some way', although there is little difference in meaning.

This measure is widely used in primary care to detect depression in both the USA and the UK – and probably in many other places as well. The authors have provided data on the best thresholds to use in detecting clinically significant depression, and in deciding on the severity of a particular episode. They point out that disability bears a linear relationship to PHQ score, so it is unclear that there would be any advantage in assessing this.

Before one turns to other ways of measuring severity, it should be remembered that before one adds extra data to the PHQ–9 it would be necessary to show that the additions produced some incremental advantage in assessing severity. The possible additions would include a measure of symptom severity, and the presence of a personal or family history of depression, but probably not a measure of impairment. Only the first of these could readily be included in the measure if numerical use was to be made of the overall score.

Bottom-up measures of depression

It is quite possible that depression manifests itself differently in different cultures, or at different ages, or between men and women. If that is so, a measure which implicitly imposes a universal definition of depression on the whole world might be mistaken.

The only way to produce a psychometrically satisfactory dimensional scale to assess the severity of a diagnosis is to evaluate a large set of potential test items with a large normal population, without skip-outs. These would then be subjected to an item-response theory (IRT) analysis, in order to select non-identical items, with good slopes and differing in the severity at which 50% of the population endorses them.

Oddly enough, no such data-set appears to exist, as IRT analysis was not greatly used in the days when the best measures were devised, and conventional factor analysis (FA) was used instead. Although this does not permit exact estimates of the discriminatory power of each potential item, FA does permit items to be discarded which have low loads on factors that seem marginal to the assessment of depression. The first stage in such a procedure should be to collect a large set of items that may characterise people with depression and carry out a conventional *item analysis* to determine which are best at discriminating between people with depression and normal people. This would lead to the creation of a smaller set of items that are to be used in the final instrument.

As can be seen from Table 13.1, some investigators have done this – but others seem to have decided *a priori* which items best characterise depression, so that their final list (column 3) is identical to their initial list (column 2). The table suggests that many scales comprise the same items that were assumed to be important from the clinical experience of the test designers, without any form of data reduction. This is especially true of some of the older scales. In the older studies, before DSM–III (American Psychiatric Association, 1980) introduced research diagnoses, investigators clearly felt free to define depression in their own idiosyncratic way, so that there was no need for data reduction. Some of these early investigators clearly had a closer approximation to the present orthodoxy than others – for example, the Beck Depression Inventory (BDI) and the Montgomery–Åsberg Depression Rating Scale (MADRS) both emerge pretty well, but the Hamilton Rating

Table 13.1 Comparison of seven better-known scales giving continuous measures of the severity of depression

Name of scale	No. of items considered	No. of items adopted	Cronbach's alpha	Comment
Hamilton Rating Scale for Depression Scale (HRSD; Hamilton, 1960, 1980)	21	17	0.46–0.85	4 items discarded because 'difficult to define' or 'difficult to differentiate'. A single general factor 'cannot be extracted' (Maier et al, 1985; Cialdella et al, 1989). One-factor conventional factor analysis explains only 36% of variance. Scale not internally consistent (Uher et al, 2008). Many items are poor contributors to the severity of depression; others have poor interrater reliability. Factor structure multidimensional with poor replicability (Bagby, 2004)
Beck Depression Inventory (BDI; Beck et al, 1961; Beck & Steer, 1984)	21	21	0.92	Highly inter-correlated first-order factors (Beck et al, 1988). Others (Storch et al, 2004; Ward, 2006; Siegert et al, 2009) claim 2 subscales: affective and somatic symptoms. An approach using M-plus (Thombs et al, 2008) argues for overall total score measuring general depression, and 2 uncorrelated factors measuring somatic (5 items) and cognitive (8 items). BDI shows robust association with severity, but poor assessment of observed mood (Bush et al, 2004)
Center for Epidemiologic Studies Depression (CES–D; Radloff, 1977)	Unknown	20	0.82[a]	Originally 4 factors: self-worth; depressed affect; positive affect; somatic symptoms. However, elsewhere than in the USA 5 papers report only 2 factors (Barlow & Wright, 1998; Cheung & Bagley, 1998; Edman et al, 1999; Meyer & Hautzinger, 2003; Lee & Chokkanathan, 2008) and 3 report 3 factors (Dick et al, 1994; Ghubash et al, 2000; Thomas & Brantley, 2004). More seriously, the proportion of false positives has been found to be high (Zich et al, 1990; Beekman et al, 1997; Batistoni et al, 2007)

Name of scale	No. of items considered	No. of items adopted	Cronbach's alpha	Comment
Montgomery–Åsberg Depression Rating Scale (MADRS; Montgomery & Åsberg, 1979)	65	10	0.61–0.91	3 studies found a 3-factor solution (Galinowski & Lehert, 1995; Suzuki *et al*, 2005; Higuchi *et al*, 2008), with dysphoria (6 items), cognitive (2 items) and neuro-vegetative symptoms (2 items); each item rated on 6-point scale. There is a robust association with severity. The coverage of 3 major areas of depression is superior to the BDI, which is strongest on cognitive items (Snaith *et al*, 1978)
Children's Depression Inventory (CDI; Kovacs, 1985)	21 from the BDI, plus 7 extra	27	0.70–0.86	Extra items added to BDI to allow for school, conduct and social problems to emerge. Original study found 5 factors: externalising; dysphoria; self-depreciation; school problems; social problems. Large community study replicated this (Craighead *et al*, 1998). A study using IRT on 779 US children between grades 3 and 6 found an invariant measure across gender and age (Carle, 2003)
Inventory of Depressive Symptoms (IDS; Rush *et al*, 1986)	28	16 (QIDS)	0.81–0.94	Rush et al (1996) found 4 factors: mood and cognition; anxious hypochondriacal; endogenous factors; atypical features. IRT used to prepare Quick Inventory of Depressive States (QIDS). Only 23 respondents were 'normals'. No data on unselected community normals. Few replications
Patient Health Questionnaire (PHQ–9; Kroenke *et al*, 2001)	9	9	0.83–0.92	The only 'top-down' measure. Three studies show only one factor (Huang *et al*, 2006; Cameron *et al*, 2008; Dum *et al*, 2008); two others (Krause et al, 2008; Richardson & Richards, 2008) show two: general depression and somatic items

a. Bush *et al*, 2004.

227

Scale for Depression (HRSD) seems less good (Uher *et al*, 2008) – and has even been described as a 'lead weight rather than a gold standard' (Bagby, 2004). Of these, only the MADRS undertook the data reduction that seems desirable in constructing a psychometric test.

Having decided upon the list of symptoms that are to be used, the investigators next determine the internal consistency of their scale using Cronbach's α (column 4) and may also determine the ability of their scale to respond to changes in their patients' clinical state. In general, most of the scales appear to have acceptable levels of internal consistency, although some studies have found unacceptably low levels for both the HRSD and the MADRS.

The next step is to determine whether the scale has the same structure in other cultures – since most of the scales are adopted in other countries. The best way of doing this is to find whether the scale has 'factor invariance' when used elsewhere than in the original country. There are some important caveats to note before firm conclusions can be drawn from disparities in data from different countries. There are many forms of multivariate analysis, and the emerging results will be partly determined by the assumptions made in each form of analysis. Different criteria for extracting factors, and whether results given are unrotated, varimax or oblique, will all necessarily affect the factor structure that emerges. Scales based on IRT are likely to produce the items most discriminant between people with depression and normal people, as well as a range of the severities at which 50% of respondents will endorse the item. Analyses conducted in community samples will provide information about the structure of depressive symptoms in normal people, while clinical samples may provide more information about the structure of more severe forms of depressive illness. Before concluding that the structure of the depressive symptoms included in a particular test is different between country A and country B, the population samples need to be selected in much the same way. Thus, minor discrepancies in the number of factors in a scale should probably be discounted.

It can therefore be seen that conclusions drawn from any discrepancies must be tentative. There seem to have been few independent studies investigating the Inventory of Depressive Symptoms, so no firm conclusions can be drawn at this stage. Despite the fact that the HRSD is almost 50 years old and extensively used, it should possibly be pensioned off now. There are better measures – the MADRS covers a good range of depressive symptoms, and both it and the BDI are highly sensitive to change.

Scales aiming to assess both depression and anxiety symptoms

There have been many such scales, and here we will only consider two older scales prepared by psychiatrists, and two newer ones prepared by clinical psychologists (see Table 13.2).

The Symptom Checklist (SCL–90) contains scales for both depression and anxiety, and there was a modest data reduction by correlation with other depression measures. As can be seen from Table 13.2, factor invariance simply does not exist, nor has the scale been validated against modern diagnostic criteria.

The Hospital Anxiety and Depression Scale (HAD), later expanded to include irritability (Snaith *et al*, 1978), was especially designed for use with patients who are also physically ill, and it excludes symptoms of depression that are commonly caused by physical illness. However, the selection of depressive items is odd and subsequent studies have not replicated the original assumptions of the authors of the scale.

The Positive and Negative Affect Scales (PANAS) come from a distinguished team of clinical psychologists, and as one would expect the method of test construction seems to have been impeccable. However, there is no attempt to relate low positive affect to the diagnosis of clinical depression, and the authors content themselves with relationships with other depression scales, such as the BDI.

The Depression, Anxiety and Stress Scales (DASS) have also been impeccably constructed. Factor invariance, while not perfect, is certainly very good. There is some evidence of a ceiling effect with the depression scale (Page *et al*, 2007) and the anxiety scale is not independent of the scale for depression – but it hardly could be. One study (Gloster *et al*, 2008) examined area under the receiver operating characteristic (ROC) curve for depression and dysthymia, and found this to be 0.79. Antony *et al* (1998) validated DASS scores against four DSM diagnoses assessed by the Structured Clinical Interview for DSM (SCID) and normal controls (see Table 13.3) and similar data are presented by Brown *et al* (1997). It can be seen that while those with major depression indeed have the highest depression scores, the three anxiety diagnoses have the lowest anxiety scores – instead, they have high 'stress' scores, although not so high as the stress scores of respondents with major depression. Furthermore, the standard deviations are fairly wide – so that there must be considerable overlap between the various diagnostic groups. In terms of Clark & Watson's (1991) tripartite theory, it would seem that the stress scale of the DASS is perhaps equivalent to the general distress or negative affect scale in the tripartite model – where the symptoms are shared between various non-psychotic diagnoses. We see from Table 13.3 that the 'stress' symptoms are greatest in major depressive disorder, panic and obsessive–compulsive disorder, rather lower in specific phobia and of course lowest among normal controls.

Conclusion

All the scales discussed will provide the researcher with a dimensional measure of depression, so that statements can be made about the severity of the disorder being described. Those who prefer international consensus

Table 13.2 Comparison of four better-known scales giving continuous measures of the severity of depression as well as a measure of anxiety

Name of scale	No. of items considered	No. of items adopted	Cronbach's alpha	Comment
Symptom Check List (SCL–90; Derogatis et al, 1976)	13 depression items	8 depression items	0.70	Derived from Hopkins Symptom Checklist. Each item rated on a 5-point distress scale. Factor invariance across gender (Derogatis & Cleary, 1977). Original 9-factor structure not confirmed by others – 11 factors (Pariente et al, 1989), 10 factors (Jerabek et al, 1982), 5 factors (Hoffmann & Overall, 1978). Different factors for different populations (Schwarzwald et al, 1991). Both Schwarzwald et al (1991) and Cyr et al (1985) argue that the scale is best thought of as a general distress scale
Hospital Anxiety Depression Scale (HAD; Snaith et al, 1978; Zigmond & Snaith, 1983)	8 depression items	7 depression items	0.71–0.80	Depression items chosen by eliminating items that may be caused by physical disease, then choosing 'anhedonic' items from a paper dealing with symptoms responding to drug therapy. Item removed had poor correlation with clinical assessment. Each item rated on 4-point frequency scale. Originally two independent factors were described, but 4 studies found 3 factors (Andersson, 1993; Leung et al, 1993; Martin & Thompson, 2000; McCue et al, 2006) and 2 studies that the factors were correlated (Moorey et al, 1991; Mykletun et al, 2001). Others found items loading on the wrong factor (Thomas et al, 2005) and total HAD score correlating better with independent measures of anxiety and depression than either of the subscales (Lisspers et al, 1997)

Name of scale	No. of items considered	No. of items adopted	Cronbach's alpha	Comment
Positive and Negative Affect Scale (PANAS; Watson et al, 1988)	65	20	0.86–0.90	Final selection of items was by choosing those with highest loads on the appropriate factor. Two factors (positive and negative affect) independent of one another in most studies, but 2 studies show they are not completely so (Crawford & Henry, 2004; Kawata, 2006); 2 studies show good factor invariance (Robles & Paez, 2003; Wang et al, 2007) but 2 others only fair factor invariance (Killgore, 2000; Gaudreau et al, 2006)
Depression, Anxiety and Stress Scales (DASS; Lovibond & Lovibond, 1993)	30 depression items	7 depression items (total for DASS: 21)	0.91–0.96	Data reduced by discarding items on sleep and appetite; then, by conventional factor analysis, choosing 7 best items. Five studies (Clara et al, 2001; Daza, 2002; Crawford & Henry, 2003; Henry & Crawford, 2005; Gloster et al, 2008) confirm the original 3-factor solution of the 3 scales, and show high correlations with other measures of anxiety and depression, in both clinical and community samples. Three studies include clinical diagnoses (Brown et al, 1997; Antony et al, 1998; Gloster et al, 2008). One small Portuguese study (Apostolo et al, 2006) found only 2 factors – anxiety and stress, and depression. Page et al (2007) argued that there is a ceiling effect in the depression scale. Brown et al (1997) argued that the correlation is only –0.45 between DASS depression and positive affect and +0.57 with negative affect in PANAS, and that the scales are themselves inter-correlated: DASS depression +0.45 with DASS anxiety and +0.66 with DASS stress

Table 13.3 Comparison of scores of diagnostic groups and controls on the 21-item Depression, Anxiety and Stress Scales (DASS)

Diagnostic group[a]	Mean (SD) DASS score		
	Stress	Depression	Anxiety
Major depressive disorder ($n = 46$)	24.30, (9.84)	29.96 (9.18)	14.04 (9.78)
Specific phobia ($n = 74$)	13.29 (11.85)	10.82 (11.25)	6.59 (6.59)
Panic disorder ($n = 67$)	16.57 (10.91)	13.19 (9.28)	12.22 (10.20)
Obsessive–compulsive disorder ($n = 54$)	17.57 (10.67)	13.34 (11.51)	8.8 (6.69)
Normal controls ($n = 49$)	3.51 (3.78)	2.12 (3.64)	1.22 (1.77)

[a] Diagnosis made using the Structured Clinical Interview for DSM (SCID).
After Antony *et al* (1998).

regarding the essential nature of depression will no doubt prefer the simple symptom-frequency counts recommended by Kroenke *et al* (2001), despite the lack of any ultimate validating criterion – except, of course, the consensus views of international psychiatrists. Until further empirical research shows that much is gained by adding extra variables – such as distress or intensity – to the measure, it must remain a simple score on the PHQ–9.

Those who prefer an approach which starts with trawling through a fairly wide range of depressive phenomena and producing a shorter scale with at least fair factor invariance should choose between the BDI and the MADRS, depending on whether they wish to use a scale with several neuro-vegetative symptoms.

Those who prefer a bottom-up approach should probably use the DASS, but if they do so they should understand that the ability of such scales to identify those with major depression is fairly limited and that, typically, few of the participants in such studies are experiencing severe depression.

References

American Psychiatric Association (1980) *Diagnostic and Statistical Manual of Mental Disorders* (3rd edition) (DSM–III). APA.

American Psychiatric Association (1994) *Diagnostic and Statistical Manual of Mental Disorders* (4th edition) (DSM–IV). APA.

Andersson, E. (1993) The Hospital Anxiety and Depression Scale: homogeneity of the subscales. *Social Behavior and Personality*, **21**, 197–204.

Antony, M. M., Bieling, P. J., Cox, B. J., *et al* (1998) Psychometric properties of the 42-item and 21-item versions of the Depression Anxiety Stress Scales in clinical groups and a community sample. *Psychological Assessment*, **10**, 176–181.

Apostolo, J. L., Mendes, A. C. & Azeredo, Z. A. (2006) Adaptation to Portuguese of the Depression, Anxiety and Stress Scales (DASS). *Revista Latino-Americana de Enfermagem*, **14**, 863–871.

Bagby, R. M. (2004) The Hamilton Depression Rating Scale: has the gold standard become a lead weight? *American Journal of Psychiatry*, **161**, 2163–2177.

Barlow, J. H. & Wright, C. C. (1998) Dimensions of the Center of Epidemiological Studies Depression Scale for people with arthritis from the UK. *Psychological Reports*, **83**, 915–919.

Batistoni, S. S., Neri, A. L. & Cupertino, A. P. (2007) Validade da escala de depressao do Center for Epidemiological Studies entre idosos brasileiros. [Validity of the Center for Epidemiological Studies Depression Scale among Brazilian elderly.] *Revista de Saude Publica*, **41**, 598–605.

Beck, A. T. & Steer, R. A. (1984) Internal consistencies of the original and revised Beck Depression Inventory. *Journal of Clinical Psychology*, **40**, 1365–1367.

Beck, A. T., Ward, C. H., Mendelson, M., *et al* (1961) An inventory for measuring depression. *Archives of General Psychiatry*, **4**, 561–571.

Beck, A. T., Steer, R. A. & Garbin, M. G. (1988) Psychometric properties of the Beck Depression Inventory: twenty-five years of evaluation. *Clinical Psychology Review*, **42**, 861–865.

Beekman, A. T. F., Deeg, D. J. H., Van Limbeek, J., *et al* (1997) Criterion validity of the Center for Epidemiologic Studies Depression Scale (CES–D): results from a community-based sample of older subjects in the Netherlands. *Psychological Medicine*, **27**, 231–235.

Brown, T. A., Chorpita, B. F., Korotitsch, W., *et al* (1997) Psychometric properties of the Depression Anxiety Stress Scales (DASS) in clinical samples. *Behaviour Research and Therapy*, **35**, 79–89.

Bush B. A. Novack T. A. Schneider J. J., *et al* (2004) Depression following traumatic brain injury: the validity of the CES-D as a brief screening device. *Journal of Clinical Psychology in Medical Settings*, **11**, 195–201.

Cameron, I. M., Crawford, J. R., Lawton, K., *et al* (2008) Psychometric comparison of PHQ-9 and HADS for measuring depression severity in primary care. *British Journal of General Practice*, **58**, 32–36.

Carle, A. C. (2003) Three latent variable model assessments of measurement bias across gender on the Children's Depression Inventory. *Dissertation Abstracts International: Section B: The Sciences and Engineering*, **64(6-B)**, 2977.

Cheung, C. K. & Bagley, C. (1998) Validating an American scale in Hong Kong: the Center for Epidemiological Studies Depression Scale (CES–D). *Journal of Psychology: Interdisciplinary and Applied*, **132**, 169–186.

Cialdella, P., Chambon, O., Boissel, J. P., *et al* (1989) La Recherche d'une Mesure Unidimensionnelle de la Depression: A Propos de L'echelle de Depression de Hamilton. [In search of a unidimensional assessment of depression: the Hamilton Rating Scale for Depression.] *Psychiatrie et Psychobiologie*, **4**, 203–210.

Clara, I. P., Cox, B. J. & Enns, M. W. (2001) Confirmatory factor analysis of the Depression–Anxiety–Stress Scales in depressed and anxious patients. *Journal of Psychopathology and Behavioral Assessment*, **23**, 61–67.

Clark, L. A. & Watson, D. (1991) Tripartite model of anxiety and depression: psychometric evidence and taxonomic implications. *Journal of Abnormal Psychology*, **100**, 316–336.

Craighead, W. E., Craighead, L. W., Smucker, M. R., *et al* (1998) Factor analysis of the Children's Depression Inventory in a community sample. *Psychological Assessment*, **10**, 156–165.

Crawford, J. R. & Henry, J. D. (2003) The Depression Anxiety Stress Scales (DASS): normative data and latent structure in a large non-clinical sample. *British Journal of Clinical Psychology*, **42**, 111–131.

Crawford, J. R. & Henry, J. D. (2004) The Positive and Negative Affect Schedule (PANAS): construct validity, measurement properties and normative data in a large non-clinical sample. *British Journal of Clinical Psychology*, **43**, 245–265.

Cyr, J. J., McKenna-Foley, J. M. & Peacock, E. (1985) Factor structure of the SCL–90–R: is there one? *Journal of Personality Assessment*, **49**, 571–578.

Daza, P. (2002) The Depression Anxiety Stress Scale–21: Spanish translation and validation with a Hispanic sample. *Dissertation Abstracts International: Section B: The Sciences and Engineering*, **62(11-B)**, 5368.

Derogatis, L. R. & Cleary, P. A. (1977) Factorial invariance across gender for the primary symptom dimensions of the SCL–90. *British Journal of Social and Clinical Psychology*, **16**, 347–356.

Derogatis, L. R., Rickels, K. & Rock, A. F. (1976) The SCL–90 and the MMPI: a step in the validation of a new self-report scale. *British Journal of Psychiatry*, **128**, 280–289.

Dick, R. W., Beals, J., Keane, E. M., *et al* (1994) Factorial structure of the CES–D among American Indian adolescents. *Journal of Adolescence*, **17**, 73–79.

Dum, M., Pickren, J., Sobell, L. C., *et al* (2008) Comparing the BDI–II and the PHQ–9 with outpatient substance abusers. *Addictive Behaviors*, **33**, 381–387.

Edman, J. L., Danko, G. P., Andrade, N., *et al* (1999) Factor structure of the CES–D (Center for Epidemiologic Studies Depression Scale) among Filipino-American adolescents. *Social Psychiatry and Psychiatric Epidemiology*, **34**, 211–215.

Galinowski, A. & Lehert, P. (1995) Structural validity of MADRS during antidepressant treatment. *International Clinical Psychopharmacology*, **10**, 157–161.

Gaudreau, P., Sanchez, X. & Blondin, J-P. (2006) Positive and negative affective states in a performance-related setting: testing the factorial structure of the PANAS across two samples of French-Canadian participants. *European Journal of Psychological Assessment*, **22**, 240–249.

Ghubash, R., Daradkeh, T. K., Al Naseri, K. S., *et al* (2000) The performance of the Center for Epidemiologic Study Depression Scale (CES–D) in an Arab female community. *International Journal of Social Psychiatry*, **46**, 241–249.

Gloster, A. T., Rhoades, H. M., Novy, D., *et al* (2008) Psychometric properties of the Depression Anxiety and Stress Scale–21 in older primary care patients. *Journal of Affective Disorders*, **110**, 248–259.

Hamilton, M. (1960) A rating scale for depression. *Journal of Neurology, Neurosurgery and Psychiatry*, **23**, 56–62.

Hamilton, M. (1980) Rating depressive patients. *Journal of Clinical Psychiatry*, **41**, 21–24.

Henry, J. D. & Crawford, J. R. (2005) The 21-item version of the Depression Anxiety Stress Scales (DASS–21): normative data and psychometric evaluation in a large non-clinical sample. *British Journal of Clinical Psychology*, **44**, 227–239.

Higuchi, H., Sato, K., Yoshida, K., *et al* (2008) No predictors of antidepressant patient response to milnacipran were obtained using the three-factor structures of the Montgomery and Åsberg Depression Rating Scale in Japanese patients with major depressive disorders. *Psychiatry and Clinical Neurosciences*, **62**, 197–202.

Hoffmann, N. G. & Overall, P. B. (1978) Factor structure of the SCL–90 in a psychiatric population. *Journal of Consulting and Clinical Psychology*, **46**, 1187–1191.

Huang, F. Y., Chung, H., Kroenke, K., *et al* (2006) Using the Patient Health Questionnaire–9 to measure depression among racially and ethnically diverse primary care patients. *Journal of General Internal Medicine*, **21**, 547–552.

Jerabek, P., Klimpl, P. & Boleloucky, Z. (1982) Factor analysis of the SCL–90 inventory. *Activitas Nervosa Superior*, **24**, 183–184.

Kawata, A. K. (2006) Measurement invariance of the Positive and Negative Affect Schedule (PANAS) in a community sample of older people. *Dissertation Abstracts International: Section B: The Sciences and Engineering*, **66(9–B)**, 5136.

Killgore, W. D. S. (2000) Evidence for a third factor on the Positive and Negative Affect Schedule in a college student sample. *Perceptual and Motor Skills*, **90**, 147–152.

Kovacs, M. (1985) The Children's Depression, Inventory (CDI). *Psychopharmacology Bulletin*, **21**, 995–998.

Krause, J. S., Bombardier, C. & Carter, R. E. (2008) Assessment of depressive symptoms during inpatient rehabilitation for spinal cord injury: is there an underlying somatic factor when using the PHQ? *Rehabilitation Psychology*, **53**, 513–520.

Kroenke, K., Spitzer, R. L. & Williams, J. B. (2001) The PHQ–9: validity of a brief depression severity measure. *Journal of General Internal Medicine*, **16**, 606–613.

Lee, A. E. Y. & Chokkanathan, S. (2008) Factor structure of the 10-item CES–D scale among community dwelling older adults in Singapore. *International Journal of Geriatric Psychiatry*, **23**, 592–597.

Leung, C. M., Ho, S., Kan, C. S., *et al* (1993) Evaluation of the Chinese version of the Hospital Anxiety and Depression Scale. *International Journal of Psychosomatics*, **40**, 29–34.

Lisspers, J., Nygren, A. & Soderman, E. (1997) Hospital Anxiety and Depression Scale (HAD): some psychometric data for a Swedish sample. *Acta Psychiatrica Scandinavica*, **96**, 281–286.

Lovibond, S. H. & Lovibond, P. F. (1993) *Manual for the Depression Anxiety Stress Scales (DASS)*. Psychology Foundation Monograph (available from the Psychology Foundation, Room 1005 Mathews Building, University of New South Wales, NSW 2052, Australia).

Maier, W., Philipp, M. & Gerken, A. (1985) Dimensionen der Hamilton-Depressionsskala (HAMD). Faktorenanalytische Untersuchungen. [Dimensions of the Hamilton Depression Scale (HAMD): a factor analytical study.] *European Archives of Psychiatry and Neurological Sciences*, **234**, 417–22.

Martin, C. R. & Thompson, D. R. (2000) A psychometric evaluation of the Hospital Anxiety and Depression Scale in coronary care patients following acute myocardial infarction. *Psychology, Health and Medicine*, **5**, 193–201.

McCue, P., Buchanan, T. & Martin, C. R. (2006) Screening for psychological distress using internet administration of the Hospital Anxiety and Depression Scale (HADS) in individuals with chronic fatigue syndrome. *British Journal of Clinical Psychology*, **45**, 483–498.

Meyer, T. D. & Hautzinger, M. (2003) The structure of affective symptoms in a sample of young adults. *Comprehensive Psychiatry*, **44**, 110–116.

Montgomery, S. A. & Åsberg, M. (1979) A new depression scale designed to be sensitive to change. *British Journal of Psychiatry*, **134**, 382–389.

Moorey, S, Greer, S, Watson, M., *et al* (1991) The factor structure and factor stability of the Hospital Anxiety and Depression Scale in patients with cancer. *British Journal of Psychiatry*, **158**, 255–259.

Mykletun, A., Stordal, E. & Dahl, A. A. (2001) Hospital Anxiety and Depression (HAD) scale: factor structure, item analyses and internal consistency in a large population. *British Journal of Psychiatry*, **179**, 540–544.

Page, A. C., Hooke, G. R. & Morrison, D. L. (2007) Psychometric properties of the Depression Anxiety Stress Scales (DASS) in depressed clinical samples. *British Journal of Clinical Psychology*, **46**, 283–297.

Pariente, P. D., Lepine, J.-P., Boulenger, J. P., *et al* (1989) The Symptom Check-List 90R (SCL–90R) in a French general psychiatric 708 outpatient sample: is there a factor structure? *European Psychiatry*, **4**, 151–157.

Radloff, L. S. (1977) The CES–D Scale: a self-report depression scale for research in the general population. *Applied Psychological Measurement*, **1**, 385–401.

Richardson, E. J. & Richards, J. S. (2008) Factor structure of the PHQ–9 screen for depression across time since injury among persons with spinal cord injury. *Rehabilitation Psychology*, **53**, 243–249.

Robles, R. & Paez, F. (2003) Study of Spanish translation and psychometric properties of the Positive and Negative Affect Scales (PANAS). *Salud Mental*, **26**, 69–75.

Rush, A. J., Giles, D. E., Schlesser, M. A., *et al* (1986) The Inventory of Depressive Symptomatology (IDS): preliminary findings. *Psychiatry Research*, **18**, 65–87.

Rush, A. J., Gullion, C. M., Basco, M. R., *et al* (1996) The Inventory of Depressive Symptomatology (IDS): psychometric properties. *Psychological Medicine*, **26**, 477–486.

Schwarzwald, J., Weisenberg, M. & Solomon, Z. (1991) Factor invariance of SCL–90–R: the case of combat stress reaction. *Psychological Assessment: A Journal of Consulting and Clinical Psychology*, **3**, 385–390.

Siegert, R. J., Walkey, F. H. & Turner-Stokes, L. (2009) An examination of the factor structure of the Beck Depression Inventory–II in a neurorehabilitation inpatient sample. *Journal of the International Neuropsychological Society*, **15**, 142–147.

Snaith, R. P., Constantopoulos, A. A., Jardine, M. Y., *et al* (1978) Clinical scale for the self-assessment of irritability. *British Journal of Psychiatry*, **132**, 164–171.

Storch, E. A., Roberti, J. W. & Roth, D. A. (2004) Factor structure, concurrent validity, and internal consistency of the Beck Depression Inventory – second edition in a sample of college students. *Depression and Anxiety*, **19**, 187–189.

Suzuki, A., Aoshima, T., Fukasawa, T., *et al* (2005) A three-factor model of the MADRS in major depressive disorder. *Depression and Anxiety*, **21**, 95–97.

Thomas, B. C., Devi, N., Sarita, G. P., *et al* (2005) Reliability and validity of the Malayalam Hospital Anxiety and Depression Scale (HADS) in cancer patients. *Indian Journal of Medical Research*, **122**, 395–399.

Thomas, J. L. & Brantley, P. J. (2004) Factor structure of the Center for Epidemiologic Studies Depression Scale in low-income women attending primary care clinics. *European Journal of Psychological Assessment*, **20**, 106–115.

Thombs, B. D., Ziegelstein, R. C., Beck, C. A., *et al* (2008) A general factor model for the Beck Depression Inventory–II: validation in a sample of patients hospitalized with acute myocardial infarction. *Journal of Psychosomatic Research*, **65**, 115–121.

Uher, R., Farmer, A., Maier, W., *et al* (2008) Measuring depression: comparison and integration of three scales in the GENDEP study. *Psychological Medicine*, **38**, 289–300.

Wang, L., Li, Z., Liu, H., *et al* (2007) Factor structure of general dimension scales of PANAS in Chinese people. *Chinese Journal of Clinical Psychology*, **15**, 565–568.

Ward, L. C. (2006) Comparison of factor structure models for the Beck Depression Inventory – II. *Psychological Assessment*, **18**, 81–88.

Watson, D., Clark, L. A. & Tellegen, A. (1988) Development and validation of brief measures of positive and negative affect: the PANAS scales. *Journal of Personality and Social Psychology*, **54**, 1063–1070.

World Health Organization (1992) *International Classification of Disease* (10th revision) (ICD–10). WHO.

Zich, J. M., Attkisson, C. C. & Greenfield, T. K. (1990) Screening for depression in primary care clinics: the CES–D and the BDI. *International Journal of Psychiatry in Medicine*, **20**, 259–277.

Zigmond, A. S. & Snaith, R. P. (1983) The Hospital Anxiety and Depression Scale. *Acta Psychiatrica Scandinavica*, **67**, 361–70.

CHAPTER 14

Symptom severity outcome measures for depression

Tom Trauer and David J. Castle

Depression is among the most prevalent of mental disorders and is one the leading causes of disability worldwide (World Health Organization, 1996). A study across six countries found that patients with higher scores for depressive symptoms had worse health, functional status, quality of life and greater use of health services across all sites (Herrman *et al*, 2002). This chapter provides an overview of the issues and methods involved in the assessment of depressive symptoms in adults and older persons; different factors and methods are required for younger consumers.[1]

Why assess outcomes?

Given its often erratic and relapsing course, the assessment of the quality and severity of depression is important for a number of reasons. These have been divided by Hickie *et al* (2002) into two groups: clinical and evaluative. The clinical reasons comprise: enhancing the involvement of consumers in their own treatment; documenting a range of clinically relevant aspects of life; improving the identification of early relapse; comparing responses to different treatments; improving understanding of short- and long-term outcomes; and alerting the clinician to a possible need to change the treatment or management. Their list of non-clinical purposes include: evaluating new treatments; contributing to assessment of cost-effectiveness; understanding variations in quality and access to services; and evaluating the impact of major health service innovations and specific policy initiatives. This is an impressive list of reasons for measuring outcomes in depression, to which we add a few of our own. Depression, like most mental disorders, has an effect beyond the index consumer. In addition to the mental pain of the condition itself, there is often 'collateral damage' to family members in terms of worry, burden of care and impaired child care, as well as to society at large in terms of lost productivity and treatment costs. Certain forms of

---

1   There are many terms for recipients of health services, including patient, consumer and user. In Australia, the preferred term is consumer, so we use that in this chapter.

outcome measure can target some of these effects. Also, it is known that not all aspects of the depressed state recover at the same rate (see below). By formally assessing domains beyond primary symptoms, one can assess wider aspects of recovery, such as social and occupational functioning.

While Hickie *et al* (2002) contend that measuring outcomes in consumers with depression and anxiety is an essential part of clinical practice, this activity does not come without some cost, and the potential benefits of assessing outcomes formally must at least offset the main immediate cost, which is clinician time. As Dinnen (2003) remarks, many clinicians resent being required to engage in 'yet another clinically irrelevant activity'. Such resistance to routine or formal outcome measurement is of course not restricted to depressive disorders (e.g. Walter *et al*, 1998; Garland *et al*, 2003). Given the now wide availability of very brief scales, the information technology to minimise the administrative burden, and an increasingly literate consumer constituency, much of the reluctance to engage in outcome measurement may be at the level of personal custom and professional culture.

Who is assessed

One of the first issues that needs to be addressed is that it is not only consumers whose principal psychiatric diagnosis is depression who may need to have the severity of their depression assessed. While depression may be a highly prevalent disorder in the general community, many individuals with other primary diagnoses will have clinically significant levels of depression as well. For example, depression is well known to co-exist with anxiety disorders, but is also highly prevalent among those with other psychiatric illnesses. In Australia, where outcome measures have been collected routinely in public mental health services since 2003, the proportions of consumers with principal diagnoses of schizophrenia, substance misuse and anxiety disorders who also had clinically significant ratings of depressed mood at the start of episodes of care in the community were 28%, 55% and 66% respectively (see http://wdst.amhocn.org, accessed 28 April 2010). Even by the time of their 3-monthly reviews, 20%, 35% and 56% had clinically significant clinician ratings of depressed mood. Needless to say, a proper assessment of mood problems is an indispensable element of the mental state examination. Thus, there is a need to monitor depression carefully in any consumers with a mental health disorder, not only those who are conspicuously depressed. One implication of this is that, ideally, measures should be sufficiently generic to be applicable to any consumer, although specialised methods may be required for those with the most severe forms. Similar issues pertain to people with physical illnesses, which also carry a high burden of depression.

Severity measures are most appropriate for tracking the progress of consumers who are in treatment, because it is they who require longitudinal assessment, unlike respondents to community surveys aimed at estimating prevalence. Survey respondents are typically assessed once, and mainly for the purpose of determining 'caseness'. So long as the severity of their condition exceeds some diagnostic threshold, they will be counted as 'cases'; the severity of their condition may be a secondary consideration. Thus, instruments that are good at discriminating cases from non-cases should be maximally sensitive at levels around the difference between a case and a non-case, while instruments that will be most useful for clinicians should be most sensitive around the higher levels observed in consumers accepted into treatment.

Context of assessment

How one assesses severity will depend on the purpose of the assessment. Given that many consumers with clinically significant depression will have multiple other, possibly related, problems as well, the assessment of depression will rarely occur in isolation. For example, one other domain that often requires parallel monitoring is the use of prescribed medications and their side-effects, as well as of unprescribed substances such alcohol and other psychoactive drugs. So, in practice a depression inventory may well be supplemented with one or more scales that assess other important areas. Alternatively, a multipurpose scale that assesses a range of psychopathology, such as the Brief Psychiatric Rating Scale (BPRS; Overall & Gorham, 1962), may be used.

Another important contextual factor is the presence of physical disease and associated problems such as loss of functioning and pain. Since moderate to severe levels of depression often have physiological, vegetative and functional correlates, it is important to understand to what extent these are consequences of the physical condition and how much of the mental state. Leaving to one side the very real conceptual issues involved, but recognising the need to avoid falling into mind/body dualism, some approaches have attempted to assess just the emotional core of the depressive state, unbiased by features of the physical state. Such methods are particularly required for older persons and for the gravely ill. In this context, it is well accepted that the Hamilton Rating Scale for Depression (HRSD; Hamilton, 1960) is more heavily weighted to physical symptoms than are some other depression scales (see Table 14.1).

By contrast, in some situations, such as research into treatment effectiveness, the focus may be firmly on the depressive phenomena themselves, which will be the primary outcomes of interest, with other features being secondary to the research question. Nevertheless, many studies of this kind will collect a range of secondary outcomes, in order to gain a more comprehensive appreciation of the treatment effect.

What to assess

As standard psychiatric texts and diagnostic systems make clear, 'depression' can manifest in a bewildering variety of ways. Comprehensive assessment using the 'bio-psychosocial' model recognises affective, cognitive and behavioural features of depression. DSM–IV–TR (American Psychiatric Association, 2000) lists nine possible symptoms, of which diverse combinations may be present in any given consumer. Narrow conceptualisations of depression recognise little more than standard signs and symptoms, but broader models may incorporate functional status, subjective quality of life and physical health. Assessments of consumers from particular ethnic backgrounds may require attention to cultural and spiritual factors as well.

Certain domains are covered in almost all depression rating instruments. Anxiety, while phenomenologically distinct from low mood, is frequently found with depression and in some systems is considered a core feature. Vaccarino *et al* (2008) found that anxiety-related symptoms generally increase with the overall severity of depression. Suicidality or tendency to self-harm is also a feature of most depression rating scales, for obvious reasons.

While a careful, detailed and lengthy assessment of many domains may be appropriate at the initial contact with a consumer, it may be impractical to do so routinely over the course of an illness. A balance must be reached between comprehensive coverage and pragmatism. When the mainstay of treatment is pharmacological, there is a temptation to focus outcome on pharmacological effects; this is understandable, because it provides a basis for corrective action, but it may overlook those aspects of outcome that are of more interest to the consumer and immediate family.

Consistent with the World Health Organization (1947) statement that health is not merely the absence of disease, some have suggested that recovery from depression is not to be assessed only by a reduction in symptoms. Fava & Mangelli (2001) have proposed that 'The route of recovery, thus, lies not exclusively in alleviating the negative, but in engendering the positive'. Joseph (2006) has pointed to the relevance of positive psychology, whereby depression and happiness are seen as opposite poles of a single dimension (in contrast to the conventional idea of depression as a unipolar concept, ranging from absent to severe).

Categorical versus dimensional approaches

Categorical methods are used to establish a diagnosis according to a defined diagnostic construct. Mostly these entail a 'tick box' approach, with a certain set of criteria needing to be endorsed in order to make a diagnosis. The most widely used diagnostic criteria for psychiatric disorders are DSM–IV (American Psychiatric Association, 1994) and ICD–10 (World Health Organization, 1992). There may be an explicit or implied hierarchy in these sorts of methods. For example, if a certain number of criteria are met, a particular diagnostic label is applied, while if more criteria are met, another diagnosis is endorsed. In the affective disorders, for example, DSM–IV–TR defines major depressive disorder as 'trumping' dysthymia.

The great virtue of the categorical approach is that it allows one to define an 'entity', to label it, and thus be able to use this to communicate with other clinicians and researchers, with the expectation of a shared understanding. This is particularly important in epidemiological studies, one of whose principal objectives is to estimate prevalence, which is the rate of cases in a given population. In this regard, if an individual is counted as having the condition, the actual level of severity becomes a secondary consideration. However, the diagnostic approach has certain limitations in clinical practice. One of these is the danger that the label becomes the predominant vocabulary, the person under the label being overlooked, and treatments being applied in largely algorithmic and formulaic fashion, rather than being individualised and holistic.

At their simplest, diagnoses are binary codes indicating the presence of the condition of interest. When recorded only in this way, outcome can be characterised as 'recovered' or 'remitted' (diagnostic criteria no longer met) or 'continuing illness' (criteria still met) or 'relapse' (criteria newly met again). This categorisation, while crude, has utility in certain situations. For example, it is reasonable to ask what proportion of consumers achieve 'recovered' status following treatment, or how many fall ill again after a period free of the condition. On the other hand, the limitation is obvious: there will be no sensitivity to small changes, or to the fluctuations in symptoms over the course of an episode of illness.

Assessment of severity will usually involve a dimensional approach, which typically involves the use of a multi-item scale that yields a score representing the degree of depression. These scores are often analysed as if they reflect an underlying dimension of severity, although strictly they may be more akin to ordinal measurement (i.e. ranks), such as absent, mild, moderate and severe. For the most part, depression has been thought of as a single dimension, although this has been questioned (Simms, 2006).

Dimensional and categorical approaches can coexist; indeed, it is common practice to identify a threshold score on a dimensional measure to discriminate cases from non-cases. But more commonly dimensional scales are used for their primary purpose of measuring the severity of symptoms, usually on a series of items which can be looked at discretely, in groups or as a total score. These scales are arguably more clinically relevant than categorical 'boxes', as they allow the clinician and the patient to determine severity of symptoms and assess treatment response and longitudinal course. Some scales are clinician rated and others are consumer self-rated; both can be useful to the clinician.

As well as tracking progress in confirmed cases, dimensional scales can also be used for screening purposes, usually in high-risk populations, as the yield of cases is higher and the performance of any screening measure is determined to a large extent by the rate of the disorder of interest in the population being assessed. An example is screening for postnatal depression: the Edinburgh Postnatal Depression Rating Scale (EPDS; Cox *et al*, 1987) was devised to assess depression in a high-risk group in whom untreated depression can have particularly devastating effects on both mother and child.

The essence of an outcome measure is its capacity to detect changes over time. Categorical approaches, such as most diagnostic approaches, are limited to detecting whether conditions that were present to some criterion are no longer present; if so, the outcome is an improvement. Dimensional approaches, which evaluate severity rather than mere presence, are better suited to detecting and quantifying the sometimes small changes that occur over the course of an episode of depression. Many depression scales, such as the Beck Depression Inventory (BDI; Beck *et al*, 1961), combine both features: the score on the multi-item scale evaluates severity, while a cut-off or threshold discriminates cases from non-cases. However, there will usually be some element of arbitrariness in the choice of the cut-off, since it is recognised that there is no distinct boundary between normal and abnormal levels of symptoms (Kurlowicz & Streim, 1998). Of course, the dimensional measure is not a substitute for the categorical diagnostic method, because the presence of certain signs and symptoms are pathognomonic, and their binary coding does not lend itself to a dimensional measurement of severity.

Leading measures

A review of depression measures noted that 280 instruments for measuring severity of depression have been published since 1918 (Santor *et al*, 2006). However, of these, only five were found to have been used with much frequency: the Beck Depression Inventory (BDI; Beck *et al*, 1961), the Hamilton Rating Scale for Depression (HRSD; Hamilton, 1960), the Montgomery–Åsberg Depression Rating Scale (MADRS; Montgomery & Åsberg, 1979), the Center for Epidemiologic Studies – Depression (CESD; Radloff, 1977) and the Symptom Checklist (SCL–90; Derogatis, 1983). Of these, the BDI and HRSD were used in about 42% of basic science studies and 63% of all treatment outcome studies (Santor *et al*, 2006, p. 146). Given the popularity of the BDI and HRSD, it is of some interest that they have been found to correlate only moderately (Sayer *et al*, 1993), which is probably due to the greater cognitive emphasis of the former and the greater physical emphasis of the latter.

Both Santor *et al* (2006) and Snaith (1993) found a marked heterogeneity among available scales. Not only do they vary in the prominence they give cognitive or physical symptoms, but they also vary in their coverage of such areas as anxiety, suicidality and loss of interest. Santor *et al* (2006, p. 143) described how some scales assess 'depression' or 'sadness' explicitly, while others do so indirectly, using such terms as 'feeling down', 'feeling blue' or 'feeling miserable'; they note that around 20% of measures of depression operationalised mood with terms other than feeling 'sad' or 'depressed'.

Clearly, there is no single 'market leader' or gold standard among depression scales, although a few scales have been used repeatedly. The choice of scale in any given situation will depend on a number of factors. Perhaps the two most important of these are the coverage of core and secondary features, and the comparability of results with other work. Table 14.1 provides an overview of the items covered by some of the leading depression rating scales. We have included those scales identified in the review of Santor et al (2006) as most commonly used, and have added the Quick Inventory of Depressive Symptomatology (QIDS), as it was used in the landmark STAR*D study (Gaynes et al, 2005) and covers all DSM–IV–TR depression items. We do not include the SCL–90, as it is not a depression-specific scale.

Self-report versus clinician rating

Typically there is low concordance between self-ratings and clinician ratings of severity. Parker et al (1997) studied self-rated and clinician-rated measures of depression and found only moderate agreement. They concluded that:

Clinical experience … reveals that many (clinician-judged) 'severely depressed' patients with psychotic and melancholic depression appear poor witnesses of the severity of their state, returning scores suggesting depression to be slight or non-existent. Conversely, many non-melancholic patients often report 'ceiling' scores that are at some variance with clinicians' estimates. Thus, patients generally have one point of reference (i.e. their own depressed state) and will for a variety of reasons perceive and seek to report their depression as severe. Clinicians, by contrast, will quantify severity according to a wider reference range. (pp. 55–56)

In addition:

many patients with psychotic and, less commonly, with melancholic depression deny or minimise being depressed, and offer other interpretations of their state… Thus, those with melancholia or psychotic depression may experience fundamental feelings (or lack of feelings) that are not well captured and quantified by self-report measures that more emphasise generic descriptions of a depressed mood. (p. 56)

With respect to family members as informants, Parker et al thought that they did not have:

sufficient experience to make comparative judgments and, like patients using self-report measures, rating more to an intrinsic subjective estimate of severity than any objective standard that reflects the wider band of 'clinical reality'. (p. 56)

Paykel & Prusoff (1973) rated at a psychiatric interview 220 patients with depression and asked them also to complete a self-report symptom inventory. Concordance between the two measures was modest, and patients with psychotic depression and those with obsessional personalities rated

Table 14.1 Dimensional depression rating scale items

	HRSD–17	MADRS	BDI	CESD	QIDS
Apparent sadness		✓			
Depressed mood/sadness	✓	✓	✓	✓	✓
Tearfulness			✓	✓	
Pessimism/self-blame/diminished self-worth/guilt	✓	✓	✓	✓	✓
Lack of enjoyment/fun		✓		✓	
Loss of interest		✓			✓
Inability to cope					
Lassitude/fatigue/feeling slowed up	✓	✓	✓	✓	✓
Suicidality/self-harm	✓	✓	✓		✓
Impaired concentration		✓		✓	✓
Hypochondriasis	✓		✓		
Psychic anxiety (e.g. worry/inner tension)	✓	✓			
Somatic anxiety	✓				
Motor agitation/restlessness	✓				✓
Motor retardation					✓
Impaired work/activities	✓		✓		
Insomnia	✓	✓	✓	✓	✓
Hypersomnia					✓
Loss of appetite	✓	✓	✓	✓	✓
Increased appetite					✓
Loss of weight	✓		✓		✓
Weight gain					✓
Sexual symptoms	✓		✓		
Lack of insight	✓				
Total number of items	17	10	21	20	16
Time period	Few days per week	At rating	7 days	7 days	7 days
Score per item	0–2, 0–4	0–6	0–3	0–3	0–3
Total range	0–48	0–60	0–63	0–60	0–27
Scoring					
not depressed	0–7	0–12	0–9	0–15	0–5
mild	8–17	13–19	10–16		6–10
moderate	18–24	20–29	17–29	16–26	11–15
severe	≥25	≥30	≥30	≥27	≥16

HRSD–17, Hamilton Rating Scale for Depression (Hamilton, 1960); MADRS, Montgomery–Åsberg Depression Rating Scale (Montgomery & Åsberg, 1979); BDI, Beck Depression Inventory (Beck *et al*, 1961); CESD, Center for Epidemiologic Studies – Depression (Radloff, 1977); QIDS, Quick Inventory of Depressive Symptomatology (Gaynes *et al*, 2005).

themselves low on self-report relative to interview assessments. Similarly, Paykel *et al* (1973) compared assessments of depression based on patients' self-reports and clinical interview. Concordances were again modest and the findings were interpreted as supporting the value of the use of multiple assessments. Prusoff *et al* (1972) found that concordance between clinical assessment and self-report was particularly low during the acute episode but generally improved at follow-up; hence self-reports, while unreliable estimates of severity in the acute phase, may be valuable in the assessment of recovery. The results of these studies suggest that, while self-reports are important and valuable in characterising the pattern of symptoms, they are less effective in quantifying severity in the way it is understood by clinicians, which incorporates forms of evidence (e.g. observation, other informants) that may not be accessed directly by the consumer.

Craig & Van Natta (1976) noted that:

The actual agreement found between self-report and observer ratings in those studies which look at this question has been relatively modest, leading to the suggestion that self-report ratings in depressed patients may not be a reliable estimate of the severity of symptoms in an in-patient population. (p. 561)

In their own study of 65 psychiatric in-patients, they found only modest correlations between observer ratings and self-ratings of patients with depressive neurosis and practically no statistically significant correlations for patients with schizophrenia. They noted that:

Several variables have been implicated as affecting this concordance. Some authors have suggested that patients and raters may differ in their concepts of depression (i.e. symptom vs. syndrome) and this may affect their level of agreement. In support of this, Pilowsky reported that more experienced clinicians had lower levels of concordance (psychiatrists, $r = 0.57$; psychologists, $r = 0.59$) with patient self-reports than less experienced raters (medical students, $r = 0.97$) and suggest that the less experienced rater may have a concept of depression closer to that of the patients. (p. 561)

They also refer to:

the findings of earlier studies which showed highest correlations between self-reports and observer ratings for verbal depressive behavior with lower agreement for non-verbal items. (p. 563)

The relationship between depression and quality of life

As outcomes in mental health, depression and quality of life (QoL) are highly related. The effective treatment of depression is promoted on the grounds that it improves consumers' QoL. The question then arises of whether QoL measures (considered in Chapter 8) can be used to evaluate outcome for consumers with depression. An advantage of this may be that many QoL scales can be used with people without identified mental health problems, whereas depression scales generally have face validity only for people who have experienced, or are experiencing, depression. Also, many QoL scales have population norms, which offer the prospect of judging whether a consumer's QoL has returned to 'normal'. QoL has been used as an outcome measure in studies of the course of depression. Beusterien *et al*

(1996) used the Medical Outcomes Study Short Form Health Status Survey (SF–36; Ware & Sherbourne, 1992), the most widely used QoL measure in health and medical research, in a study of older patients with depression. They found that it correlated well with standard psychiatric measures and was responsive to changes in severity over the course of 6 weeks. This led them to conclude that the SF–36 'is useful for estimating the burden of depression and in monitoring changes in functional health and well-being over time among the depressed elderly'.

The core of the depressive state and subjective QoL depend on an experiential judgement of personal well-being. The question is whether depression and subjective QoL are separate entities, or simply two sides of the same coin. Katschnig (2006) found that:

When examining the myriad of health-related QoL instruments available today, it becomes evident that most of them include items that can straightforwardly be considered psychopathological symptoms, mainly from the field of depression and anxiety. (p. 7)

This suggests that the close association between QoL and depression may be more artefact than reality, in the sense that the depressive state may be directly affecting the judgement of the broader areas of life commonly assessed in QoL instruments. As Katschnig points out, consumers experiencing a depressive episode will commonly evaluate their social functioning and living conditions as worse than they appear to independent observers (Beck, 1976) or even to the consumers themselves after they recover (Morgado *et al*, 1991); and an opposite effect occurs in mania.

Since QoL can be conceptualised as the gap between expectation and achievement (Calman, 1984), a further problem can occur when individuals with long-standing health and social problems adjust their aspirations downward in order to reduce cognitive dissonance. This can lead to relatively preserved subjective well-being in the presence of poor objective life circumstances, as judged independently. Sainfort *et al* (1996) found better agreement between consumers and providers on clinical factors such as symptoms and functioning than on social factors such as relationships and occupation.

This has led to advice not to rely exclusively on self-reported well-being when judging the QoL of persons with mental conditions that affect their mood state. QoL should be 'differentiated at least according to three components: psychological well-being/satisfaction, functioning in social roles and contextual factors (both social and material)' (Katschnig, 2006, p. 9), only the first of which is derived solely from direct consumer experience. The other two should be evaluated or corroborated by other informants. This conceptualisation allows the recovery of QoL to be better understood, because 'certain components of QoL change at different speeds: subjective well-being responds quickly to medication, functioning in social roles more slowly, and social support and material living conditions more slowly still' (p. 11).

Selected findings

In a study illustrating the link between categorical and dimensional approaches, Lowe *et al* (2004) classified medical out-patients into three groups (major depression, other depression, and no depression) and followed them for about a year. The nine-item Patient Health Questionnaire (PHQ–9; Kroenke *et al*, 2001), a brief measure of depression, and the Diagnostic Structured Interview for DSM–IV Axis I Disorders (SCID; First *et al*, 1995) were administered at the beginning and end of follow-up. Using depression diagnoses from the SCID, they allocated participants to 'improved', 'unchanged' and 'worse' groupings, and showed that the PHQ–9 could effectively detect depression status and change over time.

Mulder *et al* (2003) compared the relative ability of a number of depression and related scales to detect change in a study of two antidepressants. The scales were the HRSD–17, HRSD–27, MADRS, SCL–90, the Clinical Global Impression Scale (see below) and the Social Adjustment Scale (SAS; Cooper *et al*, 1982). They found that all the measures were moderately or highly correlated with each other as well as with the clinician's global impression. However, the MADRS was the most effective in dividing the sample into responders and non-responders.

Some studies have looked at alternative ways of assessing depression. Kaye (2001), noting that traditional outcome measures are closely tied to diagnostic entities, examined the use of 'target symptoms' (the specific problems for which the patient is seeking help) in a group of older persons suffering from major depressive disorder. Target symptoms correlated well with BDI score.

Mallick *et al* (2003) explored the utility of depression-free days (DFDs) as a summary measure of response and remission. DFDs correlated as expected with HRSD score and differentiated sustained versus non-sustained response.

Berk *et al* (2008) argued that the Clinical Global Impression Scale (CGI; Guy, 1976) meets most of the criteria for a clinical outcome measure, and proceeded to use it with all admissions, about half for depressive disorders, to a private psychiatric hospital over 2 years. The CGI was effective in classifying severity at both admission and discharge, and in classifying the changes between 'very much improved' and 'very much worse'. Admission, discharge and change ratings on the CGI showed significant and monotonic relationships with the locally mandated outcome measure, the Health of the Nation Outcome Scales (HoNOS; Wing *et al*, 1998).

Conclusion

This chapter has reviewed issues pertinent to the measurement of the severity of depression. While there are hundreds of rating scales available, only a handful are widely used, and those cover the main domains of depressive symptoms adequately but with differing emphases (see Table 14.1). A virtue of choosing an already widely used scale lies in the ability to compare and contrast the findings of different studies.

An important consideration is whether to use categorical or dimensional scales: the latter have definite advantages in terms of tracking symptom change over time, and are not explicitly wedded to a set of diagnostic criteria.

Another issue is the use of self-report or observer-rated scales: if feasible, the use of both might be preferred, as different perspectives are brought to bear on the issue, and both are legitimate views. The low concordance between the two perspectives may be seen as a problem; alternatively, it may be regarded as a useful source of information in its own right.

A point not adequately covered in the literature is the use of 'third party' informant ratings (e.g. by family members) for depression symptoms. Certainly informants can add a useful perspective to the assessment, but there is a potential difficulty if their perspective is at odds with that of the consumer.

Finally, the use of proxy measures of depression, notably quality of life, cannot be seen as an adequate substitute for specific depression rating scales. Having said this, measurement of levels of disability and quality of life are important extra considerations in the full assessment of the consumer with depression.

References

American Psychiatric Association (1994) *Diagnostic and Statistical Manual of Mental Disorders* (4th edition) (DSM–IV). American Psychiatric Association.

American Psychiatric Association (2000) *Diagnostic and Statistical Manual of Mental Disorders* (4th edition, text revision) (DSM–IV–TR). American Psychiatric Association.

Beck, A. T. (1976) *Cognitive Therapy and the Emotional Disorders*. International University Press.

Beck, A. T., Ward, C. H., Mendelson, M., *et al* (1961) An inventory for measuring depression. *Archives of General Psychiatry*, **4**, 561–571.

Berk, M., Ng, F., Dodd, S., *et al* (2008) The validity of the CGI severity and improvement scales as measures of clinical effectiveness suitable for routine clinical use. *Journal of Evaluation in Clinical Practice*, **14**, 979–983.

Beusterien, K. M., Steinwald, B. & Ware, J. E., Jr (1996) Usefulness of the SF–36 Health Survey in measuring health outcomes in the depressed elderly. *Journal of Geriatric Psychiatry and Neurology*, **9**, 13–21.

Calman, K. C. (1984) Quality of life in cancer patients – an hypothesis. *Journal of Medical Ethics*, **10**, 124–127.

Cooper, P., Osborn, M., Gath, D., *et al* (1982) Evaluation of a modified self-report measure of social adjustment. *British Journal of Psychiatry*, **141**, 68–75.

Cox, J. L., Holden, J. M. & Sagovsky, R. (1987) Detection of postnatal depression: development of the 10-item Edinburgh Postnatal Depression Scale. *British Journal of Psychiatry*, **150**, 782–786.

Craig, T. J. & Van Natta, P. A. (1976) Recognition of depressed affect in hospitalized psychiatric patients: staff and patient perceptions. *Diseases of the Nervous System*, **37**, 561–566.

Derogatis, L. R. (1983) *SCL–90–R Administration, Scoring, and Procedures Manual – II*. Clinical Psychometric Research.

Dinnen, A. H. (2003) Measuring outcomes in patients with depression and anxiety: an essential part of clinical practice. *Medical Journal of Australia*, **178**, 48.

Fava, G. A. & Mangelli, L. (2001) Assessment of subclinical symptoms and psychological well-being in depression. *European Archives of Psychiatry and Clinical Neuroscience*, **251** (suppl. 2), 47–52.

First, M. B., Spitzer, R. L., Gibbon, M., *et al* (1995) *Structured Clinical Interview for DSM–IV Axis I Disorders, Non-Patient Version (SCID–V–NP)*. Biometrics Research Department.

Garland, A. F., Kruse, M. & Aarons, G. A. (2003) Clinicians and outcome measurement: what's the use? *Journal of Behavioral Health Services and Research*, **30**, 393–405.

Gaynes, B. N., Rush, A. J., Trivedi, M., *et al* (2005) A direct comparison of presenting characteristics of depressed outpatients from primary vs. specialty care settings: preliminary findings from the STAR*D clinical trial. *General Hospital Psychiatry*, **27**, 87–96.

Guy, W. (1976) *ECDEU Assessment Manual for Psychopharmacology – Revised*. US Department of Health, Education, and Welfare, Public Health Service, Alcohol, Drug Abuse, and Mental Health Administration, NIMH Psychopharmacology Research Branch, Division of Extramural Research Programs.

Hamilton, M. (1960) A rating scale for depression. *Journal of Neurology, Neurosurgery and Psychiatry*, **23**, 56–62.

Herrman, H., Patrick, D. L., Diehr, P., *et al* (2002) Longitudinal investigation of depression outcomes in primary care in six countries: the LIDO Study. 1 Functional status, health service use and treatment of people with depressive symptoms. *Psychological Medicine*, **32**, 889–902.

Hickie, I. B., Andrews, G. & Davenport, T. A. (2002) Measuring outcomes in patients with depression or anxiety: an essential part of clinical practice. *Medical Journal of Australia*, **177**, 205–207.

Joseph, S. (2006) Measurement in depression: positive psychology and the statistical bipolarity of depression and happiness. *Measurement: Interdisciplinary Research and Perspectives*, **4**, 156–161.

Katschnig, H. (2006) How useful is the concept of quality of life in psychiatry? In *Quality of Life in Mental Disorders* (2nd edition) (eds H. Katschnig, H. Freeman & N. Sartorius), pp. 3–17. Wiley.

Kaye, J. L. (2001) Target complaints as a measure of outcome in psychotherapy with the depressed elderly. *Dissertation Abstracts International: Section B: The Sciences and Engineering*, **62**(5-B), 2488.

Kroenke, K., Spitzer, R. L. & Williams, J. B. (2001) The PHQ–9: validity of a brief depression severity measure. *Journal of General Internal Medicine*, **16**, 606–613.

Kurlowicz, L. H. & Streim, J. E. (1998) Measuring depression in hospitalized, medically ill, older adults. *Archives of Psychiatric Nursing*, **12**, 209–218.

Lowe, B., Kroenke, K., Herzog, W., *et al* (2004) Measuring depression outcome with a brief self-report instrument: sensitivity to change of the Patient Health Questionnaire (PHQ–9). *Journal of Affective Disorders*, **81**, 61–66.

Mallick, R., Chen, J., Entsuah, A., *et al* (2003) Depression-free days as a summary measure of the temporal pattern of response and remission in the treatment of major depression: a comparison of venlafaxine, selective serotonin reuptake inhibitors, and placebo. *Journal of Clinical Psychiatry*, **64**, 321–330.

Montgomery, S. A. & Åsberg, M. (1979) A new depression scale designed to be sensitive to change. *British Journal of Psychiatry*, **134**, 382–389.

Morgado, A., Smith, M., Lecrubier, Y., *et al* (1991) Depressed subjects unwittingly overreport poor social adjustment which they reappraise when recovered. *Journal of Nervous and Mental Disease*, **179**, 614–619.

Mulder, R. T., Joyce, P. R., Frampton, C., *et al* (2003) Relationships among measures of treatment outcome in depressed patients. *Journal of Affective Disorders*, **76**, 127–135.

Overall, J. E. & Gorham, D. R. (1962) The Brief Psychiatric Rating Scale. *Psychological Reports*, 10, 199–222.

Parker, G., Roussos, J., Hadzi-Pavlovic, D., *et al* (1997) Plumbing the depths: some problems in quantifying depression severity. *Journal of Affective Disorders*, 42, 49–58.

Paykel, E. S. & Prusoff, B. A. (1973) Response set and observer set in the assessment of depressed patients. *Psychological Medicine*, 3, 209–216.

Paykel, E. S., Prusoff, B. A., Klerman, G. L., *et al* (1973) Self-report and clinical interview ratings in depression. *Journal of Nervous and Mental Disease*, 156, 166–182.

Prusoff, B. A., Klerman, G. L. & Paykel, E. S. (1972) Concordance between clinical assessments and patients' self-report in depression. *Archives of General Psychiatry*, 26, 546–552.

Radloff, L. (1977) The CES–D scale: a self report depression scale for research in the general population. *Applied Psychological Measurement*, 1, 385–401.

Sainfort, F., Becker, M. & Diamond, R. (1996) Judgments of quality of life of individuals with severe mental disorders: patient self-report versus provider perspectives. *American Journal of Psychiatry*, 153, 497–502.

Santor, D. A., Gregus, M. & Welch, A. (2006) Eight decades of measurement in depression. *Measurement*, 4, 135–155.

Sayer, N. A., Sackheim, H. A., Moeller, J. R., *et al* (1993) The relations between observer-rating and self-report of depressive symptomatology. *Psychological Assessment*, 5, 350–360.

Simms, L. J. (2006) The future of depression measurement research. *Measurement: Interdisciplinary Research and Perspectives*, 4, 169–174.

Snaith, P. (1993) What do depression rating scales measure? *British Journal of Psychiatry*, 163, 293–298.

Vaccarino, A. L., Evans, K. R., Sills, T. L., *et al* (2008) Symptoms of anxiety in depression: assessment of item performance of the Hamilton Anxiety Rating Scale in patients with depression. *Depression and Anxiety*, 25, 1006–1013.

Walter, G., Cleary, M. & Rey, J. M. (1998) Attitudes of mental health personnel toward rating outcome. *Journal of Quality in Clinical Practice*, 18, 109–115.

Ware, J. E. & Sherbourne, C. D. (1992) The MOS 36-item Short Form Health Status Survey (SF–36): I. Conceptual framework and item selection. *Medical Care*, 30, 473–483.

Wing, J. K., Beevor, A. S., Curtis, R. H., *et al* (1998) Health of the Nation Outcome Scales (HoNOS). *British Journal of Psychiatry*, 172, 11–18.

World Health Organization (1947) *Constitution of the World Health Organization*. WHO.

World Health Organization (1992) *The ICD–10 Classification of Mental and Behavioural Disorders*. WHO.

World Health Organization (1996) *The Global Burden of Disease*. Harvard University Press.

CHAPTER 15

Outcome measures for people with personality disorders

Paul Moran and Rohan Borschmann

Personality disorders are common conditions, associated with significant burden to the individual, those around him or her and society as a whole. This chapter first briefly examines the classification and epidemiology of personality disorders, before it goes on to review current research on outcome measures for personality disorders, the instruments used in their assessment and the outcome measures used in randomised controlled trials of interventions for borderline personality disorder.

Definition and classification of personality disorders

The concept of abnormal personality was recognised by many ancient cultures, including the Ancient Greeks, Chinese and the Celts, although the modern usage of the concept of 'personality disorder' can be traced to the eighteenth century (Tyrer *et al*, 1991).

The diagnostic features of all personality disorders are listed in Box 15.1. Although the clinical features of personality disorders describe characteristics that any individual may possess in varying degrees from time to time, it is the enduring, inflexible and dysfunctional nature of such personality traits that distinguishes those who have personality disorders from those who do not.

Box 15.1 Core diagnostic features of all personality disorders

- Maladaptive patterns of behaviour, thinking, emotions and perceptions.
- Enduring and pervasive disturbance that is not limited to episodes of mental illness.
- Considerable personal distress and/or significant problems in personal, occupational and/or social functioning.
- Early manifestations (e.g. conduct disorder) in childhood.

Table 15.1 The classification of personality disorders in ICD–10 and DSM–IV

ICD–10 personality disorder	DSM–IV personality disorder
Paranoid	Paranoid
Schizoid	Schizoid
No equivalent	Schizotypal
Dissocial	Antisocial
Emotionally unstable	
impulsive type	*No equivalent*
borderline type	Borderline
Histrionic	Histrionic
No equivalent	Narcissistic
Anankastic	Obsessive–compulsive
Anxious	Avoidant
Dependent	Dependent
Other specific	Not otherwise specified

While ICD–10 (World Health Organization, 1992) continues to retain personality disorder within the main rubric of mental disorders, DSM has, since its third revision in 1980, placed personality disorders on a separate axis, Axis II (American Psychiatric Association, 1980). Table 15.1 lists the specific personality disorders classified by ICD–10 and DSM–IV (American Psychiatric Association, 1994). DSM–IV recognises three 'clusters' of personality disorder:

- cluster A (the 'odd or eccentric' types) – paranoid, schizoid and schizotypal personality disorder
- cluster B (the 'dramatic, emotional or erratic' types) – histrionic, narcissistic, antisocial and borderline personality disorders
- cluster C (the 'anxious and fearful' types) – obsessive–compulsive, avoidant and dependent.

For five categories of personality disorder, there is an exact correspondence between ICD–10 and DSM–IV. For three categories, there are differences in nomenclature between the two systems: ICD–10 uses the terms 'anankastic', 'dissocial' and 'anxious', while DSM–IV uses the terms 'obsessive–compulsive', 'antisocial' and 'avoidant', respectively. DSM–IV classifies borderline personality disorder as a specific category, while ICD–10 includes it as a subcategory of emotionally unstable personality disorder. Finally, the DSM–IV category of narcissistic personality disorder has no equivalent in ICD–10 and while the DSM–IV personality disorders include the schizotypal personality disorder, ICD–10 classifies it under 'Schizophrenia, schizotypal and delusional disorders'.

The current classification of personality disorder is not well supported by empirical data (Widiger & Simonsen, 2005). First, population-based studies indicate that abnormal personality traits are likely to be distributed continuously throughout the population, rather than in a bimodal fashion, as implied by the categorical distinction of personality disorder (Livesley *et al*, 1992). Second, the DSM categories are defined using a set of criteria, none of which is necessary or sufficient for diagnosis alone and of which only a set number need to be present. This results in considerable heterogeneity in the clinical features of patients with the same personality disorder diagnosis (Livesley, 2001). Third, the criteria for some personality disorder subtypes overlap. For example, the borderline personality disorder criterion of 'frantic efforts to avoid abandonment' can be hard to distinguish from the dependent personality disorder criterion of 'excessive lengths to obtain nurturance'. Such criterion overlap is partially responsible for the excessive co-occurrence of these two disorders. Finally, the current categories do not provide adequate coverage of the full range of personality psychopathology. Moreover, the current taxonomies fail to acknowledge personality strengths which could be capitalised upon during treatment.

A dimensional approach to the classification of abnormal personality would solve many of these problems and has therefore attracted widespread support (Widiger & Frances, 1994). However, there are doubts about the clinical utility of a dimensionally based scheme, as it is hard to apply in practice and clinicians seem to prefer using prototypical categorical schemes (Rottman *et al*, 2009). Clearly, further work is required to refine the classification of personality disorder in a way which is both scientifically valid and clinically useful (Skodol & Bender, 2009).

The epidemiology and public health impact of personality disorders

A recently published World Health Organization study conducted in 13 countries in Western Europe, Asia, Africa, the Americas and the Middle East found that the population prevalence of personality disorder was approximately 6% (Huang *et al*, 2009). Other cross-sectional surveys have delineated the sociodemographic correlates of personality disorders. Personality disorders are commoner in younger people and overall are equally distributed between males and females, although the sex ratio for specific types of personality disorder is variable (e.g. antisocial personality disorder is commoner among males). Community surveys have also found that those with a personality disorder are more likely to suffer from alcohol and drug problems (Grant *et al*, 2004) and are more likely to experience adverse life events, such as relationship difficulties, housing problems and long-term unemployment (Coid *et al*, 2006*a*).

In primary care, the prevalence of personality disorder exceeds 20% of attenders (Moran *et al*, 2000) and, in this setting, personality disorder is associated with poorer outcome for the treatment of common mental disorders (Patience *et al*, 1995) and increased health service costs (Rendu *et al*, 2002). The prevalence of personality disorder is even higher in secondary care, particularly among individuals receiving treatment for substance misuse, eating disorders and self-harm. The highest prevalence of personality disorder is found in criminal populations, where in England and Wales the prevalence of any personality disorder is nearly 80% among male remand prisoners and over 60% in the male sentenced population (Singleton *et al*, 1998).

The needs of people with personality disorder vary enormously. Many people with a personality disorder are able to negotiate life reasonably successfully. However, others suffer considerably and place a heavy burden on those around them (Hayward *et al*, 2006). It is now well established that personality disorders are associated with suicidal behaviour, although the magnitude of risk varies considerably between specific categories of disorder (Cheng *et al*, 1997). In addition, both men and women with personality disorder have an elevated mortality rate through death by homicide or accident (Hiroeh *et al*, 2001). Although for the past decade or more UK policy-makers have been heavily preoccupied with the putative link between personality disorders and violence (Mullen, 1999), much of the evidence for the association between personality disorders and violence is derived from cross-sectional studies, for which it is difficult to exclude selection bias (Coid *et al*, 2006b). Comparatively little research has examined the strength of a longitudinal association between personality disorder and violence, although at least one longitudinal study has shown that comorbid personality disorder elevates the risk of violence in people with severe mental illness (Moran *et al*, 2003a). In addition, studies of birth cohorts have shown that antisocial personality disorder is a risk factor for future offending (Hodgins *et al*, 1996).

As suggested above, people with personality disorders are frequent users of both primary and secondary health services. In primary care, personality disorder is associated with frequent attendance (Moran *et al*, 2001) and greater health and non-health costs – an effect which appears to be mediated by the excess prevalence of comorbid depression and anxiety among attenders with a personality disorder (Rendu *et al*, 2002). At the level of secondary care, people with cluster B personality disorders have been shown to use psychiatric services heavily (Perry *et al*, 1987). American data from the Collaborative Longitudinal Personality Disorders Study showed that treatment-seeking patients with borderline personality disorder report greater use of psychiatric medication, hospitalisation, psychotherapy, day care and social care than do patients with major depressive disorder (Bender *et al*, 2001).

People with personality disorders are more likely to suffer from other psychiatric problems during their lifetime. People with cluster A personality disorders are more likely to have episodes of comorbid psychotic illness, those with cluster B personality disorders are more vulnerable to substance use disorders, and cluster C personality disorders are highly comorbid with anxiety disorders (Hayward & Moran, 2008). The presence of comorbid personality disorder invariably complicates the management of mental illness and this is one of the main reasons for routinely assessing premorbid personality. The task, though, of distinguishing whether presenting symptoms are those of an underlying personality disorder or a comorbid mental disorder can be difficult and assessment should involve the use of a structured interview.

The assessment of personality disorder

The assessment of personality disorder is a skilled exercise which needs to be undertaken with an awareness of the various biases which can distort the information obtained. Acute disturbance in mental state can lead to the overidentification of personality pathology. For example, acute symptoms of depression may wrongly lead to a diagnosis of anxious or dependent personality disorder. Therefore, attention needs to be paid to a patient's current symptom state when assessing the presence of personality disorder. Assessments should incorporate frequent reminders that the questions refer to the patient's 'normal self' and the use of an informant is one way of minimising the influence of current mental state (Mann *et al*, 1981). In addition to the presence of mental illness, the patient's gender and cultural background can lead to biased assessments of personality. Women significantly outnumber men in the diagnoses of dependent, histrionic and borderline personality disorders and this has led to the suggestion that these disorders represent no more than exaggerated sex role stereotypes (Russell, 1995). Definitions of personality disorders emphasise their impact on society. However, cultures vary and personality characteristics considered abnormal in one cultural setting may be seen as adaptive in another setting. Clinicians should therefore be cautious before diagnosing personality disorders in people from sociocultural backgrounds different to their own. Nonetheless, the World Health Organization's Mental Health Surveys have shown that it is possible to assess personality disorder in different nations, languages and cultures (Loranger *et al*, 1994; Huang *et al*, 2009).

Before the introduction of multi-axial classification in DSM–III, personality disorder assessment was entirely reliant on clinical assessment – an intuitive but unreliable approach (Mellsop *et al*, 1982). DSM–III placed personality disorders on a separate axis (Axis II) and this paved the way for the development of more systematic measures. A large number of assessments are now available for professionals interested in assessing personality pathology and these fall into one of two categories: self-report questionnaires and semi-structured clinical interviews. Examples of self-report questionnaires include the International Personality Disorder Examination Screen (IPDE–S; Lenzenweger *et al*, 1997), the Personality Diagnostic Questionnaire–Revised (PDQ–R; Hyler *et al*, 1992) and the Structured Clinical Interview for DSM–IV Axis II Personality Disorders screen (SCID; Ekselius *et al*, 1994). Although the sensitivity of these questionnaires is generally high, when compared with a structured interview their specificity is often poor. Therefore, their main use is in screening and they should not be used to make a definitive diagnosis of personality disorder. A further drawback of questionnaires is that they often require the ability of the respondent to concentrate on long sets of questions.

A number of reliable structured interviews have been developed for the purposes of assessing personality disorder. Some assess only one category of personality disorder, for example the Diagnostic Interview for Borderlines (Gunderson et al, 1981), while others provide a comprehensive assessment of all personality disorder subtypes, and these include the Structured Clinical Interview for DSM–IV Personality Disorders (First et al, 1997), the International Personality Disorder Examination (Loranger et al, 1996), the Personality Assessment Schedule (Tyrer et al, 1979) and the Standardised Assessment of Personality (Moran et al, 2003b). Standardised interviews for the assessment of personality disorders generally achieve good interrater reliability, although test–retest reliability is poorer and is influenced by the length of the follow-up interval. While structured interviews provide a detailed assessment, they carry the disadvantage of being time-consuming (typically taking 1–2 hours) and administration requires training.

A recent development in the assessment of abnormal personality has been the advent of 'mini-interviews', such as the Standardised Assessment of Personality–Abbreviated Scale (SAPAS). The SAPAS is quick, simple to use and displays good psychometric performance as a screening measure (Moran et al, 2003b; Hesse et al, 2008).

Do personality features change over time?

By definition, people with personality disorders have enduring disturbance and one would therefore expect to see little change in their characteristics over time. However, findings from longitudinal studies of clinical populations in both Europe and America contradict this assertion. The Collaborative Longitudinal Personality Disorders Study (Gunderson et al, 2000) is a prospective study comparing the course of four DSM–IV personality disorders – schizotypal (STPD), borderline (BPD), avoidant (AVPD) and obsessive–compulsive (OCPD) – with each other and with major depressive disorder (MDD). The 668 participants were recruited from a range of clinical settings and have been followed up at 6 months, 1 year and annually thereafter. At 2 years, blinded independent ratings of diagnostic status were undertaken in order to examine diagnostic stability (Grilo et al, 2004). Adjusted kappa values for the four categories of personality disorder were as follows: STPD 0.56; BPD 0.50; AVPD 0.53; OCPD 0.51 (all P values < 0.0001). Approximately half the participants had lost their diagnosis of personality disorder by 24 months, although those with a personality disorder had a significantly lower remission rate than did participants with MDD.

The McLean Study of Adult Development is a longitudinal study of the course of BPD (Zanarini *et al*, 2005*a*). It has followed 290 patients with BPD (and 72 patients meeting another Axis II disorder), all of whom were initially in-patients at McLean Hospital, Massachusetts. Follow-ups of diagnostic status, symptoms and social functioning took place at 2, 4 and 6 years after recruitment and were conducted by a researcher who was blind to baseline diagnosis. Of the 95% of the patients with BPD who were reassessed at 2 years, 35% met criteria for remission from BPD (defined as no longer meeting diagnostic criteria). By 6 years, about 75% met criteria for remission and, in addition, recurrences of BPD were rare. The authors also detected differences in the speed with which certain types of BPD symptoms improved: while impulsive behaviour resolved relatively quickly, affective symptoms (anger, anxiety and depression) were significantly less likely to resolve over time. Although the generalisability of the findings is limited to treated samples of people with BPD, the authors concluded that the prognosis of BPD is better than had been previously recognised and that affective symptoms may represent core features of the temperament of people with BPD.

Data from Europe also support the idea that the features of personality disorder can change with time. Seivewright *et al* (2002) assessed the personality status at baseline and at 12 years of 202 patients with a DSM–III anxiety disorder originally enrolled in a randomised controlled trial. All the participants had had drug and psychological treatment for an anxiety disorder or dysthymia. The personality traits of participants in the cluster B group became significantly less pronounced over 12 years, but those in the cluster A group and the cluster C group became more pronounced. The measure of agreement between baseline and 12-year personality clusters was poor or slight ($\kappa = 0.14$, 95% Cl 0.04–0.23) and the authors concluded that the assumption that personality characteristics do not change with time is incorrect.

Outcome domains in personality disorder research

So, if people with personality disorder can change (a process which, as we shall see below, can in the case of BPD be accelerated with treatment), what are the best outcome domains to focus on? Because personality disorders affect both the individual and society, a wide range of outcome domains could be assessed. For example, in studies of offenders with a personality disorder, reconviction is the most commonly used outcome measure, but this does not constitute either symptomatic or personality change and as an outcome is vulnerable to the vagaries of the criminal justice system (Bateman & Fonagy, 2000). Similarly, a large number of outcomes are reported in intervention studies for BPD, owing to its multi-symptom nature (National Institute for Health and Clinical Excellence, 2009). Moreover, the choice of outcomes used in personality disorder research has historically reflected variables of interest to clinicians (symptoms, behaviour, social adjustment) and policy-makers (cost, offending behaviour, wider societal effects), but not service users. Ideally, biomedical outcomes should be complemented by measures that focus on the service user's concerns (Fitzpatrick *et al*, 1998), as clinical measures do not account for all the variance in an individual's quality of life (Perkins, 2001).

Comparatively little research has examined the views of service users and staff about what constitutes an 'appropriate' outcome domain in the treatment of personality disorder. Crawford *et al* (2008) conducted a Delphi study to assess the opinions of service providers, academic experts and service users about the treatment provided by specialist personality disorder services in the UK. Quality of life was ranked highest by all three groups. Expert authors and service providers placed social function as the next most important outcome, with service users opting for reduction in symptoms of mental distress. The authors concluded that service outcomes should be assessed in terms of improved quality of life and social functioning, and reductions in mental distress. Moran (2005) conducted qualitative interviews with a sample of service users with a cluster B personality disorder (sampled purposively from a range of adult mental health settings) in order to determine their experience of receiving care. A purposive sample of staff was also interviewed in order to determine experiences of delivering care to service users with a personality disorder. Thematic content analysis revealed that both groups identified improved quality of life as the single most important goal of treatment. On the basis of these two studies, it may therefore be reasonable to conclude that quality of life should be an outcome measure of the utmost priority to researchers interested in personality disorder. However, a systematic review of clinical trials of the treatment of BPD identified only two trials which included quality of life as an outcome measure (British Psychological Society & Royal College of Psychiatrists, 2009).

The fact that we lack an agreed set of outcomes for the treatment of personality disorder is more than simply a problem for those conducting systematic reviews: it creates real problems in clinical practice. For example, in the management of a service user with BPD, it is not uncommon for staff to hold the view that a desired outcome of an intervention should be that the service user is better able to manage crises without resorting to self-harm. Such a view is clinically reasonable, given the strong association between self-harm and suicide (Cooper *et al*, 2005). On the other hand, in the event of a situational crisis, service users may simply want to feel calmer and have learnt (invariably over a long period of time) that the most effective way of reducing the level of arousal is to harm themselves (Sachsse *et al*, 2002). Under such circumstances, it may be unrealistic to establish the cessation of self-harm as an immediately achievable goal for treatment. In addition, disagreement over an issue as critical as this could seriously harm the therapeutic alliance, which would ultimately limit engagement in treatment (Fischer *et al*, 2002) and paradoxically increase the risk that service users pose to themselves. Under such circumstances, a more realistic goal might be to formulate a crisis plan which: acknowledges the service user's current need to self-harm; encourages a range of alternative, healthy strategies for the short-term management of distress (e.g. distraction techniques, talking to a friend); and advises the service user how to seek prompt medical help in the event of self-harm.

Randomised controlled trials of the effectiveness of treatment for BPD

From a treatment perspective, BPD has been the most extensively researched category of personality disorder. As defined in DSM–IV, BPD is a complex and severe condition which manifests in a pervasive pattern of instability in interpersonal relationships and self-image and marked impulsivity. The condition is thought to occur globally, with a median prevalence of 0.7%, although its prevalence is far higher in general psychiatric settings, where it is the most commonly presenting type of personality disorder. Before the publication of DSM–III in 1980, and the boost this gave to research into personality disorder, the majority of clinicians held rather pessimistic views about the treatment of BPD. Attitudes are slowly changing with the emergence of positive findings from a series of randomised controlled trials examining the effectiveness of psychological treatments for the disorder. It is beyond the scope of this chapter to provide a comprehensive review of this literature. Nevertheless, an account of outcome measures for personality disorder would be incomplete without reference to some of the more prominent trials in this field, as they exemplify some of the challenges encountered in measuring treatment outcome for personality disorders.

Linehan et al (1991) examined the effectiveness of dialectical behaviour therapy (DBT) compared with treatment as usual for 63 chronically para-suicidal women who met criteria for BPD. The treatment lasted 1 year, with assessment every 4 months. Over the follow-up period, those allocated to the control group engaged in self-harm significantly more often. There were, however, no between-group differences on measures of depression, hopelessness, suicide ideation or 'reasons for living'. Eight subsequent trials have replicated the positive effects of DBT and, of all treatments for BPD (particularly where the focus of the intervention is on reducing self-harm), it has amassed the largest evidence base (British Psychological Society & Royal College of Psychiatrists, 2009).

Bateman & Fonagy (1999) examined the effectiveness of mentalisation-based therapy (MBT; an intervention designed to increase self-reflective capacity) when delivered in the context of day hospital treatment. Forty-four patients were randomly allocated to receive either day hospital treatment with MBT or general psychiatric treatment. MBT consisted of a combination of individual and group psychotherapy and was for a maximum of 18 months. The researchers measured a large range of outcomes at 18 months, including frequency of suicide attempts and acts of self-harm, the number and duration of in-patient admissions, the use of psychotropic medication, and self-report measures of depression, anxiety, general symptom distress, interpersonal function and social adjustment. Patients who were treated with MBT showed a statistically significant decrease on all measures, in contrast to the control group. An 8-year follow-up of 41 of patients enrolled in the original trial showed that patients allocated to DBT sustained significantly better outcome on measures of suicidality, diagnostic status (i.e. still meeting criteria for BPD or not), use of services and medication, and global function, compared with those treated with standard psychiatric care (Bateman & Fonagy, 2008). However, both groups continued to show significant deficits in social and occupational functioning.

Although the two trials described above demonstrated treatment effectiveness in terms of reduced acts of self-harm, neither conclusively demonstrated efficacy for all aspects of BPD. Given that BPD consists of a constellation of disparate affective, cognitive and behavioural symptoms and lacks a single defining feature, this is perhaps an inevitable difficulty. Nevertheless, Giesen-Bloo *et al* (2006) attempted to address the problem by comparing the effectiveness of two prolonged out-patient treatments, both of which aimed at 'achieving full recovery from BPD'. The two treatments were schema-focused therapy (SFT; a type of cognitive therapy) and transference-focused psychotherapy (TFP; a type of psychodynamic psychotherapy). According to the authors:

both treatments intend to bring about a structural change in patients' personality, which should be apparent not only from a decrease in self-destructive behaviors but also from reduced pathologic personality features, reduced general psychopathologic dysfunction, and increased quality of life.

In a multicentre trial, 88 patients with BPD were randomly allocated to receive twice-weekly SFT or TFP, delivered over 3 years. The authors used a range of outcome measures, including the Borderline Personality Disorder Severity Index (specified as the primary outcome), quality of life, general psychopathological dysfunction, and measures of SFT/TFP personality concepts. Patient assessments were made before randomisation and then every 3 months for 3 years. After 3 years of treatment, survival analyses demonstrated that significantly more SFT patients recovered or showed reliable clinical improvement on the Borderline Personality Disorder Severity Index. SFT patients also showed greater increases in quality of life than TFP patients and the authors concluded that SFT was more effective than TFP.

All three trials highlight some important general principles about the assessment of change in personality disorders:

1   Given that personality disorders lack a core defining feature, no single outcome measure can adequately capture the complexity of psychopathology. Consequently, outcome assessment needs to cover multiple domains. The most important candidate outcome domains for BPD are listed in Table 15.2.

Table 15.2 Potential outcomes reported by intervention studies in people with borderline personality disorder

Domain	Outcome to be measured
Social functioning	Interpersonal functioning
	Social adjustment
General well-being	Quality of life
User experience	Experience of care
	Satisfaction with care
	Perceived coercion
	Engagement in treatment
Harm	Death
	Suicide
	Accidents
	Side-effects of treatment
Behaviours	Impulsivity
	Self-harm
	Violence to others
	Substance misuse
	Disordered eating
Emotional symptoms	Depression
	Anxiety
	Anger
Cognitive symptoms	Suicidal ideation
	Hopelessness
	Reasons for living
	Paranoid ideation
	Self-esteem
Service use	In-patient admissions
	General practitioner contacts
	Criminal justice system contacts
Diagnosis	Meeting (or not meeting) diagnosis based on DSM–IV criteria

Adapted from British Psychological Society & Royal College of Psychiatrists (2009).

2   Outcomes should ideally be assessed at multiple points in time in order to delineate a clearer picture of change (Perry & Sanlian, 2002).

3   Given the fact that, on the whole, therapeutic change in individuals with personality disorder occurs at a comparatively slow pace, follow-up needs to occur over long periods (i.e. years rather than months).

4   While symptomatic improvement is detectable over time, social impairment appears to be a lingering feature of personality disorder (Skodol et al, 2005; Zanarini et al, 2005b) and social function should therefore be part of any comprehensive longitudinal assessment of outcome.

Conclusion

The accurate assessment of outcome for personality disorders represents a considerable challenge. The absence of core defining pathology means that multi-domain assessments are required and should include measures of quality of life and social functioning. In the light of proposed taxonomic changes which will take effect with DSM–V, categorical assessments of personality disorder should be complemented by a dimensional measure of personality, such as the Neuroticism–Extroversion–Openness Personality Inventory (NEO–PI; Costa & McCrae, 1992). Symptomatic change over time, while important to capture in any longitudinal study, may, however, simply reflect exacerbation or attenuation of comorbid mental illness (the prevalence of which is elevated among those with a personality disorder) and is not a reliable way of assessing core change in personality. Moreover, change should be assessed over comparatively long periods. A range of instruments, both self-report and observer rated, have been developed to assess a large number of outcome measures and selecting the appropriate instrument will ultimately depend on many factors, including the type of personality disorder, the length of follow-up, the availability of resources, and the duration and setting of treatment.

References

American Psychiatric Association (1980) *Diagnostic and Statistical Manual of Mental Disorders* (3rd edition) (DSM–III). American Psychiatric Association.

American Psychiatric Association (1994) *Diagnostic and Statistical Manual of Mental Disorders* (4th edition) (DSM–IV). American Psychiatric Association.

Bateman, A. & Fonagy, P. (1999) Effectiveness of partial hospitalization in the treatment of borderline personality disorder: a randomized controlled trial. *American Journal of Psychiatry*, **156**, 1563–1569.

Bateman, A. & Fonagy, P. (2000) Effectiveness of psychotherapeutic treatment of personality disorder. *British Journal of Psychiatry*, **177**, 138–143.

Bateman, A. & Fonagy, P. (2008) 8-year follow-up of patients treated for borderline personality disorder: mentalization-based treatment versus treatment as usual. *American Journal of Psychiatry*, **165**, 631–638.

Bender, D. S., Dolan, R. T., Skodol, A. E., et al (2001) Treatment utilization by patients with personality disorders. *American Journal of Psychiatry*, **158**, 295–302.

British Psychological Society & Royal College of Psychiatrists (2009) *Borderline Personality Disorder: The NICE Guideline on Treatment and Management*. British Psychological Society & Royal College of Psychiatrists.

Cheng, A. T., Mann, A. H. & Chan, K. A. (1997) Personality disorder and suicide. A case–control study. *British Journal of Psychiatry*, **170**, 441–446.

Coid, J., Yang, M., Tyrer, P., et al (2006a) Prevalence and correlates of personality disorder in Great Britain. *British Journal of Psychiatry*, **188**, 423–431.

Coid, J., Yang, M., Roberts, A., et al (2006b) Violence and psychiatric morbidity in a national household population – a report from the British Household Survey. *American Journal of Epidemiology*, **164**, 1199–1208.

Cooper, J., Kapur, N., Webb, R., et al (2005) Suicide after deliberate self-harm: a 4-year cohort study. *American Journal of Psychiatry*, **162**, 297–303.

Costa, P. T., Jr & McCrae, R. R. (1992) *Revised NEO Personality Inventory (NEO–PI) and NEO Five Factor Inventory (NEO–FFI)*. Psychological Assessment Resources, Inc.

Crawford, M., Price, K., Rutter, D., et al (2008) Dedicated community-based services for adults with personality disorder: Delphi study. *British Journal of Psychiatry*, **193**, 342–343.

Ekselius, L., Lindstrom, E., Von Knorring, L., *et al* (1994) SCID II interviews and the SCID Screen questionnaire as diagnostic tools for personality disorders in DSM–III–R. *Acta Psychiatrica Scandinavica*, **90**, 120–123.

First, M. B., Gibbon, M., Spitzer, R. L., *et al* (1997) *The Structured Clinical Interview for DSM–IV Axis II Personality Disorders (SCID–II)*. American Psychiatric Press.

Fischer, E. P., Shumway, M. & Owen, R. R. (2002) Priorities of consumers, providers, and family members in the treatment of schizophrenia. *Psychiatric Services*, **53**, 724–729.

Fitzpatrick, R., Davey, C., Buxton, M. J., *et al* (1998) Evaluating patient-based outcome measures for use in clinical trials. *Health Technology Assessment*, **2**, 1–74.

Giesen-Bloo, J., van Dyck, R., Spinhoven, P., *et al* (2006) Outpatient psychotherapy for borderline personality disorder: randomized trial of schema-focused therapy vs transference-focused psychotherapy. *Archives of General Psychiatry*, **63**, 649–658.

Grant, B. F., Stinson, F. S., Dawson, D. A., *et al* (2004) Co-occurrence of 12-month alcohol and drug use disorders and personality disorders in the United States: results from the National Epidemiologic Survey on Alcohol and Related Conditions. *Archives of General Psychiatry*, **61**, 361–368.

Grilo, C. M., Sanislow, C. A., Gunderson, J. G., *et al* (2004) Two-year stability and change of schizotypal, borderline, avoidant, and obsessive–compulsive personality disorders. *Journal of Consulting and Clinical Psychology*, **72**, 767–775.

Gunderson, J. G., Kolb, J. E. & Austin, V. (1981) The diagnostic interview for borderline patients. *American Journal of Psychiatry*, **138**, 896–903.

Gunderson, J. G., Shea, M. T., Skodol, A. E., *et al* (2000) The Collaborative Longitudinal Personality Disorders Study: development, aims, design, and sample characteristics. *Journal of Personality Disorders*, **14**, 300–315.

Hayward, M. & Moran, P. (2008) Comorbidity of personality disorders and mental illnesses. *Psychiatry*, **7**, 105–109.

Hayward, M., Slade, M. & Moran, P. A. (2006) Personality disorders and unmet needs among psychiatric inpatients. *Psychiatric Services*, **57**, 538–543.

Hesse, M., Rasmussen, J. & Pedersen, M. K. (2008) Standardised assessment of personality – a study of validity and reliability in substance abusers. *BMC Psychiatry*, **8**, 7.

Hiroeh, U., Appleby, L., Mortensen, P. B., *et al* (2001) Death by homicide, suicide, and other unnatural causes in people with mental illness: a population-based study. *Lancet*, **358**, 2110–2112.

Hodgins, S., Mednick, S. A., Brennan, P. A., *et al* (1996) Mental disorder and crime. Evidence from a Danish birth cohort. *Archives of General Psychiatry*, **53**, 489–496.

Huang, Y., Kotov, R., de Girolamo, G., *et al* (2009) DSM–IV personality disorders in the WHO World Mental Health Surveys. *British Journal of Psychiatry*, **195**, 46–53.

Hyler, S. E., Skodol, A. E., Oldham, J. M., *et al* (1992) Validity of the Personality Diagnostic Questionnaire–Revised: a replication in an outpatient sample. *Comprehensive Psychiatry*, **33**, 73–77.

Lenzenweger, M. F., Loranger, A. W., Korfine, L., *et al* (1997) Detecting personality disorders in a nonclinical population. Application of a 2-stage procedure for case identification. *Archives of General Psychiatry*, **54**, 345–351.

Linehan, M. M., Armstrong, H. E., Suarez, A., *et al* (1991) Cognitive–behavioral treatment of chronically parasuicidal borderline patients. *Archives of General Psychiatry*, **48**, 1060–1064.

Livesley, W. J. (2001) Conceptual and taxonomic issues. In *Handbook of Personality Disorders* (ed. W. J. Livesley), pp. 3–38. Guilford Press.

Livesley, W. J., Jackson, D. N. & Schroeder, M. L. (1992) Factorial structure of traits delineating personality disorders in clinical and general population samples. *Journal of Abnormal Psychology*, **101**, 432–440.

Loranger, A. W., Sartorius, N., Andreoli, A., *et al* (1994) The International Personality Disorder Examination. The World Health Organization/Alcohol, Drug Abuse and Mental Health Administration International Pilot Study of Personality Disorders. *Archives of General Psychiatry*, **51**, 215–224.

Loranger, A. W., Sartorius, N. & Janca, A. (1996) *Assessment and Diagnosis of Personality Disorders: The International Personality Disorder Examination (IPDE)*. Cambridge University Press.

Mann, A. H., Jenkins, R., Cutting, J. C., et al (1981) The development and use of a standardized assessment of abnormal personality. *Psychological Medicine*, **11**, 839–847.

Mellsop, G., Varghese, F., Joshua, S., et al (1982) The reliability of Axis II of DSM–III. *American Journal of Psychiatry*, **139**, 1360–1361.

Moran, P. (2005) *Differential Access to Services for Individuals with Severe Personality Disorder*. National R&D Programme on Forensic Mental Health.

Moran, P., Jenkins, R., Tylee, A., et al (2000) The prevalence of personality disorder among UK primary care attenders. *Acta Psychiatrica Scandinavica*, **102**, 52–57.

Moran, P., Rendu, A., Jenkins, R., et al (2001) The impact of personality disorder in UK primary care: a 1-year follow-up of attenders. *Psychological Medicine*, **31**, 1447–1454.

Moran, P., Walsh, E., Tyrer, P., et al (2003a) Impact of comorbid personality disorder on violence in psychosis: report from the UK700 trial. *British Journal of Psychiatry*, **182**, 129–134.

Moran, P., Leese, M., Lee, T., et al (2003b) Standardised Assessment of Personality – Abbreviated Scale (SAPAS): preliminary validation of a brief screen for personality disorder. *British Journal of Psychiatry*, **183**, 228–232.

Mullen, P. E. (1999) Dangerous people with severe personality disorder. British proposals for managing them are glaringly wrong-and unethical. *BMJ*, **319**, 1146–1147.

National Institute for Health and Clinical Excellence (2009) *Borderline Personality Disorder: Treatment and Management*. NICE.

Patience, D. A., McGuire, R. J., Scott, A. I. F., et al (1995) The Edinburgh Primary Care Depression Study: personality disorder and outcome. *British Journal of Psychiatry*, **167**, 324–330.

Perkins, R. (2001) What constitutes success? The relative priority of service users' and clinicians' views of mental health services. *British Journal of Psychiatry*, **179**, 9–10.

Perry, J. C. & Sanlian, N. H. (2002) Outcome measurement in personality disorders. In *Outcome Measurement in Psychiatry: A Critical Review* (eds W. W. Ishak, T. Burt & L. I. Sederer), pp. 235–257. American Psychiatric Publishing.

Perry, J. C., Lavori, P. W. & Hoke, L. (1987) A Markov model for predicting levels of psychiatric service use in borderline and antisocial personality disorders and bipolar type II affective disorder. *Journal of Psychiatric Research*, **21**, 215–232.

Rendu, A., Moran, P., Patel, A., et al (2002) Economic impact of personality disorders in UK primary care attenders. *British Journal of Psychiatry*, **181**, 62–66.

Rottman, B. M., Ahn, W. K., Sanislow, C. A., et al (2009) Can clinicians recognize DSM–IV personality disorders from five-factor model descriptions of patient cases? *American Journal of Psychiatry*, **166**, 427–433.

Russell, D. (1995) *Women, Madness and Medicine*. Blackwell.

Sachsse, U., Von der Heyde, S. & Huether, G. (2002) Stress regulation and self-mutilation. *American Journal of Psychiatry*, **159**, 672.

Seivewright, H., Tyrer, P. & Johnson, T. (2002) Change in personality status in neurotic disorders. *Lancet*, **359**, 2253–2254.

Singleton, N., Meltzer, H. & Gatward, R. (1998) *Psychiatric Morbidity Among Prisoners in England and Wales*. TSO (The Stationery Office).

Skodol, A. E. & Bender, D. S. (2009) The future of personality disorders in DSM–V? *American Journal of Psychiatry*, **166**, 388–391.

Skodol, A. E., Pagano, M. E., Bender, D. S., et al (2005) Stability of functional impairment in patients with schizotypal, borderline, avoidant, or obsessive–compulsive personality disorder over two years. *Psychological Medicine*, **35**, 443–451.

Tyrer, P., Alexander, M. S., Cicchetti, D., et al (1979) Reliability of a schedule for rating personality disorders. *British Journal of Psychiatry*, **135**, 168–174.

Tyrer, P., Casey, P. & Ferguson, B. (1991) Personality disorder in perspective. *British Journal of Psychiatry*, **159**, 463–471.

Widiger, T. & Frances, A. (1994) Towards a dimensional model for the personality disorders. In *Personality Disorders and the Five Factor Model of Personality* (eds P. Costa & T. Widiger), pp. 19–39. American Psychological Association.

Widiger, T. A. & Simonsen, E. (2005) Alternative dimensional models of personality disorder: finding a common ground. *Journal of Personality Disorders*, **19**, 110–130.

World Health Organization (1992) *The ICD–10 Classification of Mental and Behavioural Disorders*. WHO.

Zanarini, M. C., Frankenburg, F. R., Hennen, J., *et al* (2005a) The McLean Study of Adult Development (MSAD): overview and implications of the first six years of prospective follow-up. *Journal of Personality Disorders*, **19**, 505–523.

Zanarini, M. C., Frankenburg, F. R., Hennen, J, *et al* (2005b) Psychosocial functioning of borderline patients and Axis II comparison subjects followed prospectively for six years. *Journal of Personality Disorders*, **19**, 19–29.

CHAPTER 16

The Schedules for Clinical Assessment in Neuropsychiatry and the tradition of the Present State Examination

John K. Wing and Traolach S. Brugha

The principles underlying the creation and long-term development of the Present State Examination (PSE), now incorporated, with its glossary of definitions of symptoms and other components, in a shell known as the Schedules for Clinical Assessment in Neuropsychiatry (SCAN), are derived from standards of clinical assessment gradually developed from the late 18th century onwards. A form of 'mental state examination' is now an established part of the standard curriculum in most medical schools. To conduct such an examination requires the clinician to meet a demanding list of requirements. The first essential is a sound grasp of clinical psycho-pathology. This confers an ability to recognise, and distinguish within and between, an extensive range of symptoms, such as delusions, hallucinations, obsessional ruminations, irrational fears of harmless stimuli and feelings of excessive guilt. A technique of 'cross-examination', based on the glossary of differential definitions of symptoms, must be learned in the first place by observing experienced practitioners interviewing their patients. It is only after completing a comprehensive clinical symptom base that diagnostic pro-cedures should, if needed, be brought into play with the help of algorithms

This chapter was written for the second edition in 1999, following Professor John Wing's retirement as Unit Head of the Medical Research Council's Social Psychiatry Unit, where I worked and trained under John until 1987. Sadly, John died on 18 April 2010. The chapter marks the early phase of a successful era of new studies using the Schedules for Clinical Assessment in Neuropsychiatry (SCAN); it is based on measurement principles developed in earlier decades by John and other colleagues. For this reason, the chapter appears in its original form and marks out part of John's great contribution to our subject. Interested readers will be able to find numerous examples in the published literature of the use of SCAN in methodological, clinical and epidemiological studies throughout the world since that time. Consideration is now being given to adapting SCAN to the newly emerging clinical classification systems of DSM–V and ICD–11 and the associated computer applications that support the SCAN system. Although enormous progress has been made in the intervening years in clinical, neuroscientific knowledge, the need for systematic, reliable clinical description of psychopathology has not diminished. Readers interested in obtaining training in SCAN in their own language can approach the appropriate World Health Organization SCAN reference training centre via http://www.whoscan.org/.

T. S. Brugha, University of Leicester

laid down in international standards, as well as those of any other system in local use. These specifics differentiate SCAN from methods such as fully structured questionnaires or self-report forms, which have other purposes.

The aims of SCAN

The three central aims of SCAN can be summarised very simply, in one sentence. They are to provide comprehensive, accurate and technically specifiable means of describing and classifying clinical phenomena in order to make comparisons. Making comparisons is at the heart of all clinical, educational and scientific activities.

The first, clinical, aim is to promote and use high-quality clinical observation. The PSE is designed to allow comparison of each respondent's experiences and behaviour against the examiner's glossary-defined concepts by a process of controlled clinical 'cross-examination'. The resulting outputs in the form of single symptoms, profiles, scores and rule-based categories of disorder can be compared with each other wherever in the world they are elicited. Thus, they can be used as a comparable base for clinical audit, needs assessment and monitoring the progress of individual respondents. It is essential to understand that the SCAN database is not tied exclusively to systems such as ICD–10 (World Health Organization, 1992) or DSM–IV (American Psychiatric Association, 1994). All the items required for these internationally based systems, and the algorithms necessary to derive their diagnoses, are included. However, the SCAN database and glossary include large numbers of symptoms culled from the experience of its many authors, and from the literature of many decades, which are not tied to any particular system of categorisation.

The second aim is educational and developmental: to improve clinical concepts by teaching a common clinical language. This makes it feasible to compare and learn from the usage of different clinical schools. It is not necessary to agree with such a standard of reference in order to appreciate its value as a basis for communication, quantification and comparison. Differences between clinical schools of thought do exist and are taught. Comparison between them by means of a common standard of reference provides a basis for informed development. SCAN itself benefits from such comparisons. However, modifications must be made in carefully defined stages, following periods long enough to provide a substantial and generally agreed basis for change.

The third, scientific, aim is to accelerate the accumulation of knowledge. Using standard technical procedures in research projects makes the results more precise and comparable, thus leading to more rapid agreement on useful theoretical lines for further hypothesis testing. This is true of all types of scientific research – biological, epidemiological and psychosocial.

Together, the three aims can facilitate the accumulation of knowledge for clinical purposes of all kinds, including primary, secondary and tertiary prevention and high-quality health service management and planning.

The precursors of SCAN

The basic aims and rationale of the PSE were first conceived in studies carried out by the Medical Research Council's Social Psychiatry Research Unit in the late 1950s and early 1960s (Wing, 1960, 1961, 1962). A paper outlining the principles, based on studies of symptoms associated with 'neurotic' and 'psychotic' disorders, was published by five clinicians (Wing *et al*, 1967). Most of the key characteristics of subsequent editions were anticipated in this paper. Three sample sections of the Schedule derived from the studies (PSE–5), covering obsessional symptoms, delusions of bodily control and non-social speech, were included as an appendix to the paper and bear a close resemblance to their present-day counterparts.

Four revisions (respectively the seventh to the tenth editions), each related to major international research projects and systems of diagnosis, amplified and improved the format while preserving the basic principles. Two projects were particularly influential. PSE–7 and PSE–8 were used in the US–UK Diagnostic Study (Cooper *et al*, 1972) and PSE–8 in the International Pilot Study of Schizophrenia (IPSS; World Health Organization, 1973, 1979). Reliability was satisfactory in both projects and in others conducted elsewhere (e.g. Kendell *et al*, 1968; Luria & McHugh, 1974; Cooper *et al*, 1977; Wing *et al*, 1977; Luria & Berry, 1979; Rogers & Mann, 1986; Lesage *et al*, 1991).

Both large international projects concentrated on the differential diagnosis between schizophrenia and other, particularly affective, disorders. The central result of the US–UK study was that the team of research psychiatrists, examining hospital patients on both sides of the Atlantic, diagnosed far fewer schizophrenic disorders than their counterparts in the UK. The PSE profiles confirmed that New York hospital diagnoses of schizophrenia were substantially broader. This had no implications for validity in the strict sense but it did indicate that the boundaries of the disorder were, at that time, drawn so differently that the results of studies into causes, treatments and outcomes would not be comparable between New York and London if based on hospital diagnoses.

The IPSS investigators formed a larger and more diverse group than those of the US–UK study. They came from psychiatric departments in Åarhus, Agra, Cali, Ibadan, London, Moscow, Prague, Taipei and Washington, DC. The results, however, were very similar. The PSE symptom profiles showed that centres in Moscow and Washington used a broader definition of schizophrenia than the other seven. The case for an instrument such as the PSE was thus abundantly reinforced.

In addition, the experience of these projects indicated a need for three major improvements in SCAN itself:

- the glossary of differential definitions should be updated and expanded as a basis for training courses
- additional schedules would be needed to allow the rating of previous episodes of disorder and possible causes and pathologies

- algorithms for classifying from PSE item profiles into ICD–9 diagnostic categories should be created in order to give a standard of reference in addition to (not as a substitute for) clinical diagnosis, since at that time the international diagnostic systems did not provide 'official' algorithms.

These features were incorporated into PSE–9, which was short: only 140 items, derived from the 500 items of its predecessor. Each was given a differential definition in the glossary, which, together with a specified method of clinical examination, continued to be at the heart of the system. A Syndrome Checklist for previous episodes, an Aetiology Schedule, the CATEGO–4 computer program and a computer-assisted version of the text were added, filling in most of the gaps in the earlier systems. The principles were laid down in a reference manual (Wing et al, 1974).

Further innovations included a set of scales that allowed the ratings of specified groups of symptoms to be summed, and an Index of Definition (ID) that provided a means of differentiating eight levels of confidence that sufficient symptoms were present to allow a diagnosis of one of the 'functional' categories of ICD–9, an important indicator for general population studies (Wing, 1976; Wing et al, 1978). Three other modifications were also found useful: a change rating scale using PSE items for monitoring clinical progress over time (Tress et al, 1987), a technique for ascertaining lifetime prevalence (McGuffin et al, 1986), and a brief form using only ten items to identify 'non-cases', which worked with remarkable success (Cooper & McKenzie, 1981).

Publishing the full PSE–9 and its accessories for the first time in 1974, after 15 years of development, provided an opportunity to state the aims of the system, summarise its limitations and advantages, and specify the relationships between the PSE text and glossary (Wing, 1983). These have not changed since. The interesting and difficult problems encountered during translation into many different languages have not changed either (Sartorius, 1998).

The PSE/CATEGO–4 system was used in numerous studies and translations in many corners of the world, both in sample population surveys and in experimental research, for example: Henderson et al (1979), Orley & Wing (1979), Urwin & Gibbons (1979), Knights et al (1980), Bebbington et al (1981), Okasha & Ashour (1981), Sturt (1981), Dean et al (1983), Mavreas & Bebbington (1988), Huxley et al (1989), Brugha et al (1990), Lehtinen et al (1990, 1991), Pakaslahti (1994).

One unexpected problem, appreciated only after long experience, was that many users tended to regard the computerised output from PSE–9 only in terms of a single diagnosis, rather than as a rich and varied psychometric profile. This was far from the authors' intention (Wing, 1983, 1994). A central principle is that the system cannot 'make a diagnosis' in the sense that a clinician can. Those who use it are responsible for interpreting the data according to their judgement of the adequacy of the interview, the quality of the data recorded and the choice of outputs from the computer analysis. Most of these outputs are profiles of scores or pre-final categories. A 'final' category can be derived and interpreted as a diagnosis only if the clinician so decides, but that decision is made by him or her, not by the PSE, and still less by the computer.

Rose (1992) made the point that diagnosis 'splits the world in two': those who have a disorder and those who do not. But most problems have continuous distributions. The PSE was not originally designed as a diagnostic instrument, although in the course of its development as a comprehensive clinical tool it came to provide a database capable (in addition to its basic psychometric properties) of expanding to exploit the more exacting algorithms presented by the DSM and ICD series. Both systems will undoubtedly change in further editions, perhaps markedly. The symptoms of patients are much less likely to vary from those familiar now.

Preparation for SCAN

More than 15 years of experience with the PSE–9 system provided a mass of suggestions for improvement. Preparations for a tenth edition were started in 1980 in anticipation of ICD–10 (Jablensky et al, 1983). The major emphasis of collaborators and correspondents was on broadening the content, both by returning to the larger item pool of PSE–7 and PSE–8, and by adding new sections to cover somatoform, dissociative and eating disorders, alcohol and drug use, and cognitive impairments. Similar work was also begun in preparation for the use of DSM–III criteria in the Epidemiologic Catchment Area studies (Romanoski et al, 1988).

A second suggestion was that an extra rating point was needed to extend the 0–1–2 scales of severity used for most PSE–9 items, to provide a mild or 'subclinical' level, especially for use in population surveys. There is some evidence that this could be useful, by allowing clinically inexperienced trainees to rate as present items that are only marginally significant clinically (Dean et al, 1983; Brugha et al, 1999c). It has, however, introduced a difficulty when comparing PSE–9 with PSE–10 studies. Users of PSE–9 had made it clear that they would wish relevant items in PSE–10 to be convertible into PSE–9 equivalents, so that the CATEGO computer program could be applied to produce output comparable with data from earlier studies.

A third, very obvious, requirement was for a better technique for rating previous episodes of disorder, adding other items relevant to the history and to aetiology, and processing all the resulting information by means of one set of computer programs.

Finally, the widespread acceptance and use of DSM–III–R, and subsequently DSM–IV, meant that the SCAN databases must contain all the clinical and course criteria specified in their manuals, as well as those being developed for ICD–10, and that the new algorithms must contain all three sets of classifying rules. This was the right decision, but it enhanced the risk that

SCAN could be regarded as principally a diagnostic instrument, whereas the first intention remains to provide a broad and up-to-date clinical database fitted to serve much broader purposes. It also added to the delays.

An early version of SCAN, containing an expanded PSE and glossary as its major components, was devised to meet these stringent requirements and used in a study of long-stay day care in south-east London (Brugha *et al*, 1988).

These experiences, together with suggestions from international reviewers whose opinions were canvassed by a task force established by the World Health Organization and the US Alcohol, Drug Abuse and Mental Health Administration, led to further additions and modifications (Wing *et al*, 1990). The February 1988 prototype was used in international field trials to test reliability between interviewer and observer and between two interviewers over time, and also its general practicality in use across a wide range of disorders. Subsequent changes in the sections dealing with the use of alcohol and other drugs, eating and obsessional disorders, and cognitive impairments, led to further trials (Wing *et al*, 1998, chapter 8). SCAN was redesigned in the light of all these conclusions and a sequence of further drafts ensued. All contained the updated Item Group Check List and Clinical History Schedule as well.

Finally, many additions were needed to cover the development and successive publication of algorithms for the major international diagnostic systems. All the new items and instructions (including course criteria and attributions of cause) in ICD–10 Diagnostic Criteria for research and the texts of DSM–III–R and IV, had to be included. A computer-assisted PSE (CAPSE) was devised and went through similar modifications. In the event, three consecutive versions of SCAN were published by the World Health Organization: one printed by Design Locker (1992) but not used in formal trials; one by American Psychiatric Press (version 2.0; Wing *et al*, 1990); the third printed by Cambridge University Press (1999). This last is the definitive version 2 (World Health Organization Division of Mental Health, 1999). It incorporates PSE–10.2 and CAPSE–2.

The structure of SCAN

The full list of SCAN version 2 components is as follows:

- the SCAN manual, comprising –
  - PSE–10.2, sections 1–25
  - Item Group Checklist (IGC), section 26
  - Clinical History Schedule (CHS), section 27
- the SCAN glossary
- the computer-assisted PSE–10.2 (CAPSE–2 with WHO SCAN I shell)
- the SCAN training materials
- the SCAN reference manual (Wing *et al*, 1998).

Present State Examination (PSE, tenth edition)

PSE–10.2 is the largest part of the SCAN manual, taking up the first 25 of its 27 sections. Each section is devoted to a particular type of symptom or sign or other clinical feature. The phenomena of disorders in subchapters F0–F5 of ICD–10 and their equivalents in DSM–III–R and DSM–IV are all included, as part of the comprehensive database, as follows:

- F0: Dementia, including symptomatic mental disorders
- F1: Mental and behavioural disorders due to psychoactive substance use
- F2: Schizophrenia, schizotypal and delusional disorders
- F3: Mood disorders
- F4: Neurotic, stress-related and somatoform disorders
- F50–51: Eating disorders, non-organic sleep disorders

Some sections have optional checklists attached, covering items related to disorders that require specific time relationships, for example to psychosocial trauma, as in the stress and adjustment disorders. Other checklists allow a more extended range of items to be rated than is provided for in the main text, as is done, for example, for the somatoform symptoms.

A caveat must be repeated here, to reinforce earlier statements that PSE–10.2 contains numerous items that are not present in the two international systems, and that the complete database is intended to support projects independently of whether a diagnosis is required or not.

Item Group Checklist (IGC, section 26)

The IGC provides a simple means of rating information obtained from case records and informants, including the respondent's account of previous episodes. The Item Groups are not diagnostic syndromes and do not contain the items necessary for all the algorithms for ICD or DSM disorders. The resulting classification is therefore approximate compared with that of the PSE, but it is a useful supplement and can substitute in situations where the PSE cannot be fully completed.

Users of the IGC must have been trained in the use of PSE–10 and its glossary, and have become completely familiar with the structure of SCAN. This provides a substantial degree of operationalisation for rating Item Groups, each of which is composed of designated PSE–10 items.

Clinical History Schedule (CHS, section 27)

The CHS is an optional section but is recommended because of the opportunity it offers to match personal details and historical information against data recorded elsewhere in SCAN. It also provides the investigator with an opportunity to record any relevant points on ICD–10 subchapters F1 (dementias), F6 (personality disorders) and F9 (disorders with onset in childhood), which are not covered in detail in the PSE. Interviewing the patient is not generally suited to eliciting the problems associated with these disorders. For example, a full developmental history – essential for the diagnosis of autistic spectrum disorders such as Asperger syndrome – is not included.

The SCAN glossary

The glossary is at the heart of the SCAN system. It consists of differential definitions of items in the SCAN text: that is, a definition not only of what the item signifies but also of what it excludes. This 'item concept' is learned during training and thereafter carried in the examiner's mind. Virtually every item in SCAN is defined in the glossary, not only those representing symptoms but also those concerned with time relationships, precipitants, clinical course, attribution of cause and so on. It provides a common clinical language, in which interviewers, whatever their own school of thought and wherever in the world they are working, can communicate with each other and make useful comparisons.

Computer applications

Computer programs are provided to facilitate data entry, data analysis and output of the results for individual respondents. Data analysis is both top down, in terms of rule-based categories such as the disorders in ICD–10, and bottom up, in the sense that the items, item groups and dimensional scores provide alternative descriptive profiles. The computer applications can provide an immediate output as each interview is completed. In its present form the SCAN I shell also provides a standard statistical output (in SPSS PC) and outputs from ICD–10 and DSM–IV. Up-to-date details can be obtained from the WHO SCAN training centres listed on the SCAN website (http://www.whoscan.org).

SCAN training

Training centres, recognised by the World Health Organization because they have a critical mass of staff experienced in the use of SCAN for clinical and research purposes and knowledgeable about translation problems, have been set up worldwide, for example in China, Denmark, Luxembourg, Germany, India, Russia, Spain, the UK and the USA. A core element is standard in all centres but details are adapted to local circumstances. Further information can be obtained from the training centres, as above.

Further work

The developmental version of SCAN (printed as SCAN–2.0) was used in a number of community surveys, most notably to interview people screened from a first-stage UK national sample to identify people with all grades of mental illness (Jenkins *et al*, 1997). A further study compared two lay-administered diagnostic interviews (the CIDI and CISR) with SCAN–1 in a representative random sample of adults in 2000 households (Brugha *et al*, 1999a,b). The target disorders were current anxiety, depressive and obsessional disorders. As similar studies have suggested, the results show that fixed interview schedules, allowing no informed cross-questioning, have poor concordance with instruments like SCAN.

Because of the successive changes made between the prototype and the versions used in field trials, further studies will be required to establish current reliability, structure and usefulness. In particular, work is needed on test–retest reliability in the general population and in primary care, together with work on sections that have not been fully tested, such as those on the somatoform, stress and adjustment disorders. International projects are coordinated from the World Health Organization's headquarters in Geneva. Other developments include versions dedicated to particular research settings, such as the survey form referred to above, and a short form more suited to service and professional training purposes.

The importance of high-quality psychiatric epidemiological data has been emphasised by the report on the Global Burden of Disease from the World Bank (Murray & Lopez, 1997). The use of mathematical modelling techniques will make it possible for high-quality data from SCAN re-appraisal interviews to re-weight and estimate prevalence rates originally derived from large surveys (Kessler, 1999; Brugha *et al*, 2001). Close collaboration between developers of semi-structured and fully structured survey measures therefore continues to be necessary.

Conclusion

The development and successive improvement of a series of instruments culminating in SCAN–2, incorporating PSE–10.2 as its major component, began in the late 1950s because of the need for better tools for clinical measurement, categorisation and diagnosis. The underlying principles had long been decided by the time of first publication of PSE–9 in 1974. They remain the same in PSE–10.2. Based on the glossary of differential definitions, the aims are to provide comprehensive, accurate and technically specifiable means of describing and classifying clinical phenomena in order to make comparisons. In so far as it fulfils these aims, SCAN can be used to enhance clinical work, promote clinical training and advance knowledge through its use in biomedical, epidemiological and psychosocial research.

References

American Psychiatric Association (1994) *Diagnostic and Statistical Manual of Mental Disorders* (4th edition) (DSM–IV). American Psychiatric Association.

Bebbington, P. E., Hurry, J., Tennant, C., et al (1981) Epidemiology of mental disorders in Camberwell. *Psychological Medicine*, **11**, 561–580.

Brugha, T. S., Wing, J. K., Brewin, C. R., et al (1988) The problems of people in long-term psychiatric day-care. An introduction to the Camberwell High Contact Survey. *Psychological Medicine*, **18**, 443–456.

Brugha, T. S., Bebbington, P., Macarthy, B., et al (1990) Gender, social support and recovery from depressive disorders: a prospective clinical study. *Psychological Medicine*, **20**, 147–156.

Brugha, T. S., Bebbington, P., Jenkins, R., et al (1999a) Cross validation of a household population survey diagnostic interview: a comparison of CIS–R with SCAN ICD–10 diagnostic categories. *Psychological Medicine*, **29**, 1029–1042.

Brugha, T. S., Bebbington, P. E. & Jenkins, R. (1999b) A difference that matters: comparisons of structured and semi-structured diagnostic interviews of adults in the general population. *Psychological Medicine*, **29**, 1013–1020.

Brugha, T. S., Nienhuis, F. J., Bagchi, D., et al (1999c) The survey form of SCAN: the feasibility of using experienced lay survey interviewers to administer a semi-structured clinical assessment of psychotic and non-psychotic disorders. *Psychological Medicine*, **29**, 703–712.

Brugha, T. S., Jenkins, R., Taub, N. A., et al (2001) A general population comparison of the Composite International Diagnostic Interview (CIDI) and the Schedules for Clinical Assessment in Neuropsychiatry (SCAN). *Psychological Medicine*, **31**, 1001–1013.

Cooper, J. E. & McKenzie, S. (1981) The rapid prediction of low scores on a standardized psychiatric interview (PSE). In *What is a Case?* (eds J. K. Wing, P. Bebbington & L. N. Robins), pp. 143–151. Grant McIntyre.

Cooper, J. E., Kendell, R. E., Gurland, B. J., et al (1972) *Psychiatric Diagnosis in New York and London*. Oxford University Press.

Cooper, J. E., Copeland, J. R. M., Brown, G. W., et al (1977) Further studies on interviewer training and inter-rater reliability of the PSE. *Psychological Medicine*, **7**, 517–523.

Dean, C., Surtees, P. G. & Sashidharan, S. P. (1983) Comparison of research diagnostic systems in an Edinburgh community sample. *British Journal of Psychiatry*, **142**, 247–256.

Henderson, S., Duncan-Jones, P., Byrne, D. G., et al (1979) Psychiatric disorder in Canberra. A standardized study of prevalence. *Acta Psychiatrica Scandinavica*, **60**, 355–374.

Huxley, P., Raval, H., Korer, J., et al (1989) Psychiatric morbidity in the clients of social workers. Clinical outcome. *Psychological Medicine*, **19**, 189–198.

Jablensky, A., Sartorius, N., Hirschfeld, R., et al (1983) Diagnosis and classification of mental disorders and alcohol- and drug-related problems. A research agenda for the 1980s. *Psychological Medicine*, **13**, 907–921.

Jenkins, R., Lewis, G., Bebbington, P., et al (1997) The national psychiatric morbidity surveys of Great Britain – initial findings from the household survey. *Psychological Medicine*, **27**, 775–789.

Kendell, R. E., Everitt, B., Cooper, J. E., et al (1968) Reliability of the PSE. *Social Psychiatry*, **3**, 123–129.

Kessler, R. C. (1999) The WHO International Consortium in Psychiatric Epidemiology. Initial work and future directions. *Acta Psychiatrica Scandinavica*, **99**, 2–9.

Knights, A., Hirsch, S. R. & Platt, S. D. (1980) Clinical change as a function of brief admission to hospital in a controlled study using the PSE. *British Journal of Psychiatry*, **137**, 170–180.

Lehtinen, V., Lindholm, T., Veijola, J., et al (1990) The prevalence of PSE–CATEGO disorders in a Finnish adult population cohort. *Social Psychiatry and Psychiatric Epidemiology*, **25**, 187–192.

Lehtinen, V., Joukamaa, M., Jyrkinen, T., et al (1991) *Mental Health and Mental Disorders in the Finnish Adult Population*, pp. 308–342. Social Institute.

Lesage, A. D., Cyr, M. & Toupin, J. (1991) Reliable use of the PSE by psychiatric nurses of psychotic and non-psychotic patients. *Acta Psychiatrica Scandinavica*, **83**, 121–124.

275

Luria, R. E. & Berry, R. (1979) Reliability and descriptive validity of the PSE syndromes. *Archives of General Psychiatry*, **36**, 1187–1195.

Luria, R. E. & McHugh, P. R. (1974) Reliability and clinical utility of the Wing PSE. *Archives of General Psychiatry*, **30**, 866–871.

Mavreas, V. G. & Bebbington, P. E. (1988) Greeks, British Greek Cypriots and Londoners. A comparison of morbidity. *Psychological Medicine*, **18**, 433–442.

McGuffin, P., Katz, R. & Aldrich, J. (1986) Past and present state examination. The assessment of 'lifetime ever' psychopathology. *Psychological Medicine*, **16**, 461–466.

Murray, C. J. L. & Lopez, A. D. (1997) Alternative projections of mortality and disability by cause, 1990–2020. Global burden of disease study. *Lancet*, **349**, 1498–1504.

Okasha, A. & Ashour, A. (1981) Psycho-demographic study of anxiety in Egypt. The PSE in its Arabic version. *British Journal of Psychiatry*, **139**, 70–73.

Orley, J. & Wing, J. K. (1979) Psychiatric disorders in two African villages. *Archives of General Psychiatry*, **36**, 513–520.

Pakaslahti, A. (1994) Predictors of working disability in first admission schizophrenic patients. *Psychiatrica Fennica*, **25**, 150–168.

Rogers, B. & Mann, S. A. (1986) The reliability and validity of PSE assessments by lay interviewers. A national population survey. *Psychological Medicine*, **16**, 689–700.

Romanoski, A. J., Nestad, G., Cahal, R., *et al* (1988) Inter-observer reliability of a 'Standard Psychiatric Examination' for case ascertainment (DSM–III). *Journal of Nervous and Mental Disease*, **176**, 63–71.

Rose, G. (1992) *The Strategy of Preventive Medicine*. Oxford University Press.

Sartorius, N. (1998) SCAN translation. In *Diagnosis and Clinical Measurement in Psychiatry. An Instruction Manual for the Scan System* (eds J. K. Wing, N. Sartorius & T. B. Üstün), pp. 44–57. Cambridge University Press.

Sturt, E. (1981) Hierarchical patterns in the distribution of psychiatric symptoms. *Psychological Medicine*, **11**, 783–794.

Tress, K. H., Bellenis, C., Brownlow, J. H., *et al* (1987) The PSE change rating scale. *British Journal of Psychiatry*, **150**, 201–207.

Urwin, P. & Gibbons, J. L. (1979) Psychiatric diagnosis in self poisoning patients. *Psychological Medicine*, **9**, 501–507.

Wing, J. K. (1960) The measurement of behaviour in chronic schizophrenia. *Acta Psychiatrica et Neurologica*, **35**, 245–254.

Wing, J. K. (1961) A simple and reliable sub-classification of chronic schizophrenia. *Journal of Mental Science*, **107**, 862–875.

Wing, J. K. (1962) Institutionalism in mental hospitals. *Journal of Social and Clinical Psychology*, **1**, 38–51.

Wing, J. K. (1976) A technique for studying psychiatric morbidity in in-patient and out-patient series and in general population samples. *Psychological Medicine*, **6**, 665–671.

Wing, J. K. (1983) Use and misuse of the PSE. *British Journal of Psychiatry*, **143**, 111–117.

Wing, J. K. (1994) Relevance of psychiatric epidemiology to clinical psychiatry. *International Review of Psychiatry*, **6**, 259–264.

Wing, J. K., Birley, J. L. T., Cooper, J. E., *et al* (1967) Reliability of a procedure for measuring and classifying 'present psychiatric state'. *British Journal of Psychiatry*, **113**, 499–515.

Wing, J. K., Cooper, J. E. & Sartorius, N. (1974) *The Description and Classification of Psychiatric Symptoms. An Instruction Manual for the PSE and CATEGO System*. Cambridge University Press.

Wing, J. K., Nixon, J M., Mann, S. A., *et al* (1977) Reliability of the PSE (ninth edition) used in a population survey. *Psychological Medicine*, **7**, 505–516.

Wing, J. K., Mann, S. A., Leff, J. P., *et al* (1978) The concept of a 'case' in psychiatric population surveys. *Psychological Medicine*, **8**, 203–217.

Wing, J. K., Babor, T., Brugha, T., *et al* (1990) SCAN: Schedules for Clinical Assessment in Neuropsychiatry. *Archives of General Psychiatry*, **47**, 589–593.

Wing, J. K., Sartorius, N. & Üstün, T. B. (eds) (1998) *Diagnosis and Clinical Measurement in Psychiatry. A Reference Manual for the SCAN System*. Cambridge University Press.

World Health Organization (1973) *The International Pilot Study of Schizophrenia (IPSS)*. WHO.

World Health Organization (1979) *Schizophrenia. An International Follow-up Study*. WHO.

World Health Organization (1992) *The ICD–10 Classification of Mental and Behavioural Disorders*. WHO.

World Health Organization Division of Mental Health (1999) SCAN Schedules for Clinical Assessment in Neuropsychiatry Version 2.1. Available through WHO SCAN Training Centres (http://www.whoscan.org).

Part IV
International approaches
to outcome assessment

CHAPTER 17

Psychiatric assessment instruments developed by the World Health Organization

Norman Sartorius, Aleksandar Janca, Shekhar Saxena
and T. Bedirhan Üstün

Over the past four decades the World Health Organization (WHO) has produced a number of assessment instruments intended for national and cross-cultural psychiatric research. WHO instruments have been tested and used in many collaborative studies, involving more than 100 centres in different parts of the world. This chapter reviews the main WHO instruments for the assessment of:

- psychopathology
- disability and burden
- quality of life
- health services and systems
- environment and risks to mental health.

Instruments for qualitative research are also examined, before the principles used in the development of WHO instruments, their translation and their use across cultures and settings are discussed.

The WHO occupies a unique position in the field of healthcare and represents a neutral platform that can be used to bring about international collaboration in research. It has a mandate to promote and conduct research in the field of health and standardise diagnostic procedures and instruments (WHO, 2005). Over the years the WHO has gained experience in the management of international collaborative research projects and has produced reliable methods for their conduct in different cultures and settings (Sartorius, 1989). The development of cross-culturally applicable and reliable methods for the assessment of problems related to mental health has been one of the major activities in the WHO Mental Health Programme. Many of these methods have been described in scientific publications, released for general use and applied in various research projects worldwide (Sartorius, 1993). This chapter outlines the basic characteristics of the main instruments produced and used in the studies coordinated by the WHO Mental Health Programme. The specific characteristics of the instruments described – their format, area of assessment, main users, training requirements and available translations – are summarised in

Tables 17.1–17.5. More details about these and other WHO instruments can be found in the catalogue of assessment instruments used in the studies coordinated by the WHO Mental Health Programme (Janca & Chandrashekar, 1993), available from the WHO on request.

Instruments for the assessment of psychopathology

Alcohol Use Disorders Identification Test

The Alcohol Use Disorders Identification Test (AUDIT; Babor *et al*, 1989) is a brief structured interview aimed at identifying people whose alcohol consumption has become harmful to their health. It consists of ten questions: three on the amount and frequency of drinking, three on drinking behaviour and four on problems or adverse psychological reactions related to alcohol. The instrument can be interviewer- or self-administered, and the average administration time is 1–2 minutes. If the respondent is defensive or uncooperative, the clinical screening procedure (CSP) may be used to complement AUDIT. CSP contains a listing of indirect questions and clinical signs likely to indicate the harmful consequences of alcohol use.

AUDIT has been tested in a WHO collaborative project on the early detection of people with harmful alcohol consumption. High reliability of the constituent scales, as well as high face validity and the ability to distinguish light drinkers from those with harmful drinking have been reported (Saunders & Aasland, 1987; Saunders *et al*, 1993*a,b*).

Composite International Diagnostic Interview

The Composite International Diagnostic Interview (CIDI; WHO, 1993*a*) is a highly standardised diagnostic instrument for the assessment of mental disorders according to the definitions and criteria in ICD–10 (WHO, 1992) and DSM–III–R (American Psychiatric Association, 1987). A version of CIDI that would accommodate DSM–IV criteria (American Psychiatric Association, 1994) was released in 1995.

CIDI is primarily intended for use in epidemiological studies of mental disorders in general populations. The instrument consists of fully spelled-out questions and of a probing system aimed at assessing the clinical significance and psychiatric relevance of reported phenomena. No clinical judgement is required in coding and recording respondents' answers, and the schedule can be competently administered by a lay or clinician interviewer after 1 week's training. The average administration time is 90 minutes. CIDI is accompanied by a set of supporting materials that includes manuals and computer programs for data entry, correction and scoring of ICD–10 and DSM diagnoses.

A number of versions and modules of CIDI have been produced for specific research purposes (Janca *et al*, 1994*a*), including a computerised

Table 17.1 WHO instruments for the assessment of psychopathology

Instrument	Format	Area	User	Training	Languages
Alcohol Use Disorders Identification Test	Structured	Harmful alcohol use	Health or research worker	Not required	English, Japanese, Norwegian, Romanian, Spanish
Composite International Diagnostic Interview	Structured	ICD–10, DSM–III–R and DSM–V mental disorders	Lay interviewer	Essential	Arabic, Chinese, Dutch, English, French, German, Greek, Icelandic, Italian, Japanese, Kannada, Russian, Serbian, Spanish
ICD–10 Symptom Checklist for Mental Disorders	Semi-structured	ICD–10 mental disorders	Psychiatrist or psychologist	Not required	Chinese, English, Estonian, German, Italian, Japanese, Kannada, Portuguese, Russian, Spanish
International Personality Disorder Examination	Semi-structured	ICD–10, DSM–III–R and DSM–IV personality disorders	Psychiatrist or psychologist	Essential	Dutch, English, Estonian, French, German, Greek, Hindi, Japanese, Kannada, Norwegian, Swahili, Tamil
Schedules for Clinical Assessment in Neuro-psychiatry	Semi-structured	Symptoms and signs of mental disorders	Psychiatrist or psychologist	Essential	Chinese, Danish, Dutch, English, French, German, Greek, Italian, Kannada, Portuguese, Spanish, Turkish, Yoruba
Standardized Assessment of Depressive Disorders	Semi-structured	Depressive disorders	Psychiatrist or psychologist	Essential	Bulgarian, Farsi, French, German, Hindi, Japanese, Polish, Turkish,
Schedules for Clinical Assessment of Acute Psychotic States	Semi-structured	Acute psychotic states	Psychiatrist or psychologist	Essential	Czech, Danish, English, Hindi, Yoruba
Social Description	Semi-structured	Social history	Social worker	Essential or psychologist	Chinese, Czech, Danish, English, Hindi, Russian, Spanish, Yoruba
Self-Reporting Questionnaire	Question-naire	Neurotic and psychotic symptoms	Self-administered	Not applicable	Amharic, Arabic, Bahasa (Malaysia), Bengali, English, French, Hindi, Italian, Kiswahili, Njanja Lusaka, Portuguese, Spanish, Tagalog

version of CIDI (CIDI Auto; WHO, 1993c) and the Substance Abuse Module (Robins *et al*, 1990).

CIDI has been extensively tested in two field trials involving 20 centres, 12 languages and about 1200 respondents. The field trials showed that the instrument is generally acceptable and appropriate, and a reliable diagnostic tool for use across cultures and settings (Robins *et al*, 1988; Cottler *et al*, 1991; Wittchen *et al*, 1991; Janca *et al*, 1992).

The latest version of the CIDI has been developed for the World Mental Health (WMH) survey and it includes a screening module and 40 sections that focus on 22 ICD–10 and DSM–IV mental disorders and related functioning, treatment, risk factors and consequences. The WMH–CIDI is accompanied by an elaborate CD-based set of training materials designed to teach interviewers how to administer the instrument as well as to teach supervisors how to monitor the quality of data collection (Kessler & Ustun, 2004).

ICD–10 Symptom Checklist for Mental Disorders

The ICD–10 Symptom Checklist for Mental Disorders (Janca *et al*, 1994b) is a semi-structured instrument intended for clinicians' assessment of psychiatric symptoms and syndromes in the F0–F6 categories of ICD–10. The instrument requires the clinician user to examine the patient or case notes in order to rate the presence or absence of symptoms that are necessary to make a firm diagnosis in the ICD–10 system. The Checklist also lists symptoms and states that, according to ICD–10 criteria, have often been found to be associated with a syndrome (e.g. alcohol misuse in patients with mania) or that should be assessed independently from the syndrome (e.g. intellectual dysfunction in patients with organic mental disorder). The symptom lists are accompanied by instructions intended to help the user to consider differential diagnoses. The possibility of recording onset, severity and duration of the syndrome, as well as number of episodes (where applicable), is also provided. The Checklist is accompanied by the ICD–10 Symptom Glossary for Mental Disorders (Isaac *et al*, 1994). The Glossary provides brief definitions of the symptoms and terms used in the Checklist.

The ICD–10 Symptom Checklist for Mental Disorders was used at one of the sites participating in the field trials of ICD–10, and preliminary results showed good psychometric properties for the instrument. The average administration time is 15 minutes and the interviewer/observer reliability is acceptable (kappa = 0.72; Janca *et al*, 1993).

International Personality Disorder Examination

The International Personality Disorder Examination (IPDE; WHO, 1993b) is a semi-structured interview schedule designed for the assessment of personality disorders according to ICD–10 and DSM–IV criteria. It is designed for use by clinicians who have received training in its use. The IPDE covers the following six areas of the respondent's personality and behaviour: work, self, interpersonal relationships, affects, reality testing and impulse control. The last six items in the schedule are scored without questioning and are based on the interviewer's observation of the respondent during the interview. The IPDE requires that a behaviour or a trait be present for at least 5 years before it should be considered a manifestation of personality or a symptom of personality disorder and that at least one criterion of personality disorder be fulfilled before the age of 15 years. The information about the respondent obtained by reliable informants can also be recorded and is used in the final scoring of the diagnosis. The final scoring, which may be done clerically or by computer, is used in making ICD–10 and/or DSM–IV diagnoses; a dimensional score can also be calculated.

Because of the length of the interview (2–3 hours) the IPDE has been produced in two versions, one for ICD–10 and the other for DSM–IV diagnoses. Both versions of the instrument are accompanied by a user manual, screener, hand-scoring sheets and computer-scoring programs.

The IPDE has been tested in a WHO-coordinated field trial in which 14 centres from 11 countries participated. The results indicated good acceptability, high interrater reliability and satisfactory temporal stability for the criteria and diagnoses assessed by the interview (Loranger *et al*, 1991, 1994).

Schedules for Clinical Assessment in Neuropsychiatry

Schedules for Clinical Assessment in Neuropsychiatry (SCAN; WHO, 1994; see also Chapter 16 of the present volume) is a semi-structured clinical interview schedule designed for clinicians' assessment of the symptoms and course of adult mental disorders. SCAN comprises an interview schedule, namely the tenth edition of the Present State Examination (PSE; Wing *et al*, 1974), a glossary of differential definitions, the Item Group Checklist (IGC) and the Clinical History Schedule (CHS). The SCAN glossary is an essential part of SCAN and provides differential definitions of SCAN items and a commentary on the SCAN text. A reference manual for SCAN facilitates the use of the instrument (Wing *et al*, 1998). Part I of the SCAN covers non-psychotic symptoms, such as physical health, worrying, tension, panic, anxiety and phobias, obsessional symptoms, depressed mood and ideation, impaired thinking, concentration, energy, interests, bodily functions, weight, sleep, eating disorders, and alcohol and drug misuse; part II covers psychotic and cognitive disorders, as well as abnormalities of behaviour, speech and affect.

The average administration time of SCAN is 90 minutes. When using SCAN, the clinician interviewer (e.g. psychiatrist or clinical psychologist) decides whether a symptom has been present during the specified time and to what degree of severity. One or two periods are selected to cover the main phenomena necessary for diagnosis. The periods usually include the 'present state' (i.e. the month before examination) and the 'lifetime before' (i.e. any time previously). Another option is to rate the 'representative episode', which may be chosen because it is particularly characteristic of the patient's illness.

A set of computer programs (CATEGO) is used for processing SCAN data and for the scoring and diagnoses according to ICD–10 and DSM–IV criteria. A computerised version of SCAN (CAPSE) is also available. It assists the interviewer in applying SCAN and allows direct entry of ratings at the time of the interview. Questions and ratings are displayed on the screen; if needed, SCAN glossary definitions can also be referred to.

SCAN has been tested in WHO-organised field trials involving 20 centres in 14 countries. The field trials indicated good feasibility and reliability of the instrument, comparable to those obtained in testing the PSE–9 (Wing et al, 1990).

An adaptation of the SCAN – the Diagnostic Interview for Psychosis (DIP) – has recently been developed, evaluated and used in the Australian National Study of Low Prevalence (Psychotic) Disorders. The DIP is intended for use by interviewers with a clinical background and was designed to occupy the ground between fully structured, lay-administered schedules and semi-structured, psychiatrist-administered interviews. It encompasses several domains, including: demographic information; social functioning and disability; a diagnostic module comprising symptoms, signs and history ratings; and patterns of service use and patient-perceived service need. The DIP generates diagnoses according to several diagnostic systems using the OPCRIT computerised diagnostic algorithms and can be administered either via computer diagnostic systems or on hard-copy (Castle et al, 2006).

Standardised Assessment of Depressive Disorders

The Standardised Assessment of Depressive Disorders (SADD) is a semi-structured clinical interview schedule aimed at assessing the symptoms and signs of depressive disorders. Part 1 of the instrument covers the basic sociodemographic patient data. Part 2 contains a checklist of 39 symptoms and signs characteristic of depression and is accompanied by a glossary that provides definitions of symptoms and signs to be assessed, a listing of possible probes, and examples of answers for each symptom. The checklist also includes a number of open-ended questions for recording rare or culture-specific symptoms of depression, as well as items related to the history of the patient (e.g. number of episodes, precipitating factors, presence of mental disorders in relatives). Part 3 of the instrument serves to record the diagnosis and severity of the patient's condition.

The ratings in SADD refer to the week preceding the interview and to any other time before the current episode. The administration of the instrument takes a short time if the clinician has examined the patient previously. If the case is 'fresh', the time taken to obtain the necessary information and rate it is longer (typically 45–60 minutes). SADD has been tested in the

WHO Collaborative Study on the Standardised Assessment of Depressive Disorders and has been found to be easy to use and acceptable to both psychiatrists and patients. The reliability of the sociodemographic, symptom checklist and history sections of the instrument has been found to be high (Sartorius *et al*, 1980, 1983).

Schedule for Clinical Assessment of Acute Psychotic States

The Schedule for Clinical Assessment of Acute Psychotic States (SCAAPS) is a semi-structured interview schedule for clinicians' recording of information about patients with acute psychotic states. Such information is collected from different sources, such as the clinical interview of the patient, key informants and medical records. The instrument also offers the possibility of recording the follow-up diagnostic evaluation of the patient.

SCAAPS consists of six parts. Part A contains the screening criteria for acute psychotic states (e.g. onset of symptoms within 3 months of the initial assessment); part B comprises items related to the psychiatric history and social description of the patient; part C contains a 19-item symptom checklist covering symptoms from worrying and anxiety to symptoms reflecting stressful life events; part D serves to record the initial diagnostic evaluation and the results of the 1-year follow-up assessment; part E covers the treatment, course and outcome of the disorder; part F is intended for narrative summaries of the initial examination, and 3-month and 1-year follow-up. The average duration of the SCAAPS interview is 120 minutes.

The instrument has been used in the WHO Collaborative Studies on Acute Psychoses and has been found to be a cross-culturally appropriate tool for collecting data about acute psychotic states in different parts of the world (Cooper *et al*, 1990).

Social Description

The Social Description (SD) is a schedule with open-ended questions aimed at collecting information in a systematic manner about the social history of the psychiatric patient. It is intended for research purposes and can be used by social workers or clinicians. It covers the following areas: residence and household; education of the patient; work activities of the patient; children; marital status; education and occupation of the spouse; education and occupation of the parents; education and occupation of the head of the current household; religion; patient's childhood setting; daily and leisure activities; birth order of the patient and siblings; a thumbnail sketch by the interviewer, who has to rate on a five-point scale the current socioeconomic status of the patient, the patient's family background, and the patient's current social isolation within the framework of his/her respective culture. The average administration time is 120 minutes.

The SD was used in the WHO International Pilot Study of Schizophrenia and was found to be a useful means for collecting the social history of patients in different cultures and settings (WHO, 1973). It has since been used in a modified form in several other WHO studies, such as the Collaborative Determinants of Outcome of Severe Mental Disorders (Jablensky *et al*, 1992).

Self-Reporting Questionnaire

The Self-Reporting Questionnaire (SRQ) is an instrument designed for screening the presence of psychiatric illness in patients contacting primary care settings. It can be self-administered (or interviewer administered with illiterate or semi-literate patients) and its administration time is 5–10 minutes. The questionnaire consists of 24 questions, 20 of which are related to neurotic symptoms and 4 of which relate to psychotic symptoms. Each of the 24 questions is scored 1 or 0: a score of 1 indicates that the symptom was present during the past month; a score of 0 indicates that it was absent. Depending on the criteria, culture and language, different cut-off scores are selected in different studies, but most often the cut-off is 7. A score of 7 or above indicates the existence of a probable psychological problem. The SRQ is accompanied by a user's guide (Beusenberg & Orley, 1994) that describes the instrument, its use and scoring, and also summarises the results of reliability and validity studies.

The SRQ has been tested in over 20 studies (including the WHO Collaborative Study on Strategies for Extending Mental Health Care and the WHO Study on Mental Disorders in Primary Health Care), and has been found to be an appropriate, reliable and valid case-finding tool for use in primary care, particularly in low-income countries (Harding *et al*, 1980, 1983; WHO, 1984).

Instruments for the assessment of disability and burden

World Health Organization Psychiatric Disability Assessment Schedule

World Health Organization Psychiatric Disability Assessment Schedule (WHO/DAS) is a semi-structured instrument designed for the evaluation of the social functioning of patients with mental disorders (Üstün *et al*, 2010). Such an evaluation can be done by a psychiatrist, psychologist or social worker. The information about the functioning of the patient is collected from the patient, key informant(s) or written records. The instrument has been developed in accordance with the principles underlying the WHO *International Classification of Impairments, Disabilities and Handicaps* (WHO, 1980).

The WHO/DAS consists of 97 items grouped in five parts. Part 1 comprises items related to the patient's overall behaviour, and includes

Table 17.2 WHO instruments for the assessment of disability, burden and quality of life

Instrument	Format	Area	User	Training	Languages
WHO Psychiatric Disability Assessment Schedule	Semi-structured	Disability due to mental and other disorders	Psychiatrist, psychologist, or social worker	Essential	Arabic, Bulgarian, Chinese, Croatian, Danish, English, French, German, Hindi, Japanese, Russian, Serbian, Spanish, Turkish, Urdu
WHO Short Disability Assessment Scale	Rating scale	Disability due to mental and/or physical disorders	Psychiatrist or psychologist	Not required	Arabic, Chinese, Czech, Danish, Dutch, English, German, Hindi, Italian, Japanese, Kannada, Portuguese, Romanian, Russian, Spanish
WHO Psychological Impairments Rating Schedule	Semi-structured	Psychological and behavioural deficits	Psychiatrist or psychologist	Essential	Arabic, Bulgarian, Croatian, English, French, German, Serbian, Turkish
Broad Rating Schedule	Semi-structured	Psychotic symptoms and related disability	Psychiatrist or psychologist	Not required	Bulgarian, Chinese, Czech, Danish, English, German, Hindi, Japanese, Russian, Yoruba
Family Interview Schedule	Structured	Family perception of patient	Psychiatrist, psychologist, social worker or nurse	Essential	Bulgarian, Chinese, Czech, Danish, English, German, Hindi, Japanese, Russian, Yoruba
Social Unit Rating	Semi-structured	Burden of mental illness or the family	Lay interviewer	Essential	Arabic, English, French, Hindi, Portuguese, Spanish
Burden Assessment Schedule	Questionnaire	Burden on care-givers	Self-administered	Not applicable	English, Hindi
WHO Quality of Life Assessment Instrument	Questionnaire	Quality of life	Self-administered	Not applicable	Croatian, Dutch, English, French, Russian, Shona, Spanish, Tamil
Subjective Well-Being Inventory	Questionnaire	Feelings of well-being	Self-administered	Not applicable	English, Hindi

ratings of self-care, underactivity, slowness and social withdrawal. Part 2 serves to assess the patient's social role performance, and covers participation in household activities, marital role, parental role, sexual role, social contacts, occupational role, interests and information, and behaviour in emergencies or out-of-the ordinary situations. Part 3 is for the assessment of the patient's social functioning in the hospital, including ward behaviour, nurses' opinions, occupations and contact with the outside world. Part 4 covers modifying factors related to the patient's dysfunction (specific assets, specific liabilities, home atmosphere and outside support). Parts 5 and 6 serve for a global evaluation of the patient and a summary of the ratings and scoring, respectively. Items in Parts 1 and 2 of the WHO/DAS are rated on a six-point scale: no dysfunction, minimal dysfunction, obvious dysfunction, serious dysfunction, very serious dysfunction and maximum dysfunction. The patient's current functioning (past month) is rated against the presumed 'average' or 'normal' functioning of a person of the same sex, comparable age and similar socioeconomic background. The average administration time is 30 minutes. A guide to the use of WHO/DAS and an explanation of certain key terms (e.g. psychological burden, social skills, impairment) accompany the instrument.

WHO/DAS has been tested and used in the WHO Collaborative Study on the Assessment and Reduction of Psychiatric Disability and has been found to be a reliable and valid tool for the assessment and cross-cultural comparison of psychiatric disability (Jablensky et al, 1980).

WHODAS 2.0

The current version of this instrument has been abbreviated as WHODAS 2.0 and represents a generic assessment tool developed as a companion to the WHO's *International Classification of Functioning, Disability and Health: ICF* (WHO, 2001). It has been designed for the standardised measurement of health and disability across cultures, and captures levels of functioning in the following six life domains:

1   Understanding and communicating with the world (cognition)
2   Moving and getting around (mobility)
3   Self-care (attending to one's hygiene, dressing, eating and staying alone)
4   Getting along with people (interpersonal interactions)
5   Life activities (domestic responsibilities, leisure and work)
6   Participation in society (joining in community activities).

For all six domains WHODAS 2.0 provides a profile and a summary measure of functioning and disability that is reliable and applicable across cultures in all adult populations. WHODAS 2.0 is a common metric of the impact of any health condition in terms of functioning. As a generic measure, WHODAS 2.0 is not specific to any one disease but is used to compare disability due to different diseases.

WHODAS 2.0 has proven useful for assessing health and disability levels in the general population and in specific groups (e.g. persons with a range of different mental and physical health conditions). Furthermore, WHODAS 2.0 allows the designing of health and health-related interventions and the monitoring of their impact.

As mentined above, WHODAS 2.0 is based on the conceptual framework of the ICF. All domains were developed from a comprehensive set of ICF items and map directly onto ICF's 'Activity and participation' component. As in the ICF, WHODAS 2.0 places health and disability on a continuum. Disability is defined as a decrement in functioning. WHODAS 2.0, like the ICF, is aetiologically neutral, that is, independent of the background disease or previous health conditions. This feature makes it possible to focus directly on functioning and disability and allows the assessment of functioning separately from the disease conditions.

There are several different versions of WHODAS 2.0, which are intended for different modes of administration. The main versions are the full and the short versions, with 36 and 12 questions, respectively. The 12-item version explains 81% of the variance of the more detailed 36-item version. For both versions general population norms are available.

Short Version (WHODAS–S)

The WHODAS–S has been developed as a component of the multi-axial presentation of the ICD–10 *Classification of Mental and Behavioural Disorders* (WHO, 1997). It is a simple scale intended for the recording of the clinicians' assessment of disablement caused by mental and physical disorders. The ratings refer to specific areas of functioning, such as personal care (e.g. personal hygiene, dressing, feeding), occupation (e.g. function in paid activities, studying, home-making), family and household (e.g. interaction with spouse, parents, children and other relatives) and the broader social context (e.g. performance in relation to community members, participation in leisure and other social activities). The scale provides anchor-point definitions for six ratings, ranging from 0 (no dysfunction) to 5 (maximum dysfunction). Administration of WHODAS–S takes 5 minutes if the clinician knows the patient and has examined him or her.

WHODAS–S has been tested in WHO-coordinated field trials of the ICD–10 multi-axial classification that involved about 70 centres from more than 25 countries. The trials indicated good acceptance of the instrument by clinicians belonging to different psychiatric schools and traditions (Janca *et al*, 1996*a*).

World Health Organization Psychological Impairments Rating Schedule

The World Health Organization Psychological Impairments Rating Schedule (WHO/PIRS) is a semi-structured instrument intended for clinicians' assessment of selected areas of psychological and behavioural deficits in patients with functional psychotic disorder. The main areas covered by the instrument concern negative symptoms, social skill and communication, and an overall impression of the patient and his or her personality. WHO/PIRS should be administered after a PSE interview, preferably by the same clinician. The average administration time is 25 minutes.

The instrument consists of 97 items grouped in ten sections. Part A includes items and scales for rating observed behaviour of the patient. Part B includes a pattern assembly, three Rorschach cards and a letter-deletion test aimed at eliciting the patient's performance when presented with standard tasks.

WHO/PIRS was used in the WHO Collaborative Study on Impairments and Disabilities Associated with Schizophrenic Disorders and was found to be a reliable assessment tool (test–retest reliability kappa = 0.79; Jablensky et al, 1980).

Broad Rating Schedule

The Broad Rating Schedule (BRS) has been developed for use in a long-term follow-up study of patients given a diagnosis of schizophrenia, and serves to summarise the follow-up findings. The schedule uses information from all available sources, including the patient, informant and medical or other records. The severity of psychotic symptoms and disabilities is rated for the previous month on a scale ranging from absent to severe. Symptoms, as well as disabilities, are also rated on a modified version of the DSM–III–R Global Assessment of Functioning (GAF) Scale, which ranges from 1 (persistent danger of severely hurting oneself or others, or persistent inability to function in almost all areas) to 90 (absent or minimal symptoms, or good functioning in all areas, interested and involved in a wide range of activities, etc.). The instrument also contains sections on participants who have died or are lost to follow-up. The ratings of these sections are based on the best judgement of the clinician using all available information. The BRS should be rated after completion of the interview of the patient and informant and a review of the records. Clinicians do not need specific training in the use of the schedule.

Family Interview Schedule

The Family Interview Schedule (FIS) is a structured instrument for the assessment of family members' perceptions of the patient's psychiatric problems and their consequences for the patient and family. It was developed for use in the WHO Long-Term Follow-Up Study of Schizophrenia. The source of information for this schedule should be a permanent member of the patient's family.

The schedule is divided into the following sections: I, symptoms and social behaviour; II, impact; III, stigma; IV, service providers; V, attribution. The section on symptoms and social behaviour covers the day-to-day behaviour and responsibilities of the patient in the past month (e.g. helping with household chores). The section on impact ascertains involvement of family members in helping the patient as well as their difficulties in managing and coping with problems caused by the patient's psychiatric problems. The section on stigma consists of a list of experiences the family member has had because of the patient's psychiatric problems (e.g. that neighbours treated him or her differently). The service providers section of the instrument is aimed at assessing the help provided to the patient and the family by doctors, nurses and other health professionals. The section on attribution is intended to record the family member's views (based on the information obtained from carers) on the causes of the patient's psychiatric problems.

The FIS is accompanied by a visual analogue' measure, that is, a graphic presentation of the scale ranging from 'almost never or not at all' to 'almost always or a lot'. The FIS takes 30–45 minutes to administer. The user (psychiatrist, psychologist, social worker or nurse) should be trained in its administration.

Social Unit Rating

The Social Unit Rating (SUR) is a semi-structured interview aimed at recording the effect of a patient's illness on his or her immediate living group. It consists of 20 items that cover basic sociodemographic information about the patient (e.g. occupation, education, employment), time residing in a given area, time residing in the present household, composition of the social unit, main sources of income, total weekly income and sources of help for the social unit. The rest of the items relate to the pre-illness status of the social unit and to the effect of the patient's illness on the social unit.

Any lay interviewer can administer the SUR after appropriate training. The administration time is 30–45 minutes. The SUR was used in the WHO Collaborative Study on Strategies for Extending Mental Health Care and has been found to be a useful means of assessming the effects of mental illness on the family or household of the patient (Giel *et al*, 1983).

Burden Assessment Schedule

The Burden Assessment Schedule (BAS) is a 20-item questionnaire that assesses and quantifies the subjective role burden of caring for a patient with chronic psychosis, as perceived by carers and, in particular, spouses. The two key areas of concern (which reflect carers' main feelings about their caring role) are impact on relations with others and perceived severity of the disease. Each question related to these areas of concern is rated on a scale ranging from 'not at all' to 'very much'. An example of such a question is 'Does caring for the patient make you feel tired and exhausted?' The BAS was developed and tested in India using an ethnographic exploration method; it demonstrated good acceptability and reliability of the instrument (Sell *et al*, 1998).

Instruments for the assessment of quality of life

World Health Organization Quality of Life Assessment Instrument

The WHO Quality of Life Assessment Instrument (WHOQOL; WHOQOL Group, 1994) allows an enquiry into the perception of individuals of their own position in life in the context of the culture and value systems in which they live and in relation to their goals, expectations, standards and concerns. The instrument covers the following six broad domains of the quality of life: physical, psychological, level of independence, social relationships, environment and spiritual. Within each, a series of facets of the quality of life summarises that particular domain. For example, the psychological domain includes the facets: positive feelings; thinking, learning, memory and concentration; self-esteem; body image and appearance; and negative feelings. Response scales in the instrument are concerned with the intensity, frequency and subjective evaluation of states, behaviour and capacities. The WHOQOL provides a profile that consists of an overall quality-of-life score, scores for each of the six broad domains, scores for individual facets of the quality of life and, within facets, separate scores for the recording of the respondent's perception of his or her condition and quality of life.

The WHOQOL exists in two versions: the 100-item WHOQOL–100, and the 26-item WHOQOL–Bref. Information on psychometric properties of these two WHOQOL versions is available in the international literature (WHOQOL Group 1998*a,b*; Saxena *et al*, 2001) as well as in the manuals available from the WHO website (http://www.who.int/mental_health/resources/evidence_research/en/index.html).

Besides WHOQOL–100 and WHOQOL–Bref, which are generic assessment instruments, the WHO has also developed WHOQOL–HIV versions to assess quality of life in persons with HIV and AIDS (WHOQOL HIV Group 2003*a,b*, 2004). A version (WHOQOL–SRPB) for the systematic assessment of quality of life specifically in relation to spirituality, religious and personal beliefs has also been developed (WHO SRPB Group, 2006).

Subjective Well-Being Inventory

The Subjective Well-Being Inventory (SUBI) is a questionnaire for the assessment of subjective well-being. It can be self-administered or interviewer administered and is designed for research purposes. The questionnaire consists of 40 items designed to measure feelings of well-being (or lack of it) as experienced by an individual in relation to concerns such as health or family. The items in SUBI represent the following factors in the structure of subjective well-being: general well-being – positive effect; expectation–achievement congruence; confidence in coping; transcendence; family group support; social support; primary group concern; inadequate mental mastery; perceived ill-health; deficiency in social contacts; general well-being – negative effect. SUBI is accompanied by the 'stepwise ethnographic exploration' procedure, which can be used to assess that SUBI is appropriate for use in the cultural setting in which the study will take place. The instrument has been used in research projects carried out by the WHO Regional Office for South-East Asia and has been found to be culturally applicable for the quantitative measurement of subjective well-being (Sell & Nagpal, 1992).

Instruments for the assessment of health services and systems

Pathways Interview Schedule

The Pathways Interview Schedule is a semi-structured instrument designed for the systematic gathering of information on the routes and sources of care used by patients before they see a mental health professional. The instrument can be administered by a psychiatrist, psychologist, social worker or nurse, and its average administration time is 10 minutes. An instruction manual describing how to use the instrument is available.

The Pathways Interview Schedule consists of seven sections. Section A covers basic information about the centre and the mental health professional. In section B the basic information about the patient is recorded (e.g. age, sex, marital status, social position, history of care by any mental health service). Section C covers the details of the first carer (e.g. who he/she was, who suggested that care, the main problem presented, when it began, the main treatment offered, duration of patient's journey to first carer). Sections D, E and F cover similar details of the second, third and fourth carers. Section G is intended for the diagnosis of the patient according to the assessment by the mental health professional.

The instrument was used in the WHO Study on Pathways to Psychiatric Care and was found to be a simple and inexpensive method of studying a psychiatric service and routes followed by patients seeking care for psychiatric disorders (Gater et al, 1990, 1991).

Checklists for Quality Assurance in Mental Health Care

Checklists for Quality Assurance in Mental Health Care are a set of checklists accompanied by glossaries designed to assist in the development of programmes of quality assurance in mental healthcare. The checklists are based on recommendations of a group of experts in mental healthcare and

Table 17.3 WHO instruments for the assessment of health services

Instrument	Format	Area	User	Training	Languages
Pathways Interview Schedule	Semi-structured	Sources of care	Health or research worker	Not required	Arabic, Bahasa (Indonesian), Chinese, Czech, English, French, Japanese, Kannada, Korean, Portuguese, Spanish, Turkish, Urdu
Checklists for Quality Assurance in Mental Health Care:					
Mental Health Policy Checklist	Semi-structured	Mental healthcare (policy)	Health or administrative worker	Not required	Chinese, English, French, Italian, Portuguese, Spanish
Mental Health Programme Checklist	Semi-structured	Mental healthcare (programme)	Health or administrative worker	Not required	Chinese, English, French, Italian, Portuguese, Spanish
Primary Health Care Facility Checklist	Semi-structured	Mental healthcare (primary-care facility)	Health or administrative worker	Not required	Chinese, English, French, Italian, Portuguese, Spanish
Outpatient Mental Health Facility Checklist	Semi-structured	Mental healthcare (out-patient facility)	Health or administrative worker	Not required	Chinese, English, French, Italian, Portuguese, Spanish
Inpatient Mental Health Facility Checklist	Semi-structured	Mental healthcare (in-patient facility)	Health or administrative worker	Not required	Chinese, English, French, Italian, Portuguese, Spanish
Residential Facility for the Elderly Mentally Ill Checklist	Semi-structured	Mental healthcare (residential facility for the elderly mentally ill)	Health or administrative worker	Not required	Chinese, Czech, Danish, English, Hindi, Russian, Spanish, Yoruba
WHO Child Care Facility Schedule	Semi-structured	Quality of child care facility	Health or administrative worker	Not required	English, French, Greek, Portuguese
WHO Assessment Instrument for Mental Health Systems	Structured	Quality of mental health system	Mental health expert	Required	English, French, Portuguese, Russian, Spanish

have been tested in a field trial that included ten countries in all the WHO regions (Bertolote, 1994).

Six sets of checklists and glossaries are available:

Mental Health Policy Checklist

The aim of this instrument is to assess national mental health policies and to assist in the development of country programmes of quality assurance in mental health. The checklist has 21 items enquiring about issues such as the existence of a written mental health policy and operational programmes. The rest of the items are grouped into the following categories: decentralisation, intersectoral action, comprehensiveness, equity, continuity, community participation and periodic reviews of mental health policy. The average administration time is 75 minutes. The instrument can also be used to assess the policy of smaller population units (e.g. a federal state).

Mental Health Programme Checklist

This is an instrument for the assessment of a country's mental health programmes and for assisting in the development of programmes of quality assurance in mental health. The checklist consists of 32 items, covering areas such as whether there are written national, regional and local mental health programmes, the range of actions for promotion of mental health, treatment, rehabilitation and prevention of mental disorders, and so on. The rest of the items are grouped into the following sections: plan of work, monitoring and evaluation, and community participation in the planning, implementation and evaluation of mental health actions/programmes. The glossary provides descriptions of these items. The average administration time of the checklist is 30 minutes.

Primary Health Care Facility Checklist

The aim of this instrument is to assess primary healthcare facilities that deliver mental healthcare and to assist in the development of programmes of quality assurance of mental healthcare in such facilities. The instrument consists of a checklist, glossary, scoring instructions and list of references. The checklist has 42 items covering: physical environment (e.g. reasonable space available, adequate supply of basic drugs); administrative arrangements (e.g. written procedures available for the protection of confidentiality of patients and staff records); care process (e.g. written treatment plans for each patient, followed by all staff); interaction with families (e.g. family members are encouraged to be involved in the patient's treatment programme); and outreach (e.g. contact is regularly made with other health facilities, social agencies, patients' employers, etc.). The average administration time is 60 minutes.

Outpatient Mental Health Facility Checklist

This instrument is used to assess out-patient mental health facilities in a given country or set-up, and to assist in the development of programmes of quality assurance in mental health in such facilities. It consists of a checklist, glossary and scoring instructions. The checklist comprises 53 items and covers areas such as: physical environment (e.g. the facility has been officially inspected and meets local standards for the protection of the health and safety of patients and staff); administrative arrangements (e.g. a written policy on philosophy and model of care is available and priorities have been defined); care process (e.g. every patient is evaluated in terms of biological, psychological and social functioning); interaction with families (e.g. home visits for improving caring and coping skills of families of selected patients are carried out); and outreach (e.g. a standard information form is always sent to another facility whenever a patient is referred to it). The average administration time is 60 minutes.

Inpatient Mental Health Facility Checklist

The aim of this instrument is to assess in-patient mental health facilities in a given country or set-up, and to assist in the development of programmes of quality assurance in mental health in such facilities. It consists of 77 items covering areas such as physical environment, administrative arrangements, staffing, care process, interaction with families, discharge and follow-up. A glossary provides descriptions of items to be assessed. Scoring instructions are also available. The average administration time is 20 minutes.

Residential Facility for the Elderly Mentally Ill Patients Checklist

This is an instrument used to assess residential facilities for elderly people with a mental illness and assist in the development of programmes of quality assurance in mental health in such facilities. The checklist consists of 69 items that cover the physical environment, administrative arrangements, care process, and interaction with families and community. The glossary provides a description of these items and instructions for their scoring are also given. The average administration time is 75 minutes.

World Health Organization Child Care Facility Schedule

The WHO Child Care Facility Schedule (WHO CCFS; WHO, 1990a) is an observer-rated schedule aimed at assessing the quality of child care in day-care programmes for children. It can be administered by a research or administrative worker, who should be familiar with recording and rating procedures. The average administration time is 90 minutes.

The instrument consists of 80 items covering the following areas that define good-quality child care: physical environment (e.g. the indoor environment is spacious enough for the number of children present and is attractive and pleasant); health and safety (e.g. the facility meets local standards for protection of the health and safety of children in group settings); nutrition and food service (e.g. meal times are used by staff to promote good nutrition); administration (e.g. at least annually, staff conduct a self-study to identify strengths and weaknesses of the programme); staff–family interaction (e.g. parents and other family members are encouraged to be involved in the programme in various ways and there are no rules prohibiting their unannounced visits); staff–children interaction (e.g. staff respect the cultural backgrounds of the children and adapt the learning situation to preserve their heritage and acquaint other children with the cultural legacy of all members of the group); observable child behaviour (e.g. children respect the needs, feelings and property of others, for example by taking turns and sharing toys); and curriculum (e.g. the daily schedule is planned to provide a variety of activities, including those that are indoor/outdoor, quiet/active, etc.).

The WHO CCFS contains a glossary which defines each of the items to be observed and rated. The instrument is also accompanied by a user manual and a list of relevant references. Field studies of the WHO CCFS have been carried out in Greece, the Philippines and Nigeria, and the instrument has been found to be cross-culturally acceptable and reliable in terms of the percentage agreement between raters (Tsiantis *et al*, 1991).

WHO Assessment Instrument for Mental Health Systems

The WHO Assessment Instrument for Mental Health Systems (WHO–AIMS) is a comprehensive assessment tool designed to assess mental health systems in middle- and low-income countries. For the purpose of this instrument, a mental health system is defined as all the activities whose primary purpose is to promote, restore or maintain mental health. The mental health system is conceptualised to include all organisations and resources focused on improving mental health. WHO–AIMS can be used for an entire country, or for a region, state, or province within a large country. Although it was specifically designed for use in low- and middle-income countries, most of the items are relevant and applicable to resource-poor settings within high- income countries. In addition, the instrument may also be useful for high-income countries where there is a desire to achieve a comprehensive picture of the mental health system outside psychiatric services. WHO–AIMS provides essential information for mental health policy development and service delivery. It allows countries to develop information-based mental health policy and plans, with clear baseline information and targets.

The instrument covers six domains: policy and legislative framework; mental health services; mental health in primary care; human resources; public information and links with other sectors; and monitoring and research. These domains address the ten recommendations of the *World Health Report 2001* through 28 facets and 155 items. All six domains need to be assessed to form a basic, yet broad, picture of a mental health system, with a focus on health sector activities.

The instrument primarily consists of input indicators (resources that are used to develop or modify systems and services) and process indicators (assessment of utilisation of services). Supporting documentation (answers to frequently asked questions, guidance on data collection, and definitions of frequently used terms), a data-entry program and a template for writing country reports are included in the instrument. Data for WHO–AIMS are collected by a team based within the country, with active technical support from the WHO. More information on WHO–AIMS can be found in a published paper (Saxena *et al*, 2007) and at WHO's WHO–AIMS website (http://www.who.int/mental_health/evidence/WHO-AIMS/en/index. html). A large number of country reports developed with the WHO–AIMS data are also available on this website.

Instruments for the assessment of environment and risks

Axis III Checklist

The Axis III Checklist was produced in the framework of the development of the ICD–10 multi-axial schema (WHO, 1997) and is intended for clinicians' assessment of Axis III, that is, contextual (environmental/circumstantial and personal lifestyle/life management) factors contributing to the presentation or course of the ICD–10 mental and/or physical disorder(s) recorded on Axis I of the schema. The contextual factors listed under Axis III represent a selection of ICD–10 Z00–Z99 categories, that is, 'Factors influencing health status and contact with health services' (Chapter XXI of ICD–10). The following groups of contextual factors are covered by Axis III and assessed by the Checklist: negative events in childhood (e.g. removal from home in childhood, Z61.1); problems related to education and literacy (e.g. underachievement in school, Z55.3); problems related to the primary support group, including family circumstances (e.g. disruption of family by separation or divorce, Z63.5); problems related to the social environment (e.g. social exclusion and rejection, Z60.4); problems related to housing or economic circumstances (e.g. homelessness, Z59.0); problems related to (un)employment (e.g. change of job, Z56.1); problems related to physical environment (e.g. occupational exposure to risk factors, Z57); problems related to psychosocial or legal circumstances (e.g. imprisonment or other incarceration, Z65.1); problems related to a family history of diseases or disabilities (e.g. family history of mental or behavioural disorders, Z81); lifestyle and life management problems (e.g. burn-out, Z73.0).

The Axis III Checklist is included in the ICD–10 Multiaxial Diagnostic Formulation Form, and the clinician is required to tick all applicable categories of Z factors and specify Z codes for each. A listing of contextual factors and the respective ICD–10 Z codes is given as an appendix to the Form. The average administration time of the Axis III Checklist is 10 minutes. The instrument was tested in the multicentre international field trials of the multi-axial presentation of ICD–10 and was found to be useful and easy to use by clinicians in different parts of the world (Janca *et al*, 1996*b*).

Table 17.4 WHO instruments for the assessment of environment and risks

Instrument	Format	Area	User	Training	Languages
Axis III Checklist	Semi-structured	Contextual factors	Psychiatrist or psychologist	Not required	Arabic, Chinese, Czech, Danish, Dutch, English, German, Hindi, Italian, Japanese, Kannada, Portuguese, Romanian, Russian, Spanish
Interview Schedule for Children	Semi-structured	Child's psychosocial environment	Psychiatrist, psychologist, social worker or nurse	Not required	English, German, Portuguese, Slovenian, Spanish
Parent Interview Schedule	Semi-structured	Child's psychosocial environment	Psychiatrist, psychologist, social worker or nurse	Not required	English, German, Portuguese, Slovenian, Spanish
Home Risk Card	Semi-structured	Child's home risk factors	Health or research worker	Not required	English, Hindi

Interview Schedule for Children

The Interview Schedule for Children (ISC; WHO, 1991) is a semi-structured instrument for the systematic collection of information on a child's psychosocial environment. The instrument has been developed as a companion to the psychosocial axis (Axis V) of the WHO *Multiaxial Classification of Child and Adolescent Psychiatric Disorders* (WHO, 1988). The ISC is accompanied by a glossary that provides descriptions of items and diagnostic guidelines for Axis V (associated abnormal psychosocial situations). However, to ensure the smooth flow of the interview, the items are in a different order from that of the glossary. The items in the schedule are as follows: abnormal immediate environment; stressful events/situations resulting from child's disorder/disability; societal stressors; chronic interpersonal stress associated with school/work; acute life events; abnormal qualities of upbringing; abnormal intrafamilial relationships; inadequate or distorted intrafamilial communication; and mental disorder, deviance or handicap in the child's primary support group.

The relevant codes for each category have to be inserted into each individual section and the results are transferred to the summary page. It is, however, recommended that the coding and scoring are not done until the interview has been completed. The instrument is intended for psychiatrists, psychologists, social workers and nurses, and its administration takes 60 minutes (van Goor-Lambo *et al*, 1990).

Parent Interview Schedule

The Parent Interview Schedule (PIS; WHO, 1990*b*) is a semi-structured instrument for the systematic collection of information about the child's psychosocial environment so that appropriate codings can be made on the psychosocial axis (Axis V) of the WHO *Multiaxial Classification of Child Psychiatric Disorders* (WHO, 1988). The instrument is accompanied by a glossary and diagnostic guidelines for the assessment of items. As in the ISC, the relevant codes have to be inserted in each individual section and the results should be transferred to the summary page after the interview. Items in the PIS are identical to those in the ISC, and similarly their order in the schedule and glossary is different to ensure the smooth flow of the interview. The instrument is intended for psychiatrists, psychologists, social workers or nurses, and its administration takes 60 minutes. The preliminary results of the Axis V field trials (van Goor-Lambo *et al*, 1990) were used in the preparation of the final version of PIS.

Home Risk Card

The Home Risk Card is a listing of risk factors that, if present at the home of a child, may indicate that the child and family need extra help and special attention. The risk factors covered by the instrument include: mother's age (under 17 years); number of children under 3 years (more than two); mother/carer ignorant of the child's needs and unresponsive to health messages (e.g. cannot answer questions about the child that mothers normally can answer); mother/carer mentally disordered or severely depressed (e.g. looks desperate, hopeless, cries easily); mother/carer neglectful or uninterested in the well-being/development of the child (e.g. shouts or hits the child for trivial reasons during home visit); disorganised, unclean house; father known to be delinquent (e.g. arrested by police), alcoholic or otherwise mentally disordered; severe marital discord (e.g. physical violence between parents); abject poverty (e.g. no change of clothing).

The Home Risk Card guides the user in noting facts about the child and household that may require adequate intervention measures. The recorded information should also be inserted into the child's health card and serve as a reminder to the health professional about the child's need for extra help and attention.

A brief set of instructions helps the user in the application of the Card, which usually takes 5–10 minutes. The Home Risk Card has been used in a project organised by the WHO Regional Office for South-East Asia and has been found to be a useful guide for the assessment of home risk factors in this region (Sell & Nagpal, 1992).

Instruments for qualitative research

A guide providing a general overview of the concepts, methods and tools commonly used in qualitative research has been produced by the WHO (Hudelson, 1994). It is an introductory guide for programme managers, project directors, researchers and others who need to make decisions concerning when and how to conduct research for programme development purposes. The guide: gives an overview of qualitative research and its potential uses; describes the most common data-collection methods used in qualitative research, and specifies their strengths and weaknesses; discusses issues of sampling, study design and report writing in qualitative research; and gives examples of several qualitative research designs used by health programmes.

For the WHO Cross-cultural Applicability Research (CAR) study on diagnostic criteria and instruments for the assessment of alcohol and drug misuse and dependence, a set of qualitative research methods and instruments was developed (Room et al, 1996). These include the following.

Exploratory Translation and Back-translation Guidelines

This is a set of specified procedures for conducting a careful translation and back-translation of an instrument so as to ensure its equivalence in different

Table 17.5 WHO instruments for the assessment of qualitative research

Instrument	Format	Area	User	Training	Languages
Exploratory Translation and Back-Translation Guidelines	Guide	Linguistic equivalence	Health or research worker	Not required	English, Greek, Kannada, Korean, Romanian, Spanish, Turkish, Yoruba
Key Informant Interview Schedule	Semi-structured	Cultural aspects of mental health	Anthropologist or ethnographer	Essential	English, Greek, Kannada, Korean, Romanian, Spanish, Turkish, Yoruba
Focus Group Interview Guide	Guide	Cultural aspects of mental health	Anthropologist or ethnographer	Essential	English, Greek, Kannada, Korean, Romanian, Spanish, Turkish, Yoruba

languages and cultures. The exploratory translation and back-translation used in the WHO CAR study comprised a series of step-by-step procedures summarised in Table 17.6.

Key Informant Interview Schedule

This is a semi-structured, exploratory, ethnographic interview schedule that covers phenomena relevant to ICD–10 and DSM–III–R definitions and criteria for substance use disorders (e.g. withdrawal, tolerance, loss of control). The questions follow a 'funnel-type structure': general topics are first discussed and then more detailed questions about specific issues are asked.

The informant's answers are noted on the schedule verbatim. However, to ensure accuracy of the notes, the key informant interviews should be tape-recorded whenever possible or an observer should be present while the interviewer asks questions and both should take notes.

The Key Informant Interview Schedule developed for the WHO CAR study has been applied in nine centres representing distinct cultures and has been found to be an appropriate method for eliciting information on culture-specific characteristics of substance use and misuse in different parts of the world (Bennett *et al*, 1993).

Table 17.6 Steps in the development of equivalent versions of instruments in different languages

Step	Procedure
1	Establishment of a (bilingual) group of experts belonging to the culture in which the instrument was developed and the culture in which it will (also) be used
2	Examination of the conceptual structure of the instrument by the expert group
3	Translation of items into the target language (or formulation of items in both languages if the instrument is produced anew)
4	Examination of translation by the bilingual group
5	Examination of the translation in unilingual groups (i.e. a group of individuals who do not know the source language of the instruments and therefore cannot guess the meaning of badly formulated items). The unilingual groups are usually moderated by a member of the bilingual expert group
6	Back-translation of the text, possibly amended by the unilingual group
7	Examination of the back-translation by a bilingual group informed by its members about the contents of discussion in the unilingual groups. Participation of members of the bilingual group in the designing of the studies to establish the metric properties (e.g. validity, reliability, sensitivity) of the instrument

Focus Group Interview Guide

This is a brief interview guide that specifies the main topics for discussion on various aspects of culture-specific characteristics of psychoactive substance use and misuse. According to the WHO CAR study protocol, the following topics have been explored by this method: what is normal and abnormal use of alcohol or drugs; the meanings of the various diagnostic terms related to the concept of alcohol or drug dependence; the similarities and differences between alcohol and drug misuse and alcohol and drug addiction; and which prevention and intervention strategies are most likely to be effective against alcohol- or drug-related problems in the culture.

A set of instructions for the selection, composition and moderation of focus groups accompanies the list of discussion topics. Techniques of recording, reconstructing, managing and analysing the information obtained through the focus groups are also specified.

Discussion

All the WHO instruments have been developed in the context of collaborative and cross-cultural studies. In some instances an instrument that was already in use in one cultural setting was selected as the initial draft, which was then developed further; in other instances the development of the instrument started from a draft produced by an international group of experts representing several cultural settings and disciplines. All the instruments exist in more than one language and the vast majority have been used in more than one country. This was not accidental: the WHO has in fact made it its aim to produce instruments for cross-cultural and collaborative work that will serve as a part of a common language, helping researchers and other experts from different countries to understand one another, to work together and to compare the results of their studies, even when these are not performed at a particular time following a commonly agreed protocol.

The decision to develop instruments suitable for international, cross-cultural and collaborative work has had several consequences. First, the development of the instruments took more time than it would take to develop an instrument for use in a single country or language.

Second, certain characteristics of patients, their sociocultural surroundings and the health services that they receive are so different that it is not possible to assess them using the same instrument. In such instances guidelines about the assessment were provided, while the formulation of specific items and other measurement tasks were entrusted to groups of experts who were fully acquainted with the circumstances.

Third, the development of instruments required additional funds for face-to-face meetings of the experts involved. These meetings (usually conducted at the participating centres) proved to have important consequences. The discussions of the results of the field trials and other aspects of the research necessary to produce the instrument and assess its metric characteristics gave invaluable insights into the differences between cultures and into the feasibility of investigations in different settings. The meetings also served as an important motivator to continue the often tedious work required over a long period. An effort was made on each occasion to bring together the centre heads and younger investigators, for whom attendance at such meetings was of particular importance.

Fourth, certain constraints were imposed on the instruments by the structure of the languages in which they were produced. Certain concepts have no natural 'home' in other languages and enquiring about them can therefore become very time-consuming and difficult. In such instances it is usually better to sacrifice an item or section than to make part of the instrument awkward to use and complicate the training of interviewers. When this is not acceptable, it is usually necessary to return to the beginning and consider whether it is possible to obtain information about the topic of interest in another manner, not using assessment instruments of the type described here.

Fifth, cross-cultural differences can best be overcome if the assessments are carried out by individuals who are familiar with the culture and well trained in the use of the instruments. Most of the instruments that the WHO has developed are therefore semi-structured and have been proposed for application by a trained member of the same culture. The use of semi-structured interviews, however, requires more training than is the case for fully standardised instruments. However, the amount of extra training is much less than is necessary when non-structured assessment methods are chosen. Furthermore, semi-structured instruments share some of the advantages of the fully structured instruments (e.g. the systematic coverage of all areas of interest and simpler data processing).

Sixth, issues such as copyright, translation rights and modification procedures have to be considered, with a view to covering the different centres and languages in which the instrument has been produced.

The WHO instruments have been developed in collaboration with groups of experts in many countries. Their contribution to the production of the instruments has been invaluable, and it is certain that without their selfless and enthusiastic collaboration it would not have been possible to develop the instruments and collect the data that have been made available over the years. In the course of this work over the past four decades, most of the centres that have participated in this work have made many international contacts, gained new insights about other cultures, increased their expertise in cross-cultural work and learned about the most convenient ways of collaborating internationally. The network of centres that has come into existence and that continues to work on instruments (and collaborate in research) has been an excellent by-product of the work on instrument development.

Another by-product of the work on instruments and of other WHO-coordinated international and cross-cultural collaborative research has been the formulation of guidelines concerning ethical aspects of collaboration in the field of mental health across national borders (Sartorius, 1990). One of the principles developed is that collaboration in research – in view of the high investments and various potential disadvantages of short-term international collaborative projects – should be structured in a manner that will make it highly probable that collaboration in the collaborative network will continue after the project that started the network has been completed. This has been realised in the instance of the WHO network that continues its existing collaborative links among all centres – including those that are at present not actively involved in any particular studies.

The technology of translation used in the development of WHO instruments deserves a brief mention. The method that has been developed rests on various previous methods used to ensure equivalence of translation in collaborative mental health research (Sartorius, 1979) but has parts that have not been systematically used before. The steps used to produce equivalent versions in different languages are shown in Table 17.6. The procedure outlined is an approximation of the process described in more detail elsewhere (Sartorius & Kuyken, 1994; Sartorius, 1998). The features that deserve attention at this point are the decision to incorporate an examination of the translation by a unilingual group and the existence of bilingual/bicultural groups that can guide the process of producing equivalent versions of the instrument in different languages.

The instruments described in this paper cover the needs for data collection in a number of areas of psychiatric investigation. Other areas, however, also require attention, and it is to be hoped that the WHO will continue working on the development of instruments for these. Among them are:

1   The instruments that could be used to assess the stigma of psychiatric illness and the influence of various interventions that the health services or the society as a whole might undertake to diminish it.
2   Instruments that would be useful to measure the tolerance of individuals for their own diseases and the diseases of others.
3   Instruments that might help us to assess conditions and states such as 'burn-out' and 'malaise' and their impact on the productivity of the individuals who suffer from them and of the community as a whole.
4   Instruments that could help us to assess features of the community relevant to the provision of mental healthcare (e.g. the capacity of the community to accept sick and disabled members).
5   Instruments that could better describe the needs of individuals and communities.
6   Instruments we could use in the assessment of states that are at the borderline of normality (e.g. mild cognitive disorders, subthreshold mental disorders).
7   Instruments that could be used in international studies of impairments, disabilities and handicaps, defined in terms of the second revision of the International Classification of Impairments, Disabilities and Handicaps.

8   Instruments that could be used for evaluation of mental health systems and gaps in provision of mental healthcare in middle- and low-income countries.

The difficulties of producing an instrument satisfying all the metric requirements and dealing with an area of assessment that should be investigated because of its public health importance pale in comparison with the difficulty of ensuring that the instrument is well known, properly updated, sufficiently well learned and widely applied. It is probably to this second task that the majority of efforts should be directed if we are to contribute to a better understanding among all those concerned with mental illness and with ways of helping patients, their families and communities.

References

American Psychiatric Association (1987) *Diagnostic and Statistical Manual of Mental Disorders* (3rd edition, revised) (DSM–III–R). APA.

American Psychiatric Association (1994) *Diagnostic and Statistical Manual of Mental Disorders* (4th edition) (DSM–IV). APA.

Babor, T. F., de la Fuente, J. R., Saunders, J. B., *et al* (1989) *AUDIT, the Alcohol Use Disorders Identification Test. Guidelines for Use in Primary Health Care*. WHO.

Bennett, L. A., Janca, A., Grant, B. F., *et al* (1993) Boundaries between normal and pathological drinking: a cross-cultural comparison. *Alcohol Health and Research World*, **17**, 190–195.

Bertolote, J. (1994) *Quality Assurance in Mental Health Care: Checklists and Glossaries, Vol. I.* WHO.

Beusenberg, M. & Orley, J. (1994) *A User's Guide to the Self-Reporting Questionnaire (SRQ)*. WHO.

Castle, D. J., Jablensky, A., McGrath, J. J., *et al* (2006) The Diagnostic Interview for Psychosis (DIP): development, reliability and applications. *Psychological Medicine*, **36**, 69–80.

Cooper, I. E., Jablensky, A. & Sartorius, N. (1990) WHO collaborative studies on acute psychoses using the SCAAPS schedule. In *Psychiatry: A World Perspective, Vol. 1. Classification and Psychopathology, Child Psychiatry, Substance Use* (eds C. N. Stefanis, *et al*), pp. 185–192. International Congress Series. Excerpta Medica.

Cottler, L. B., Robins, L. N., Grant, B. F., *et al* (1991) The CIDI – Core substance abuse and dependence questions: cross-cultural and nosological issues. *British Journal of Psychiatry*, **159**, 653–658.

Gater, R., Goldberg, D. & Sartorius, N. (1990) The WHO Pathways to Care Study. In *Psychiatry: A World Perspective, Vol. 4. Social Psychiatry, Ethics and Law: History of Psychiatry and Education* (eds C. N. Stefanis, *et al*), pp. 75–78. International Congress Series. Excerpta Medica.

Gater, R., De Almeida, E., Sousa, B., *et al* (1991) The pathways to psychiatric care: a cross-cultural study. *Psychological Medicine*, **21**, 761–764.

Giel, R., de Arango, M. V., Babikir, A. H., *et al* (1983) The burden of mental illness on the family. Results of observations in four developing countries. *Acta Psychiatrica Scandinavica*, **68**, 186–201.

Harding, T. W., de Arango, M. V., Balthazar, J., *et al* (1980) Mental disorders in primary health care: a study of their frequency and diagnosis in four developing countries. *Psychological Medicine*, **10**, 231–241.

Harding, T. W., Climent, C. E., Diop, M., *et al* (1983) The WHO collaborative study on strategies for extending mental health care. II. The development of new research methods. *American Journal of Psychiatry*, **140**, 1474–1480.

Hudelson, P. M. (1994) *Qualitative Research for Health Programmes*. WHO.

Isaac, M., Janca, A. & Sartorius, N. (1994) *The ICD–10 Symptom Glossary for Mental Disorders*. WHO.

Jablensky, A., Schwarz, R. & Tomov, T. (1980) WHO collaborative study on impairments and disabilities associated with schizophrenic disorders. A preliminary communication: objectives and methods. In *Epidemiological Research as Basis for the Organization of Extramural Psychiatry. Acta Psychiatrica Scandinavica*, **62** (suppl. 286), 152–159.

Jablensky, A., Sartorius, N., Ernberg, G., *et al* (1992) Schizophrenia: manifestations, incidence and course in different cultures: a World Health Organization ten-country study. *Psychological Medicine*, monograph suppl. 201.

Janca, A. & Chandrashekar, C. R. (1993) *Catalogue of Assessment Instruments Used in the Studies Coordinated by the WHO Mental Health Programme*. WHO.

Janca, A., Robins, L. N., Cottler, L. B., *et al* (1992) Clinical observation of assessment using the Composite International Diagnostic Interview (CIDI): an analysis of the CIDI field trials-wave II at the St Louis site. *British Journal of Psychiatry*, **160**, 815–818.

Janca, A., Ustun, T. B., Early, T. S., *et al* (1993) The ICD–10 Symptom Checklist – a companion to the ICD–10 classification of mental and behavioural disorders. *Social Psychiatry and Psychiatric Epidemiology*, **28**, 239–242.

Janca, A., Ustun, T. B. & Sartorius, N. (1994a) New versions of World Health Organization instruments for the assessment of mental disorders. *Acta Psychiatrica Scandinavica*, **90**, 73–83.

Janca, A., Ustun, T. B., van Drimmelen, J., *et al* (1994b) The ICD–10 symptom checklist for mental disorders, version 2.0. WHO, Geneva.

Janca, A., Kastrup, M. C., Katschnig, H., *et al* (1996a) The World Health Organization Short Disability Assessment (WHO DAS–S). A tool for the assessment of difficulties in selected areas of functioning of patients' mental disorders. *Social Psychiatry and Psychiatric Epidemiology*, **31**, 349–354.

Janca, A., Mezzich, J. E., Kastrup, M., *et al* (1996b) Contextual aspects of mental disorders: a proposal for axis III of the ICD–10 multi-axial system. *Acta Psychiatrica Scandanavica*, **94**, 31–36.

Kessler, R. C. & Ustun, T. B. (2004) The World Mental Health (WMH) Survey Initiative version of the World Health Organization (WHO) Composite International Diagnostic Interview (WMH–CIDI). *International Journal of Methods in Psychiatric Research*, **13**, 93–121.

Loranger, A., Hirschfield, R., Sartorius, N., *et al* (1991) The WHO/ADAMHA international pilot study of personality disorders: background and purpose. *Journal of Personality Disorders*, **5**, 296–306.

Loranger, A. W., Sartorius, N., Andreoli, A., *et al* (1994) The International Personality Disorder Examination (IPDE): the WHO/ADAMHA international pilot study of personality disorders. *Archives of General Psychiatry*, **51**, 215–224.

Robins, L. N., Wing, J. E., Wittchen, H-U., *et al* (1988) The composite International Diagnostic Interview: an epidemiologic instrument suitable for use in conjunction with different diagnostic systems and in different cultures. *Archives of General Psychiatry*, **45**, 1069–1077.

Robins, L. N., Cottler, L. B. & Babor, T. (1990) *CIDI Substance Abuse Module*. Department of Psychiatry, Washington University School of Medicine.

Room, R., Janca, A., Bennett, L. A., *et al* (1996) WHO cross-cultural applicability research on diagnosis and assessment of substance use disorders: an overview of methods and selected results. *Addiction*, **91**, 199–220.

Sartorius, N. (1979) Cross-cultural psychiatry. In *Psychiatrie der Gegenwart, Vol. III* (2nd edition) (eds K. P. Kisker, I. E. Meyer, C. Muller, *et al*), pp. 711–737. Springer.

Sartorius, N. (1989) Recent research activities in WHO's mental health programme. *Psychological Medicine*, **19**, 233–244.

Sartorius, N. (1990) Cultural factors in the etiology of schizophrenia. In *Psychiatry: A World Perspective, Vol. 4. Social Psychiatry, Ethics and Law: History of Psychiatry and Education* (eds C. N. Stefanis, *et al*), pp. 33–44. International Congress Series. Excerpta Medica.

Sartorius, N. (1993) WHO's work on the epidemiology of mental disorders. *Social Psychiatry and Psychiatric Epidemiology*, **28**, 147–155.

Sartorius, N. (1998) SCAN translation. In *Diagnosis and Clinical Measurement in Psychiatry – A Reference Manual for SCAN* (eds J. K. Wing, N. Sartorius & T. B. Ustun), pp. 44–57. Cambridge University Press.

Sartorius, N. & Kuyken, W. (1994) Translation of health status instruments. In *Quality of Life Assessment: International Perspectives* (eds J. Orley & W. Kuyken), pp. 3–18. Springer.

Sartorius, N., Jablensky, A., Gulbinat, W., *et al* (1980) WHO collaborative study: assessment of depressive disorders. Preliminary communication. *Psychological Medicine*, **10**, 743–749.

Sartorius, N., Davidian, H., Ernberg, G., *et al* (1983) *Depressive Disorders in Different Cultures. Report in the WHO Collaborative Study on Standardised Assessment of Depressive Disorders.* WHO.

Saunders, J. B. & Aasland, O. G. (1987) *WHO Collaborative Project on the Identification and Treatment of Persons with Harmful Alcohol Consumption. Report on Phase 1. Development of a Screening Instrument.* WHO.

Saunders, J. B., Aasland, O. G., Arundsen, A., *et al* (1993a) Alcohol consumption and related problems among primary health care patients. WHO collaborative project on early detection of persons with harmful alcohol consumption. I. *Addiction*, **88**, 339–352.

Saunders, J. B., Aasland, O. G., Babor, T. F., *et al* (1993b) Development of the Alcohol Use Disorders Identification Test (AUDIT). WHO collaborative project on early detection of persons with harmful alcohol consumption. II. *Addiction*, **88**, 617–629.

Saxena, S., Carlson, D., Billington, R., *et al* (2001) The WHO Quality of Life Assessment Instrument (WHOQOL–Bref): the importance of its items for cross cultural research. *Quality of Life Research*, **10**, 711–721.

Saxena, S., Lora, A., van Ommeren, M., *et al* (2007) WHO's Assessment Instrument for Mental Health Systems: collecting essential information for policy and service delivery. *Psychiatric Services*, **58**, 816–821.

Sell, H. & Nagpal, R. (1992) *Assessment of Subjective Well-Being. The Subjective Well-Being Inventory (SUBI).* WHO Regional Office for South-East Asia.

Sell, H., Thara, R., Padmarati, R., *et al* (1998) *The Burden Assessment Schedule (BAS).* WHO Regional Office for South-Eastern Asia.

Tsiantis, J., Caldwell, B., Dragonas, T., *et al* (1991) Development of a WHO child care facility schedule (CCFS): a pilot collaborative study. *Bulletin of the WHO*, **69**, 51–57.

Üstün, T. B., Chatterji, S., Kostanjsek, N., *et al* (2010) Developing the World Health Oragnization Disability Assessment Schedule 2.0. *WHO Bulletin*, doi: 10.2471/BLT.09.067231.

van Goor-Lambo, G., Orley, I., Poustka, F., *et al* (1990) Classification of abnormal psychosocial situations: preliminary report of a revision of a WHO scheme. *Journal of Child Psychology and Psychiatry*, **31**, 229–241.

WHOQOL Group (1994) The development of the WHO Quality of Life Assessment Instrument (the WHOQOL). In *Quality of Life Assessment: International Perspectives* (eds J. Orley & W. Kuyken), pp. 41–57. Springer.

WHOQOL Group (1998a) Development of the World Health Organization WHOQOL–Bref quality of life assessment. *Psychological Medicine*, **28**, 551–559.

WHOQOL Group (1998b) The World Health Organization Quality of Life Assessment (WHOQOL): development and general psychometric properties. *Social Sciences and Medicine*, **46**, 1569–1585.

WHOQOL HIV Group (2003a) Initial steps to developing the World Health Organization's Quality of Life Instrument (WHOQOL) module for international assessment in HIV/AIDS. *AIDS Care*, **15**, 347–357.

WHOQOL HIV Group (2003b) Preliminary development of the World Health Organization's Quality of Life HIV instrument (WHOQOL–HIV): analysis of the pilot version. *Social Science and Medicine*, **57**, 1259–1275.

WHOQOL HIV Group (2004) WHOQOL–HIV for quality of life assessment among people living with HIV and AIDS: results from the field test. *AIDS Care*, **16**, 882–889.

WHOQOL SRPB Group (2006) A cross-cultural study of spirituality, religion, and personal beliefs as components of quality of life. *Social Science and Medicine*, **62**, 1486–1497.

Wing, J. K., Cooper, J. E. & Sartorius, N. (1974) *Measurement and Classification of Psychiatric Symptoms: An Instruction Manual for the PSE and CATEGO Programme.* Cambridge University Press.

Wing, J. K., Babor, T., Brugha, T., *et al* (1990) SCAN: Schedules for Clinical Assessment in Neuropsychiatry. *Archives of General Psychiatry*, **47**, 589–593.

Wing, J. K., Sartorius, N. & Ustun, T. B. (1998) *Diagnosis and Clinical Measurement in Psychiatry: A Reference Manual for SCAN.* Cambridge University Press.

Wittchen, H.-U., Robins, L. N., Cottler, L., *et al* (1991) Cross-cultural feasibility, reliability and sources of variance of the Composite International Diagnostic Interview (CIDI) – results of the multicentre WHO/ADAMHA field trials (wave I). *British Journal of Psychiatry*, **159**, 645–653.

World Health Organization (1973) *Report on the International Pilot Study of Schizophrenia, Vol. I.* WHO.

World Health Organization (1980) *International Classification of Impairments, Disabilities and Handicaps.* WHO.

World Health Organization (1984) *Mental Health Care in Developing Countries: A Critical Appraisal of Research Findings. Report of a WHO Study Group.* WHO.

World Health Organization (1988) *Draft Multiaxial Classification of Child Psychiatric Disorders. Axis V. Associated Abnormal Psychosocial Situations Including Glossary Descriptions of Items and Diagnostic Guidelines.* WHO.

World Health Organization (1990a) *WHO Child Care Facility Schedule With User Manual.* WHO.

World Health Organization (1990b) *Parent Interview Schedule. Draft for Comments and Field Testing.* WHO.

World Health Organization (1991) *Interview Schedule for Children. Draft for Comments and Field Testing.* WHO.

World Health Organization (1992) *The ICD–10 Classification of Mental and Behavioural Disorders: Clinical Descriptions and Diagnostic Guidelines.* WHO.

World Health Organization (1993a) *The Composite International Diagnostic Interview, Core Version 1.1.* American Psychiatric Press.

World Health Organization (1993b) *International Personality Disorder Examination.* WHO.

World Health Organization (1993c) Computerized CIDI (CIDI–Auto). WHO.

World Health Organization (1994) *Schedules for Clinical Assessment in Neuropsychiatry (SCAN).* American Psychiatric Research.

World Health Organization (1997) *Multi-axial Presentation of the ICD–10 for Use in Adult Psychiatry.* Cambridge University Press.

World Health Organization (2001) *International Classification of Functioning, Disability and Health: ICF.* WHO.

World Health Organization (2005) *Basic Documents* (45th edition). WHO.

CHAPTER 18

Measuring outcomes in mental health: implications for policy

Rachel Jenkins, Graham Mellsop and Bruce Singh

The activities and purposes of mental health services can be broadly described under four broad headings: needs assessment, inputs, processes and outcomes. During the twentieth century, the focus of service development and evaluation was largely on input and process variables, while use of outcome measures was seen as too difficult, and it was not until the 1990s that efforts were made to introduce systematic thinking about needs assessment and the measurement of outcomes (Jenkins, 1990, 1994). The strength of this book is that it illuminates the increasing number of possibilities to use outcome indicators as the main point of reference for measuring cost-effectiveness.

The approach that uses inputs as measures of service adequacy has historically focused on the number of beds available, the type and ranges of buildings and places that are provided, the numbers of staff of different disciplines and their levels of training and the amount of money injected into the service. Although this information is vital for assessing the performance of a mental health service, it is a one-sided approach. Such information may be entirely misleading if the investment, described in these terms, produces no actual benefits to patients. The input approach on its own, although frequently used and administratively convenient, can give no indication about whether services are actually achieving their goals.

The second and most common approach to assessing the performance of a mental health system is to use process measures. Examples of this approach are the determination of length of stay in hospital, bed occupancy rates, staffing levels, staff turnover rates, and the number and duration of community contacts for home treatment services. Again, this information is vital for understanding the dynamic way in which a variety of services operate, how the physical and human resource infrastructures are deployed in practice, and the distribution of these resources in different geographical and administrative sectors. This approach is the focus of performance management, which is increasingly emphasised as health services are run more and more on corporate lines. However, this can be compared to a detailed description of the functioning of an ocean liner without any reference to whether the ship is sailing in the right direction. Auditing provides service process information, and service commissioning and the management of services are often based on such process information. As with input information, however, such process measures alone cannot shed any light on whether the intended aims of the service, both as a whole and in its components, are realised in practice.

The third approach, that of measuring outcome variables, is therefore the most important. In 1990, Jenkins called for a system of outcome indicators for mental healthcare:

In order to evaluate our health care system, we need to be able to measure the baseline health of the population, and then to measure the impact of health care on that baseline. We need to be able to monitor and evaluate progress towards more effective health care and better health, to evaluate the efficacy of health promotion and illness prevention programmes, and to improve resource allocation in health care. In order to do this effectively in a valid and reproducible manner, health indicators are required. Besides the more global indicators of general health, lifestyles, quality of life and health equity, we also need indicators relevant to the different categories of illness, and to specific strategies to prevent diseases, to alleviate disability, and to restore function. (Jenkins, 1990)

Drawing on theoretical aspects of mental healthcare indicators and the various classes of outcome measures available, Jenkins drew up a preliminary system of indicators of healthcare input, process and outcome for the major categories of mental illness, including schizophrenia, affective disorders, neurosis, dementia, intellectual disability, child psychiatry, forensic psychiatry, and alcohol and drug misuse. The system was not intended to be definitive or exhaustive, but rather to form a basis for development by clinicians, researchers and planners for their own requirements.

This chapter draws together much of the progress that has been made over the last 20 years and illuminates the increasing number of possibilities to use outcome indicators as the main point of reference for measuring cost-effectiveness in mental healthcare services. These two decades have also seen revolutionary changes in the way governments approach healthcare, by setting health action targets, an approach initiated by the World Health Organization (WHO) in its 'Health for All by the Year 2000' campaign, and the more recent international health targets included in the Millennium Development Goals.

England was one of the first countries to respond, when it established its 'Health of the Nation' strategy, which set out health outcome targets in five key areas, including mental health. Three targets were selected for mental health (see Box 18.1), the first of which was a true mental health outcome target (as opposed to using inputs or process indicators as proxy measurements) and the second two targets were suicide mortality outcome targets. In order to measure the mental health outcome target, the Royal College of Psychiatrists was commissioned to develop the Health of the Nation Outcome Scale (HoNOS; Wing *et al*, 1996), which is now widely

Box 18.1 UK mental health targets

Three mental illness targets were set in the 1992 'Health of the Nation' strategy (Department of Health, 1992):

- to improve significantly the health and social functioning of people with a mental illness
- to reduce the overall suicide rate by at least 15% by the year 2000 (from 11.0 per 100 000 population in 1990 to no more than 9.4)
- to reduce the suicide rate of people with a severe mental illness by at least 33% by the year 2000 (from the lifetime estimate of 15% in 1990 to no more than 10%)

A single mental health target was set in the 1999 'Our Healthier Nation' strategy (Department of Health, 1999):

- to reduce the death rate from suicide and undetermined injury by at least a fifth by 2010, saving up to 4000 lives in total.

used in the UK, and incorporated into the Minimum data-set, which is the common standard for mental health information (Glover, 2000). In Australia the HoNOS is now required in all public and private mental health services, and is collected and reported on nationally under the Australian National Outcomes and Classification Network (see http://www.mhnocc. org/amhocn).

England built on its earlier progress by establishing the 'Our Healthier Nation' strategy in 1999, which has set a single outcome target for each of the key areas (see Box 18.1), including further suicide rate reduction. Similarly, Australia set out its Goals and Targets (Commonwealth Department of Human Services and Health, 1994).

These developments have been inspired and motivated by a desire to be able to achieve and measure real health outcomes and health gains, and to move on from the rather static approach of using process indicators as a performance measure, which has the in-built risk that, in the attempt to produce an apparently good result with a process indicator, service providers may do too much of a relatively less useful activity at the expense of achieving good health outcomes. Instead, the outcome measure data have always been intended to be directly useful at the interface between clinician and service user and at the front line, with the clinical team's planning of their therapeutic programmes.

However, these developments have happened in the course and context of an increasing need and drive to control rising costs, to deliver value for money and to audit services (Jenkins & Knapp, 1996). The setting of objectives makes clear the intended outcomes of a national health strategy and it prompts attention to be given to the design of specific strategies,

315

which leads logically to the identification of component tasks and to the assignment of these tasks. Critical to this process is the consideration of the practicality of specific targets, time-line strategies and resource allocations. However, without clear means of assessing outcomes, a programme will have only expenditure of resources with no easily discernible accomplishments. Defining measurements makes it possible to organise the feedback from results and to review and revise objectives, roles, priorities and the allocation of resources systematically.

In several countries, measures of need have been constructed to guide the allocation of healthcare resources. The measurement of outcomes is clearly related to the measurement of need and it is now widely accepted that the most useful outcome measures are simply standardised assessments which lend themselves to quantification, and which can be repeated to measure change (Mellsop & Wilson, 2006).

The idea of shifting resources to where they can meet the greatest need or, more correctly, where they will lead to the best outcomes or do the most good is not difficult to grasp. If more good can be done than is being done, if more needs can be met with the same resources, then the argument is that that is what should be done. This is the position which evidence-based medicine attempts to establish. The concept of need incorporated into this planning framework is that of capacity to benefit. The move in a number of countries to plan health services with a focus on outcomes or health gain emphasises efficiency and equity in the context of needs.

Measurement of need assesses, in a sense, the gap between the current status and the best achievable outcomes. Since 1993, a programme of national surveys of psychiatric morbidity has been established in the UK to ensure the government has continuing access to up-to-date national figures on mental health needs. To date, there have been three surveys of the general adult population (in 1993, 2000 and 2008), two surveys of children and adolescents, a survey of prisoners, a survey of looked-after children, a survey of homeless people and a survey of carers. Similarly, a number of other countries have conducted national surveys, including Australia in 1997 and 2007 (Henderson *et al*, 2000; Slade *et al*, 2009), New Zealand in 2005 (Wells *et al*, 2006), the USA (Kessler *et al*, 2005) and some other countries as part of the World Mental Health Survey (Kessler & Ustun, 2008).

Another impetus for the development of a broader range of outcome measures in mental health has come from the pharmaceutical industry (Revicki, 1967). In order to gain approval for marketing of a drug, some countries (e.g. Australia) now require cost-effectiveness studies to demonstrate the value to the community of the introduction of a new drug as compared with the established medication, particularly as, in the majority of cases, such new drugs are significantly more expensive. The evidence that the selective serotonin reuptake inhibitors are no more effective in terms of their influence on symptom levels than the tricyclics forced a rethink of the measurement of treatment outcomes. Quality of life and disability outcomes have thus received serious consideration for the evaluation of psychopharmacological treatments for serious psychiatric disorders.

The appearance of such measures in clinical outcome studies has been noted since the 1980s. Quality-of-life outcomes represent a patient-centred approach to evaluating the impact of both disease and treatment on functioning and well-being. Interest in quality-of-life outcomes and schizophrenia began with concerns about the functioning of patients with a chronic mental illness following deinstitutionalisation during the 1970s. As considered in Chapter 8, a number of instruments have now been developed to assess quality of life in patients with severe psychiatric disorder, despite criticisms that such patients are unable to provide valid and reliable assessments. The first generation of studies showed that such measures are useful for differentiating the therapeutic effects of the newer antidepressants and antipsychotic medications from the older ones.

Nowadays, the majority of clinical outcome studies of new antidepressants and antipsychotics include quality-of-life measures; and these studies have demonstrated significant improvement in patient outcome as measured by these scales, despite the fact that the effect on symptom variables is usually no different from that of the older medications. A reduction in the number of adverse side-effects has come to be seen as another important outcome measure influencing compliance. However, it is important to retain the distinction between quality of life and symptom severity and to retain symptom severity as a central outcome variable.

In the 1960s, the concept of justice entered the discussion of healthcare policy (Daniels, 1985). This was used in several different ways, sometimes to mean treating individual patients justly by observing their rights and sometimes to mean that all patients were equally entitled to equal shares in the distribution of healthcare. In addition, discussions of public health have traditionally been concerned with the utilitarian principle of maximising the total benefits for the populations involved. In fact, some would say that utility underlies all discussions of medical ethics. However, in recent years, utility has come to the fore because of the increasing importance, for public health medicine, of rationing of scarce resources. Questions of the supply and fair distribution of healthcare resources are matters related to public policy and ones that are relevant to the principles of both utility and justice. Utility is the principle concerned with the maximising of outcomes and preferences. In its original formulation it was the greatest happiness of the greatest number. The question then arises, how does one ensure the most effective use of limited resources to benefit the greatest number of the population? A related question is, which interventions will be both effective and affordable?

In many countries there has been a reassessment of the structure and organisation of mental health services, with a view to making them more effective and to achieving value for money. Many different models are being tried and common outcome measures are necessary to ensure that the lesson learnt in one country or part of a country can be used in others. There is an increasing interest in the health gain achieved by mental health promotion and prevention activities as well as treatment, rehabilitation and reduction of mortality interventions. Sharing information can also guide the way in which money can be invested in health in order to achieve the maximum health benefit.

References

Commonwealth Department of Human Services and Health (1994) *Better Health Outcomes for Australians. National Goals, Targets and Strategies for Better Health Outcomes into the Next Century.* Australian Government Publishing Service.

Daniels, N. (1985) *Just Health Care.* Cambridge University Press.

Department of Health (1992) *The Health of the Nation: A Strategy for Health in England* (Cm 1986). HMSO.

Department of Health (1999) *Our Healthier Nation: Saving Lives* (Cm 4386). TSO (The Stationery Office).

Glover, G. R. (2000) A comprehensive clinical database for mental health care in England. *Social Psychiatry and Psychiatric Epidemiology,* **35,** 523–529.

Henderson, S., Andrews, G. & Hall, W. (2000) Australia's mental health: an overview of the general population survey. *Australian and New Zealand Journal of Psychiatry,* **34,** 197–205.

Jenkins, R. (1990) Towards a system of outcome indicators for mental health care. *British Journal of Psychiatry,* **157,** 500–514.

Jenkins, R. (1994) Ageing in learning difficulties: the development of health care outcome indicators. *Journal of Intellectual Disability Research,* **38,** 257–264.

Jenkins, R. & Knapp, M. (1996) Use of health economic data by health administrators in national health systems. In *The Handbook of Mental Health Economics and Health Policy. Vol. 1: Schizophrenia* (eds M. Moscarelli, A. Rapp & N. Sartorius), pp. 503–510. Wiley.

Kessler, R. C. & Ustun, T. B. (2008) *The WHO World Mental Health Survey: Global Perspectives on the Epidemiology of Mental Disorders.* Cambridge University Press.

Kessler, R. C., Chiu, W. T., Demler, O., *et al* (2005) Prevalence, severity, and comorbidity of 12-month DSM–IV disorders in the National Comorbidity Survey Replication. *Archives of General Psychiatry,* **62,** 617–627.

Mellsop, G. W. & Wilson, J. (2006) Outcome measures in mental health services: Humpty Dumpty is alive and well. *Australasian Psychiatry,* **14,** 137–140.

Revicki, D. A. (1967) Methods of pharmaco-economic evaluation of therapies for patients with schizophrenia. *Journal of Psychiatry and Neuroscience,* **22,** 256–266.

Slade, T., Johnston, A., Oakley Browne, M. A., *et al* (2009) National Survey of Mental Health and Wellbeing: description of methods and summary of key findings. *Australian and New Zealand Journal of Psychiatry,* **43,** 594–605.

Wells, J. E., Oakley Browne, M. A., Scott, K. M., *et al* (2006) Prevalence, interference with life and severity of 12-month DSM–IV disorders in Te Rau Hinengaro: the New Zealand Mental Health Survey. *Australian and New Zealand Journal of Psychiatry,* **40,** 845–854.

Wing, J. K., Curtis, R. H. & Beevor, A. S. (1996) *HoNOS: Health of the Nation Outcome Scales. Report on Research and Development. July 1993–December 1995.* Royal College of Psychiatrists.

CHAPTER 19

Outcome measures for the treatment of depression in primary care

William E. Narrow and Farifteh F. Duffy

Major depression is highly prevalent, often chronic or recurrent, and among the most disabling and costly of illnesses, yet its burden is often unrecognised. Historically, the primary care sector of the US health system has played a large role in both the mental and physical healthcare of patients with depression (Regier *et al*, 1993; Kessler *et al*, 2003). This role is amplified by the managed care industry, which may emphasise restricted access to specialty care in its efforts to limit costs. This chapter reviews state-of-the-art research on the treatment of depression in primary care, with special attention to the measurement tools used to support outcomes assessment.

Epidemiology, service use and costs of depression in primary care

Prevalence of disorder

In the general population, the 12-month prevalence of major depressive disorder has been estimated at 6.6%, according to the US National Comorbidity Survey Replication (NCS-R; Kessler *et al*, 2003). About a quarter to a half of patients with depression are treated in primary care (Narrow *et al*, 1993; Regier *et al*, 1993; Kessler *et al*, 2003) and, accordingly, the disorder is highly prevalent in primary care, with a point prevalence estimated at 5–10% (Katon *et al*, 1992, Simon & Von Korff, 1995) among adults 18 years of age and older.

Disability

According to the World Health Organization Global Burden of Disease Study, unipolar major depressive disorder was the fourth leading cause of worldwide disability for both sexes in the 1990s (Murray & Lopez, 1996*a*). It is projected that depression will rank as the second largest contributor to the worldwide burden of disease by 2020 (Murray & Lopez, 1996b). The Medical Outcomes Study (MOS) demonstrated that physical functioning and well-being scores on the 36-item Short Form (SF–36) for patients with major depression were comparable, and in some cases significantly worse than scores for patients with other chronic medical conditions. Mental functioning and well-being scores were consistently and significantly worse for the MOS patients with depression than for patients with medical illnesses (Hays et al, 1995). Another longitudinal observational study compared primary care patients with depression during their 'worst-functioning' assessment interval with participants who did not have depression (Rost et al, 1998). The former group had scores 3.5–4 times higher than the latter on the SF–36 role limitations – physical scale and over 9 times higher scores on the role limitations – emotional scale, as well as 8–10 times more disability days in the previous month. Moreover, 45–55% had had suicidal ideation in the 6 months before the assessment. In sum, these findings point to a high degree of individual suffering and potentially enormous costs to society in terms of lost productivity.

Under-diagnosis and under-treatment

Despite the prevalence of depression and its associated disability, the disorder often goes unrecognised and untreated in primary care. The MOS found that only 46–51% of patients with depression who visited medical clinicians had their condition detected, compared with 78–87% of patients with depression who visited mental health specialists (Wells et al, 1989). Higher rates of recognition in primary care, up to 65%, have been reported when depression was diagnosed through structured diagnostic interviews, and when researchers asked clinicians directly about the presence of psychological disorders in their patients, rather than relying on diagnoses recorded in patients' charts. Patients with recognised depression appear to have more severe illness and greater disability and are more likely to receive antidepressant treatment (Simon & Von Korff, 1995). In a prospective cohort of adults treated in a primary care clinic and independently evaluated for mental disorders at baseline and at 5-year follow-up, 56% of patients with major depression and 32% of those with minor depression at baseline reported being diagnosed or treated at 5-year follow-up. Depressive disorders meeting diagnostic criteria were more likely to be detected than subthreshold conditions, i.e. major depression was more likely to be detected than minor depression. Other factors increasing the likelihood of detection included persistence of the disorder over the 5-year period, co-occurrence with anxiety disorders, and worse functional status (Jackson et al, 2007).

Among primary care physicians (including family physicians, internists, and obstetricians and gynaecologists), antidepressant medication is the preferred treatment; women physicians are twice as likely to prescribe antidepressants as male physicians (Williams *et al*, 1999). However, the prescribed treatment is often inadequate. Primary care physicians tend to prescribe inadequate dosages and duration of medication, with infrequent follow-up visits and lack of adjustment in dose according to patient response. Referrals to specialty care are often not made when needed (Katon *et al*, 1990, 1992; Lin *et al*, 1997; van der Feltz-Cornelis, 1997). The NCS–R demonstrated that among patients treated for depression in general medical settings, only 41% received treatment of at least minimal adequacy. In specialty mental health settings, 64% of patients with depression received at least minimally adequate treatment (Kessler *et al*, 2003). Patient adherence to antidepressant medication is reasonably high in the first month of treatment, with over half of patients completing a prescription. However, there is a considerable drop-off at 4 and 6 months of treatment. There is evidence that adherence is higher with non-tricyclic antidepressants (Katon *et al*, 1992; Simon *et al*, 1993, 1995a; Lin *et al*, 1995). Further complicating primary care treatments, adherence to treatment regimens for chronic physical illnesses is a particular problem when comorbid depression is present (Katon, 1996).

Service use

Several large epidemiological studies conducted over the past 25 years have documented the level of mental health service use among Americans with major depression. The Epidemiologic Catchment Area (ECA) Program of the US National Institute of Mental Health (NIMH) showed that, over 1 year, about 54% of persons with active unipolar major depression used any mental health or addiction service, with 45% using the health systems sector (comprised of the specialty and general medical sectors): 27.8% used the specialty sector and 25.3% used the general medical sector for their mental health problems (Regier *et al*, 1993). There was a large difference in the average number of mental health visits per treated person per year between the two sectors: 17.5 visits in the specialty sector and 4.2 visits in the general medical sector (Narrow *et al*, 1993).

The National Comorbidity Survey (NCS), done in the early 1990s, 7–10 years after the ECA Program, showed somewhat different results for service use. Among persons with major depression, 36.4% used any mental health service and 27.7% used services in the health systems sector, with 21.2% using specialty services and 12.1% using general medical services (Kessler *et al*, 1999). Average visit frequency was about one visit less per year than in the ECA study: 16.5 per person per year in the specialty sector and 3.4 per treated person per year in the general medical sector (Kessler *et al*, 1999). In the NCS–R, conducted in 2001–02, 57% of respondents with major depressive disorder reported receiving some type of treatment in the 12 months before interview, with 51.6% receiving care in the healthcare sector (i.e. specialty mental health sector and general medical sector): 31.6% in specialty mental health and 27.2% in general medical (Kessler *et al*, 2003).

It is difficult to explain the lower rate of service use in the general medical settings in the NCS compared with the ECA Program, with the subsequent rate in the NCS–R coming closer to what was reported in the latter. Difference in utilisation rates may be due to a true decrease in use from the time when the ECA was conducted, and a subsequent increase in depression care in the general medical sector by the time NCS–R was conducted (Kessler *et al*, 2003). Alternatively, methodological differences may account for the disparity between the three surveys (Narrow *et al*, 2002).

Persons with depression are over-represented among high users of general medical services for physical health reasons (Kessler *et al*, 1987; Katon, 1996; Lefevre *et al*, 1999; Pearson *et al*, 1999). For example, distressed high users were found to have high prevalences of chronic medical problems and illness-related disability. In addition, 24% were found to have current major depression, 17% current dysthymia and 68% had a lifetime history of major depression (Katon *et al*, 1990).

Costs of care

Based on prevalence, disability and treatment rates obtained from the NCS–R, Greenberg *et al* (2003) estimated the economic burden of depression in the USA to be $83.1 billion in the year 2000, which included $26.1 billion in direct medical costs, $5.4 billion in suicide-related mortality costs and $51.5 billion in workplace costs.

As suggested above, persons with major depression tend to be high users of general medical and mental health services, with high costs to the general medical sector. Simon *et al* (1995*b*) examined age- and sex-matched samples of attenders at a primary care health maintenance organisation (HMO) with and without depression as diagnosed by their general medical provider. They found that patients with depression had significantly higher annual healthcare costs, at a mean of $4246, than did patients without depression, at $2371. The former had higher costs for each component of care, including in-patient and out-patient care, pharmacy and laboratory, and similar results were found regardless of whether the depression was treated with antidepressant medication. Indeed, among those treated, specialty treatment of the depression accounted for less than 25% of the difference in total costs of care, with about half of the difference accounted for by non-specific increases in out-patient service use. Twofold differences in costs persisted for at least 12 months after the initiation of the treatment for depression. Similar results were found by Unützer *et al* (1997) in a large cohort of older adults. In this study, costs were about 50% higher for patients with significant depressive symptoms (as measured by the Center for Epidemiologic Studies – Depression scale) than for patients without such symptoms. Again, costs were uniformly increased across all healthcare components, and specialty care accounted for a very small portion (about 1%) of total costs. It remains to be determined whether the costs of adequately treating depression will be offset by reduced medical costs and improved work productivity (Simon & Katzelnick, 1997, Schulberg *et al*, 1998).

Randomised trials of treatment effectiveness

Based on the foundation presented above, efforts aimed at improving the care of patients with depression in primary care have had several goals – increased recognition and treatment by primary care providers, increased rates of appropriate treatment, increased patient adherence to treatment recommendations, reduction in depressive symptoms and disorder, reduction in disability, increased positive functioning and quality of life, reduced costs of non-mental (i.e. medical) healthcare and overall cost-effectiveness. This is a diverse set of goals that encompasses change in outcomes at at least three levels: provider, patient and expenditure. In this chapter we focus on the assessment of patient-level outcomes. First, in this section, state-of-the-art research studies in the USA that have examined these issues are briefly described. A description of the outcome measures used in these studies follows. All the studies had as a goal the use of treatments of proven efficacy in primary care; that is, they move beyond the more tightly controlled efficacy trials to 'real life' effectiveness trials.

The aims of the collaborative care intervention trial (Katon *et al*, 1995) were to determine whether the treatment of depression in primary care could be improved to the level of recommended treatment guidelines of the Agency for Health Care Policy and Research (AHCPR), whether this treatment improved short-term patient outcomes, and whether it was acceptable to the patients and the primary care providers. Patients from primary care clinics in a large HMO who had depression screening scores of 0.75 or more on the 20-item Symptom Checklist (SCL–20) were randomised. The intervention arm ($n = 77$) received collaborative treatment of their depression by one of two on-site psychiatrists along with the primary care provider, who had received didactic training in depression and its treatment. Antidepressant medication along with patient education were the main treatments in the intervention group, although referrals to psychotherapy could be made. The control arm ($n = 76$) received usual care from the primary care provider.

Katon *et al* (1996) subsequently adapted the collaborative care model to incorporate non-psychiatrist providers and behavioural (i.e. non-medication) treatment in similar primary care settings as utilised above. The study aims were similar to those of the previous study, namely achieving AHCPR guideline-level care, acceptability and improved outcomes. In this study, the intervention ($n = 108$) consisted of a highly structured programme given by an on-site, doctorally trained psychologist that included brief cognitively oriented psychotherapy, adherence counselling and a relapse-prevention programme. The study psychiatrist acted as a consultant and provided medication recommendations to the primary care physician based on a weekly progress report. The control group ($n = 109$) received usual care from their primary care physician.

Schulberg et al (1996) aimed to test guideline-concordant treatments, including psychotherapy, within a framework of effectiveness research. They chose patients from four ambulatory health centres, screened for depression with the Center for Epidemiologic Studies – Depression (CES–D) scale, and confirmed the diagnosis with the Diagnostic Interview Schedule (DIS) and the Hamilton Rating Scale for Depression (HRSD). There were two intervention arms. One intervention group of 93 patients received interpersonal psychotherapy from a trained psychologist or psychiatrist in 16 weekly sessions. The second intervention group of 91 patients received nortriptyline from internist or family practitioners trained in pharmacotherapy through didactic sessions and a manual. The control group of 92 patients received usual care from their primary care physicians.

The Partners in Care Study (Wells et al, 1999) has been described as the second-generation of the Patient Outcomes Research Team (PORT) initiative of the AHCPR. The main goals of Partners in Care Study are to examine the outcomes of treatment for depression in terms of patient health and satisfaction, healthcare and social costs, and quality and cost-effectiveness of care. The two experimental interventions were basic quality improvement with enhanced medication management and quality improvement with enhanced psychotherapy. These interventions were compared with usual care. Primary care clinics from seven geographically diverse managed care organisations were randomised into one of the two intervention groups or the usual care group. Patients were screened with the Composite International Diagnostic Interview (CIDI) stem questions for major depression and dysthymia. A total of 913 patients were placed in an intervention group and 443 received care as usual.

Improving Primary Care for Depression in Late Life (IMPACT) was a multicentre randomised controlled trial of a depression management programme for late-life depression (Unützer et al, 2001, 2002). The study goals were to compare the cost-effectiveness of a collaborative stepped care intervention programme with that of care as usual. Approximately 1750 adults aged 60 and over with major depression or dysthymia were randomised into the collaborative care programme or care as usual in a total of 15 primary care clinics across seven sites. The collaborative care programme involved a depression clinical specialist responsible for the coordination of care in collaboration with patients' primary care physician and a team psychiatrist, over a 1-year period. The Structured Clinical Interview for DSM (SCID) was used to determine the diagnosis of depressive disorder. The SCL–20 assessed the severity of symptoms of depression. The Sheehan Disability Scale and the Medical Outcomes Study 12-item Short-Form Health Survey (SF–12) were used to evaluate patients' functioning and disability. Data were collected at baseline and at 3, 6, 12, 18 and 24 months.

Additionally, the nine-item Patient Health Questionnaire (PHQ–9) was used for in-person or telephone follow-up every other week or more to monitor treatment response.

The Re-engineering Systems for the Treatment of Depression in Primary Care (RESPECT) randomised controlled trials were designed to compare with usual care, in primary care settings, the effectiveness of a depression management model (Oxman *et al*, 2002; Dietrich *et al*, 2004). The 'three-component model' of depression care used in the intervention arm of the RESPECT trials comprised 'a prepared practice, care management, and enhanced mental health support'. A total of five healthcare organisations were recruited, each with at least ten affiliated primary care practices; a total of 60 practices were identified. Practices were subsequently paired based on specified practice characteristics; within pairs, practices were assigned to either intervention or usual care. A total of 224 patients were treated in the intervention and 181 in the usual care sites. The PHQ–9 was used as part of initial diagnostic assessment, for monitoring treatment response, to guide change in treatment and as a common metric aiding communication between providers and care managers. The SCL–20 was also used for measuring the severity of depression. The 12-item version of the World Health Organization Disability Assessment Schedule (WHODAS 2.0, discussed below and in Chapter 17) was used for measuring the disability status of patients. The assessments took place at baseline and at 3 and 6 months. Care managers conducted 10-minute telephone follow-ups at 1, 4 and 8 weeks after the initial visit and every 4 weeks thereafter until remission. During the call barriers to adherence, means of overcoming them and treatment response (using the PHQ–9) were assessed.

A comprehensive review of the literature by Gilbody *et al* (2006) has lent support to collaborative care models of depression care as potentially effective interventions to improve quality of treatment in primary care and improve longer-term outcomes for patients. Building on principles governing the management of chronic disease, collaborative care commonly involves a non-medical specialist augmenting the primary care role, working in conjunction with the patient, the patients' primary care physician and a mental health specialist.

A different set of studies, described below, have tested the clinical as well the economic outcomes of algorithm-based treatments of depression, and the use of measurement-based approaches at critical decision points to inform clinical decision-making. The overarching goals of these studies were to treat patients to remission and recovery.

The Texas Medication Algorithm Project (TMAP) for depression aimed to compare the clinical and economic outcomes for algorithm-guided treatment for major depressive disorder (MDD–ALGO) against treatment as usual (TAU) (Rush *et al*, 2004a; Trivedi *et al*, 2004a); similar TMAP algorithms have been developed and studied for schizophrenia and bipolar disorder (Suppes *et al*, 2003; Miller *et al*, 2004). For the TMAP depression project, the algorithm-guided treatment included pre-specified medication algorithms and a pre-specified patient/family educational package, combined with clinical support. A seven-step medication algorithm for non-psychotic MDD and a five-step algorithm for psychotic MDD guided medication management in the MDD–ALGO intervention group. A total of 14 clinics in various parts of Texas were involved: four clinics provided ALGO–MDD, four clinics provided TAU for MDD patients but ALGO for either schizophrenia or bipolar disorder (TAU–MDD in ALGO) and six clinics provided TAU only (TAU–MDD in non-ALGO). A total of 181 patients were treated in ALGO–MDD clinics, 154 in TAU–MDD non-ALGO clinics and 212 in TAU–MDD in ALGO clinic sites. To collect information on patients' depressive symptoms, the Inventory of Depression Symptomatology – Clinician Rating (IDC–C$_{30}$) and the Inventory of Depression Symptomatology – Self-Report (IDC–SR$_{30}$) scales were used. Data were collected at baseline and at 3, 6, 9 and 12 months. The SF–12, data on medication side-effects and Patient Perception of Benefits were also collected during each assessment period.

The Sequenced Treatment Alternatives to Relieve Depression trial (STAR*D) was a multi-site randomised multi-step clinical trial designed to assess the effectiveness of a sequential series of treatments for major depression in generalisable samples of out-patients treated in primary care or psychiatric settings; the primary outcome studied was remission (Fava *et al*, 2003; Rush *et al*, 2004b; Trivedi *et al*, 2006). This study involved 14 centres overseeing study implementation at primary care ($n = 18$) or psychiatric out-patient ($n = 23$) clinical sites across the USA. A total of 4000 adult out-patients with non-psychotic major depressive disorder were enrolled in level 1, and started treatment with citalopram. Patients who responded to citalopram had an option of entering a 12-month naturalistic follow-up, while those who did not achieve symptomatic benefit from level 1 care became eligible for randomisation to level 2, which entailed seven treatment options. Four levels of care for treatment non-responders were developed as part of a rigorous protocol involving routine measurement of symptoms and side-effects at each visit, along with a treatment protocol describing when and how to modify treatment.

Patient-level outcome measures used in treatment effectiveness research on depression in primary care

The outcome measures used for these studies are listed in Table 19.1. For simplicity, they are grouped into five categories: symptoms, functioning/disability, adherence, satisfaction with care and health service use. This chapter concentrates on the measures in the first two categories, which generally are standard measures with extensive prior use and publications in peer-reviewed journals. In addition, a major initiative of the US National Institutes of Health to develop patient-reported outcome measures is also described.

Depressive symptoms

Hamilton Rating Scale for Depression

The Hamilton Rating Scale for Depression (HRSD; Hamilton, 1960, 1967) is frequently used to measure depression severity as an outcome of treatment. The scale is comprises 17 items that assess depression severity with four additional non-scored items used for diagnostic rather than severity purposes (Zitman *et al*, 1990). The range of items is heavily focused on somatic symptoms: depressed mood, guilt, suicide, insomnia (three items), work and interests, retardation, agitation, psychic anxiety, somatic anxiety, gastrointestinal symptoms, general somatic symptoms, loss of libido, hypochondriasis, loss of insight and loss of weight. Items are scored on a scale of 0–2 or 0–4, although operationalised scoring criteria specific to each item are not consistently provided. The scale is administered in an interview format, and use of collateral information in developing the ratings for a patient was encouraged by the developer of the scale. The interview time frame is the last few days or week. Raters must be trained in the use of the scale and must have clinical experience. To increase the scale's reliability, Hamilton (1967) recommended using two raters for each interview and summing their ratings. The HRSD takes about 30 minutes to administer.

In addition to Hamilton's original version of the scale, a different but frequently used version is the ECDEU version (Guy, 1976). Developed for the NIMH Early Clinical Drug Evaluation Unit (ECDEU) Program, this version is more structured and, unlike the original scale, provides anchor points for scoring each item (Nordgren, 1995). It also adds three items to the scale – helplessness, hopelessness and worthlessness – making it a 24-item scale. Because of concerns about the reliability of individual HRSD items (Cicchetti & Prusoff, 1983; Rehm & O'Hara, 1985), a semi structured interview guide was developed based on the ECDEU version of the instrument (Williams, 1988). This instrument, called the SIGH–D, gives initial and follow-up questions for each of the 21 items in the scale, and allows the interviewer to develop further questions as needed. This method has improved the test–retest reliability of most of the individual items, without lengthening the time of administration (Williams, 1988). A fully structured version of the HRSD, called the SI–HSRD, was developed for use in the MOS (Potts *et al*, 1990.) Although this version apparently has lower item-level test–retest reliabilities than the SIGH–D, it has been successfully administered by non-clinicians, and can be given over the telephone. It uses a past-month time frame. A 14-item version of the SI–HRSD was recommended by the developers of the scale.

The proliferation of 'versions' of the Hamilton scale necessitates careful investigation by the researcher or clinician choosing an instrument. Like-wise, when reporting results, the exact version of the scale used and any modifications must be reported, to facilitate comparisons.

Table 19.1 Outcome measures used in eight US studies of the treatment of depression in primary care

Study	Depressive and physical symptom measures	Measures of functioning or disability	Measures of treatment adherence	Measures of satisfaction with care	Measures of health service use
Katon et al (1995)	SCL–90–R depression scale; IDS; NEO Personality Inventory neuroticism scale; CDS; screen for side-effects of medication		Dosage check; whether medication was taken for 25 of last 30 days; health records for dose and duration	Satisfaction with care; perceived helpfulness of antidepressants	
Katon et al (1996)	As above plus SF–36; SCL–20 (self-administered measure of depression symptom severity)		As above plus self-report adherence		
Schulberg et al (1996); Coulehan et al (1997)	BDI; HRSD–17; DUSOI	SF–36; GAS			
Wells et al (1999)	CESD; CIDI screener for depressive disorder (omitting dysthymia stem)	SF–12 physical and mental health summary scales; current employment	Prescription medications used in past month; medication used for over 1 month in previous 6 months; appropriate use of antidepressants based on guideline dose criteria		Health service use in past 6 months; total number of medical visits; medical visits for emotional problems; mental health specialty visits; use of individual, family or group therapy by specialist
Unützer et al (2002): IMPACT trials	SCL–20; SCID (clinician-rated for diagnoses of major depression or dysthymia); PHQ–9 used for in-person or telephone follow-up every other week or more to monitor treatment response	SDS; SF–12; assessment for any existing chronic medical conditions	Patient followed up by care manager at least every other week during the project	Satisfaction with care	Cornell Services Index

Study				
Dietrich et al (2004): RESPECT trials	PHQ–9 self-administered, used as part of initial diagnostic assessment, for monitoring treatment response, to guide change in treatment, and as common metric aiding communication between providers and care managerd; SCL–20 self-administered for assessment of severity of depression	WHODAS–12		Care manager 10 min telephone follow-up at 1, 4 and 8 weeks after the initial visit and every 4 weeks thereafter until remission. During the call barriers to adherence, means of overcoming them, and treatment response (using PHQ–9) enquired about
Rush et al (2003a): TMAP	IDS–C$_{30}$ clinician-rated measure of depression symptom severity; IDS–SR$_{30}$ self-administered measure of depression symptom severity	SF–12; side-effect burden	Patient perception of benefits	
Fava et al (2003): STAR*D	Clinician-rated HRSD–17, IDS–C$_{30}$, QIDS–C$_{16}$ plus patient-rated Psychiatric Diagnostic Screening Questionnaire; QIDS–SR$_{16}$	CIRS to assess co-occurring general medical conditions; SF–12; Frequency, Intensity, and Burden of Side Effects Rating Scale (FIBSER)		16-item Quality of Life Enjoyment and Satisfaction Questionnaire; Work and Social Adjustment Scale

See text for abbreviations and references.

Beck Depression Inventory

The Beck Depression Inventory (BDI) is a 21-item rating scale that is also widely used in the assessment of depressive symptoms. Like the HRSD, there are several versions of the BDI in use; unlike the HRSD, many of these versions were developed by the original developer. The original scale (Beck *et al*, 1961) was designed to be administered by a trained interviewer and assessed symptoms on a current time frame ('right now').

A subsequent version (Beck *et al*, 1979) was released in which items were clarified to allow self-administration and easier scoring, alternative ways of asking the same question were eliminated, and double-negative statements were avoided. The time frame used in this revision is 'past week'. The items included in the scales are: mood, pessimism, sense of failure, lack of satisfaction, guilt feelings, sense of punishment, self-dislike, self-accusations, suicidal wishes, crying, irritability, social withdrawal, indecisiveness, distortion of body image, work inhibition, sleep disturbance, fatigability, loss of appetite, weight loss, somatic preoccupation and loss of libido. Items are rated on a scale of 0–3 and total scores can range from 0 to 63 (Beck & Steer, 1984.) The scale takes 'a few minutes to complete and score' (Nordgren, 1995).

The BDI and the HRSD have many obvious differences, including mode of administration, cost of administration (e.g. training interviewers and avoiding 'interviewer drift' in studies using the HSRD), length of administration and item coverage. All these factors must enter into a decision on choice of instrument. Studies comparing the two instruments have been inconclusive. Some (Moran & Lambert, 1983; Richter *et al*, 1997) concluded that the BDI is over-reactive in detecting change in response to therapeutic intervention, therefore running the risk of false positives. Others have concluded that the HRSD may be over-reactive (Edwards *et al*, 1984; Lambert *et al*, 1986). One study that directly compared the two instruments with the same patients over time found satisfactory and significant correlations between the total scores for two-thirds of the patients, and poor correlations for the remaining third. The authors found no obvious differences in personality or severity of illness that distinguished the two groups (Bailey & Coppen, 1976).

Inventory for Depressive Symptomatology and Quick Inventory of Depressive Symptomatology

The Inventory for Depressive Symptomatology (IDS; Rush *et al*, 1986, 1996) has both self-report (IDS–SR) and clinician-rated versions (IDS–C). The original scale had 28 items; two items were subsequently added to cover atypical symptoms. While not as frequently used as the HRSD and the BDI, both versions of the scale have satisfactory psychometric properties, correlate well with ratings from the HRSD and BDI, and, unlike the HRSD and BDI, cover the full range of DSM–IV depression criteria. Items are scored on a 0–3 scale. Factor analysis revealed three dimensions for each scale: cognitive/mood, anxiety/arousal, and vegetative (Rush *et al*, 1996).

The Quick Inventory of Depressive Symptomatology (QIDS), a subset of IDS, consists of the 16 items that cover the nine diagnostic symptoms for a major depressive episode, and follows the same scoring scheme as the IDS. The QIDS is also available in clinician-rated and patient-rated versions (QIDS–C and QIDS–SR, respectively). The scoring range on the QIDS (–C or –SR) is 0–27, with scores of 21 or more indicating very severe symptoms, scores of 16–20 indicating severe, 11–15 moderate, 6–10 mild, and 0–5 indicating no depression. Rush *et al* (2003*b*) have found self-rated depression assessment to be equivalent to clinician assessment for the severity of depression.

The psychometric properties and clinical utility of the IDS and QIDS have been well documented (Rush *et al*, 2003*b*, 2006; Trivedi *et al*, 2004*b*). The internal consistency of QIDS–SR is 0.85–0.92 (Rush *et al*, 2003*b*); IDS and QIDS total scores are highly correlated with HRSD and BDI total scores (Rush *et al*, 1996; Trivedi *et al*, 2004*b*).

Depression Symptom Checklist

The 90-item revised Symptom Checklist (SCL–90–R; Derogatis *et al*, 1976; Derogatis & Cleary, 1977; Derogatis, 1983) evolved from an older instrument, the Hopkins Symptom Checklist (Derogatis *et al*, 1974), as a self-report measure of psychopathology. Each of the 90 items is rated on a five-point scale of distress, from 'not at all' to 'extremely'. The SCL–90–R is scored on nine primary symptom dimensions and three global indices of psychopathology. The primary symptom dimensions are somatisation, obsessive–compulsive, interpersonal sensitivity, depression, anxiety, hostility, phobic anxiety, paranoid ideation and psychoticism. The global indices are the global severity index, the positive symptom distress index and the positive symptom total. The depression symptom dimension is composed of 13 items, reflecting a broad range of depressive symptoms, including dysphoric mood and affect, withdrawal, lack of motivation, loss of vitality, hopeless feelings, suicidal ideation, and other cognitive and somatic symptoms. The depression symptom dimension has an internal consistency coefficient of 0.90 (Derogatis *et al*, 1976).

The SCL–90–R has been criticised for inadequate factor structure and poor discriminant validity, with several investigators finding much of the covariation in symptom dimensions being accounted for by a single global distress factor. In particular, the depression dimension has been found to be highly inter-correlated with the anxiety dimension, raising doubts as to their distinguishability (Morgan *et al*, 1998). However, studies have shown that when homogeneous samples of persons with depression or anxiety are used, separate anxiety and depression dimensions can be distinguished (Cox *et al*, 1993; Morgan *et al*, 1998). This finding reinforces the extent to which anxiety and depressive symptoms coexist in unselected patient samples.

Center for Epidemiologic Studies – Depression scale

The Center for Epidemiologic Studies – Depression scale (CES–D; Radloff, 1977; Radloff & Locke, 1986) was developed at the NIMH for use in epidemiological studies of the presence and severity of depressive symptoms in general populations. It is a 20-item scale, with 16 items assessing symptoms in the negative direction (e.g. 'I felt sad') and 4 items assessing symptoms in the positive direction (e.g. 'I enjoyed life'). The latter items were included to discourage tendencies towards response set, as well as to assess positive affect. The items cover a range of depressive symptoms, including depressed mood, feelings of guilt and worthlessness, feelings of helplessness and hopelessness, psychomotor retardation, loss of appetite and sleep disturbance. Items are rated on a 0–3 scale, and the positive items are reversed before scoring, so the highest possible score is 60. The conventional cut-off score signifying significant depressive symptoms is 16 or above. The CES–D is a self-report scale and can be self-administered or interviewer administered.

Patient Health Questionnaire

The Primary Care Evaluation of Mental Disorders (PRIME–MD) instrument is patient rated and allows evaluation of eight specific DSM–IV diagnoses: major depressive syndrome, other depressive syndrome, panic disorder, other anxiety syndrome, somatoform disorder, bulimia nervosa, binge-eating disorder, and alcohol misuse (Spitzer et al, 1994). The nine-item Patient Health Questionnaire was derived from the original PRIME–MD. The PHQ–9 parallels the DSM–IV symptom criteria for depressive disorders. Each symptom is measured on a four-point scale for frequency over a 2-week period; scores range from 0 ('not at all') to 3 ('nearly every day'), with an overall score ranging between 0 and 27. Thresholds for levels of depression severity are as follows: 0–4, none; 5–9, mild; 10–14, moderate; 15–19, moderately severe; and 20–27, severe. Because of the PHQ–9's brevity, ease of administration and interpretation, dual capability of assessing DSM–IV criteria and symptom severity, and sensitivity to change over time, it has been used increasingly for screening and in the routine follow-up of patients with depression in primary care as well as psychiatry (Duffy et al, 2008; Nease et al, 2008). The psychometric properties, sensitivity to change and clinical utility of the PHQ–9 have been well documented (Kroenke et al, 2001; Kroenke & Spitzer, 2002; Löwe et al, 2004a–d, 2006). For a PHQ–9 cut-off of 10 or greater, Cronbach's alpha was 0.86–0.89; sensitivity and specificity were 88% when compared against reinterview by a mental health professional using the clinician interview guide from PRIME–MD and open-ended questions derived from the Structured Clinical Interview for DSM (Kroenke et al, 2001).

Patient-Reported Outcomes Measurement Information System

The Patient-Reported Outcomes Measurement Information System (PROMIS) initiative (Cella et al, 2007) was started in 2004 as a cooperative agreement between the NIH, six primary research sites and a statistical coordinating centre. PROMIS is a part of the NIH Roadmap for Medical Research Initiative, which was implemented to facilitate re-engineering of the clinical research enterprise and speed the movement of research discoveries from the bench to the bedside. The PROMIS initiative aims to develop a computerised adaptive testing system to assess patient-reported outcomes efficiently in both clinical research and patient care settings. These outcomes are based on the World Health Organization's tripartite model of health, comprising physical, mental and social health. They cover both symptoms and health-related quality of life and are meant to be applicable across a wide range of chronic conditions. Among the outcomes developed by PROMIS so far, several have direct relevance to depression, including pain, fatigue, sleep and wake disturbance, depressive symptoms, anxiety symptoms, and ability to participate in the social realm.

Development of the PROMIS measures started with item pools drawn from items in established questionnaires and new items written by experts. A PROMIS core questionnaire was established and administered in paper and electronic forms to a large sample of individuals suffering from a variety of chronic diseases. These collected data were then analysed and calibrated to establish the items in the PROMIS item banks. The PROMIS item bank for depression focuses on negative mood (e.g. sadness, guilt), decrease in positive affect (e.g. loss of interest), information-processing deficits (e.g. problems in decision making), negative views of the self (e.g. self-criticism, worthlessness) and negative social cognition (e.g. loneliness, interpersonal alienation). A computerised adaptive testing (CAT) system is used for administration of the PROMIS measures, although psychometrically derived fixed short forms have also been created. The CAT system is publicly available on the web. Further development of PROMIS measures is ongoing, including testing in various clinical populations and the development of measures for child and adolescent populations.

Despite the relatively recent development of the PROMIS scales for depression and related mental health conditions, several primary care research projects are integrating these scales into their protocols as outcome measures (D. Cella & S. Yount, personal communication, 2010). Findings from these studies are not yet available in the published literature.

Structured Clinical Interview for DSM–IV Axis I Disorders

The Structured Clinical Interview for DSM–IV Axis I Disorders (SCID–I) is a semi-structured clinical interview for use by trained clinicians who have experience making mental health diagnoses. As such, it is not practical for use in routine primary care practice, but it is widely used as a diagnostic tool for research in these settings. The SCID–I was developed according to DSM–IV diagnostic criteria, covering a broad spectrum of Axis I psychiatric diagnoses. It is available in research, clinical trials, and clinician versions. Based on one study, the interrater reliabilities for major depressive disorder and dysthymia as measured by the SCID–I were good. Test–retest reliability was fair for major depressive disorder and poor for dysthymia (Zanarini *et al*, 2000).

Composite International Diagnostic Interview

The Composite International Diagnostic Interview (CIDI; Robins *et al*, 1988; World Health Organization, 1997) is a fully structured diagnostic interview which is suitable for administration by trained lay interviewers. It is available in paper-and-pencil and computer-assisted versions. Responses are scored by computer algorithms to provide psychiatric diagnoses according to either DSM–IV or ICD–10 criteria. The diagnostic sections of the CIDI include phobic and other anxiety disorders, depressive and dysthymic disorders, bipolar affective disorders, schizophrenia and other psychotic disorders, eating disorders, substance use disorders, obsessive–compulsive and post-traumatic stress disorders, dementia, amnestic and other cognitive disorders, and somatoform and dissociative disorders. Diagnoses can be provided in several time frames, including lifetime, 1 year and 1 month. Because the CIDI is a modularised instrument, the diagnostic sections of interest can be selected for administration in lieu of the entire interview. Reliability and validity of the CIDI are good for depression and most other diagnoses (Andrews & Peters, 1998).

NEO Personality Inventory

The NEO Personality Inventory (Costa & McCrae, 1992) measures personality dimensions according to the five-factor model (FFM) of personality (Digman, 1990). The scale originally measured three personality domains: neuroticism, extraversion and openness to experience (hence 'NEO'). Conscientiousness and agreeableness were added in later versions to fit the FFM. The various versions of the Inventory were rigorously developed through factor analysis. Test–retest reliability and internal consistency are very good (Costa & McCrae, 1988). The current version of the Inventory is referred to as the NEO–PI–R. It is a copyrighted instrument containing 240 items, with three additional validity items. Each of the five domains contains 'facet scales'. Within the neuroticism domain, these are anxiety, hostility, depression, self-consciousness, impulsiveness and vulnerability (Costa & McCrae, 1988). The entire NEO–PI–R can be completed in 45 minutes or less, and there are versions for self-administration and administration by a rater who knows the respondent well. The NEO–PI–R has been used successfully with populations of patient with depression (Bagby *et al*, 1998, 1999).

Physical symptoms

Cumulative Illness Rating Scale

The Cumulative Illness Rating Scale (CIRS) is a clinician-administered scale for physical illness burden. It captures data on all comorbid diseases for a given patient, classifies comorbidities by 13 organ systems, and rates them according to their severity from 0 to 4. The total score, number of categories endorsed, severity and comorbidity indices all correlate strongly with clinical features, such as laboratory values, medication usage, length of in-hospital stay, functional disability, as well as post-mortem ratings (Conwell et al, 1993; Salvi et al, 2008).

Frequency, Intensity, and Burden of Side Effects Rating Scale

The Frequency, Intensity, and Burden of Side Effects Rating Scale (FIBSER) is a three-item self-administered measure that assesses the frequency and intensity of medication side-effects and interference with day-to-day functioning (Wisniewski et al, 2006). The FIBSER was developed specifically for patients with depression and is used in both research and clinical practice. Psychometrically, the internal consistency is high (Cronbach's alpha ranging from 0.91 to 0.93) and the face validity is excellent. However, FIBSER had a relatively weak correlation with the Patient Rated Inventory of Side Effects and specifically with QIDS–C (Wisniewski et al, 2006). Moreover, among patients who exited the STAR*D study due to treatment side-effects, only 55% side-effects rated on FIBSER present 75% of the time or more, only 48% rated side-effect intensity as severe to intolerable, and only 29% indicated severe impairment or inability to function due to antidepressant side-effects (Wisniewski et al, 2006); hence FIBSER did not demonstrate a strong construct validity.

Chronic Disease Score

The Chronic Disease Score (CDS; Von Korff et al, 1992) was developed from the population-based computerised prescription system of the Group Health Cooperative of Puget Sound to measure chronic disease status. The scoring system was developed with the following principles in mind: the score should increase with the number of chronic diseases under treatment; the score should increase with increasing complexity of the medication regimen used to treat a specific chronic disease; potentially life-threatening or progressive diseases should be scored higher than benign or stable diseases; medication regimens used in the score should target diseases, not symptoms (and so, for example, analgesics and sedatives should not be counted). Seventeen diseases were chosen for inclusion, each with one or more medication classes and accompanying scoring rules. For example, high cholesterol was given a score of 1 if antilipaemics were used, diabetes was given a score of 2 if either insulin or oral hypoglycaemics were used. For heart disease, three medication classes were identified and the patient scored 3 if one class was used, 4 if two classes were used, or 5 if all three classes were used.

The CDS score was found to correlate with physician ratings of disease severity, and it was predictive of hospital admissions and mortality in the following year. There was a modest association with self-reported health status and disability, and the score was not associated with depression or anxiety. Finally, the CDS showed high year-to-year stability in a population sample. For studies with suitable record systems, techniques such as the CDS and related measurements such as the Illness Scale (Mossey & Roos, 1987), which uses insurance claims data, can be used effectively at minimal cost.

Duke Severity of Illness Checklist

The Duke Severity of Illness Checklist (DUSOI; Parkerson *et al*, 1993) was developed as a generic measure of severity of illness and comorbidity. It is available in paper and computerised (Parkerson *et al*, 1994) versions and can be completed after a face-to-face medical encounter or from a review of medical records. Training is accomplished with a four-page user's manual. The Checklist requires a listing of all diagnoses and health problems which are active at the time of the interview or in the previous week. For each diagnosis or health problem, four 'severity parameters' are listed: symptom level, complications, prognosis without treatment, and treatability (i.e. need for treatment and expected response to treatment). Each parameter is then rated on a five-point scale for each diagnosis or health problem. Three main scores can be obtained from the resulting data: the DUSOI diagnosis severity of illness score, which ranges from 1 to 100; the DUSOI overall severity of illness score, which is a weighted sum of all diagnosis severities for a given patient; and the DUSOI comorbidity severity of illness, which is computed in the same way as the overall score but without the index diagnosis score. Less than 2 minutes is required to complete the computerised version of the checklist (Parkerson *et al*, 1994.)

One of the main advantages of the DUSOI is its clinical relevance: scores are computed from a clinician's impression, whether the clinician completes the checklist directly or whether the chart is audited. Interrater reliability has been moderate to excellent (Parkerson *et al*, 1994; Shiels *et al*, 1997), despite the reliance of the scale on individual judgements and uncertainties in the treatability and prognosis of many conditions. It has been suggested that reliability of the DUSOI may be improved by a more detailed training manual and more explicit criteria for rating severity within parameters (Shiels *et al*, 1997).

Functioning and disability

Sheehan Disability Scale

The Sheehan Disability Scale (SDS) is designed to assess patients' impairment at work, in social life and at home, on a ten-point visual analog scale (Leon *et al*, 1992, 1997; Sheehan *et al*, 1996). It can be used as a self-report, administered by a clinician, or completed by both. The SDS has high internal consistency (0.89), is sensitive to change following treatment, and in clinical trials it discriminates between active drug and placebo (Leon *et al*, 1992; Sheehan *et al*, 1996). Among patients with alcohol dependence, drug dependence, generalised anxiety disorder, major depressive disorder, obsessive–compulsive disorder and panic disorder, sensitivity of 0.83 and specificity of 0.69 have been found (Leon *et al*, 1997).

World Health Organization Disability Assessment Schedule 2.0

The World Health Organization Disability Assessment Schedule (WHODAS 2.0; World Health Organization, 2000) is a multidimensional questionnaire designed to measure patients' functioning and disability. It evaluates patients' difficulty in six domains of functioning: cognition, mobility, self-care, interpersonal interactions, life activities, and participation in society. This instrument is available in long (36 items) and short (12 items) versions, and in self-administered and interviewer-administered formats. The WHODAS 2.0 can be used for patients with all types of health conditions, and has been tested in clinical and general populations. The psychometric properties and clinical utility of the WHODAS 2.0 have been well documented (World Health Organization, 2000).

Global Assessment Scale

Probably the most widely used global functioning measures for mental disorders are the Global Assessment Scale (GAS; Endicott *et al*, 1976) and its modification, the Global Assessment of Functioning Scale (GAF). The GAS is itself based on an older instrument called the Health–Sickness Rating Scale (Luborsky, 1962), which was developed as a means for clinicians to judge mental health or illness along a single dimension on a 100-point scale. The GAS retains the 100-point continuum of mental illness to mental health, ranging from a score of 1 for the hypothetically sickest individual, to 100 for the hypothetically healthiest individual. The scale is subdivided into ten-point intervals, and each interval carries a description which includes representative symptoms and impairments in functioning. Diagnostic characterisations are avoided in the descriptions. The developers of the scale intended the two highest intervals (81–90 and 91–100) for 'those unusually fortunate individuals who not only are without significant psychopathology but also exhibit many positive traits often referred to as "positive mental health"' (Endicott *et al*, 1976). They wrote that most out-patients would score between 31 and 70, and most in-patients between 1 and 40. GAS ratings are based on the individual's lowest functioning level in the preceding week. In order to determine a specific rating within the chosen interval, the two adjacent intervals are examined to determine whether the individual is closer to one or the other. All sources of information can be considered in making the rating. The interrater reliability and validity of the GAS are satisfactory in a research context with proper training in the scale's use (Endicott *et al*, 1976).

Medical Outcomes Study Short Forms

Unlike the GAS, the Medical Outcomes Study Short Forms measure health profiles across a number of dimensions. Derived from the full-length MOS scale (245 items), two currently popular short forms contain 36 items (SF–36; Ware & Sherbourne, 1992) and 12 items (SF–12; Ware *et al*, 1996).

The SF–36 was designed to replace older 18- and 20-item short forms (Stewart *et al*, 1988), which had problems in comprehensiveness, content validity and floor effects (Ware & Sherbourne, 1992). The SF–36 measures eight health concepts: physical functioning (10 items), role limitations due to physical problems (4 items), bodily pain (2 items), general health perceptions (5 items), social functioning (2 items), general mental health (5 items), role limitations due to emotional problems (3 items) and vitality (4 items). An additional item, not used in any of the scales, assesses the respondent's perception of change in his or her health status in the past year. Most questions refer to the past 4 weeks, and response options vary from question to question, from yes/no responses to six-level Likert-type scales. The SF–36 can be self-administered, or administered by telephone or personal interview; different forms and instructions are used for each method of administration. The scale can be administered in 5–10 minutes (Ware & Sherbourne, 1992).

Data from the MOS were used to assess the psychometric properties of the SF–36 scales, which were embedded in the full 245-item MOS assessment. With few exceptions, the SF–36 items met acceptable levels for data completeness, scaling assumptions and scale internal consistency. Floor effects were reduced from the SF–20, but remained substantial for the two role disability scales. Ceiling effects were substantial for the role disability scales and the social functioning scale. The investigators emphasised that only the physical functioning scale met minimum standards of internal consistency on an individual patient level, with confidence intervals being unacceptably large for the other scales, so further research is needed before the SF–36 can be used for individual patient assessment and evaluation of individual treatment effects (McHorney *et al*, 1994).

Further research has identified two summary measures in the SF–36: the Physical Component Summary (PCS), comprising the physical functioning, role limitations (physical, bodily pain, and general health perceptions scales), and the Mental Component Summary (MCS), comprising the social functioning, general mental health, role limitations (emotional, and vitality scales) (Ware *et al*, 1996). Research on the SF–36 has shown that physical and mental health factors accounted for 80–85% of the reliable variance in the eight scales. Further, the PCS and the MCS were able to detect hypothesised differences in nearly all tests based on physical and mental criteria, respectively (Ware *et al*, 1996).

The SF–12 was developed in response to the need for even shorter measures than the SF–36 for use in large surveys and monitoring efforts (Ware *et al*, 1996). Items were chosen by applying separate forward step-regression analyses to the SF–36 PCS and MCS summary measures. Ten items were found to reproduce more than 90% of the variance in the PCS and MCS, and two additional items were added to represent all eight SF–36 scales. The SF–12 takes 2 minutes or less to self-administer. Reliability and validity coefficients were acceptable for the SF–12, although predictably was somewhat lower than for the SF–36 (Ware *et al*, 1996).

Conclusion

The Global Burden of Disease project estimated that unipolar major depression was the fourth-leading cause of disability-adjusted life years (DALYs) in 1990 (Murray & Lopez, 1996a) and is projected to be the second-leading cause of DALYs by the year 2020 (Murray & Lopez, 1996b). Although the scientific basis for primary prevention programmes is increasing, the early identification and treatment of depression remain the most effective method of reducing the burden of illness. The primary care sector has played an important treatment role in the past and will continue to do so in the future, for several reasons. From the patient's perspective, the stigma of mental illness or the costs and inconvenience of obtaining specialty mental health services may make primary care treatment more attractive. The uneven geographical distribution of specialty mental health services in the USA means that some patients have no access to such services, particularly in isolated and rural areas, and primary care services may be the only treatment option. Managed care organisations may also encourage the treatment of depression in primary care settings, particularly if the case is mild, in order to control costs.

Maximising the effectiveness of the treatment of depression in primary care is critical for the reasons mentioned above, and because of the problems in recognition and treatment adequacy that are known to exist when patients with the condition visit their primary care providers. In the past decade, increasing attention has been paid to the development of strategies that will improve the detection and treatment of depression in primary care settings. This has included a focus on the development of simple, brief symptom assessments that not only can be used in primary care settings, but also would have utility for specialty mental health practice. The use of scores from such instruments could facilitate communication between clinicians for depression evaluation and treatment, much as common tests such as haemoglobin H1C levels or blood pressure do for diabetes and hypertension care, respectively. The increasing emphasis being placed on measurement-based care in health policy underscores the need for such metrics for common mental disorders such as depression.

The developers of DSM–V have placed an emphasis on the potential uses of dimensional assessments of psychopathology in conjunction with the categorical diagnostic system currently in use. The measures of depression severity described in this chapter are examples of such assessments. The World Health Organization is also working, with assistance from the developers of DSM–V and others, to develop a diagnostic manual of mental disorders for use in primary care across the world. The goal is for this manual to be linked to the ICD–11 and DSM–V descriptions of mental disorders, thus allowing seamless communication between the general medical and specialty sectors. Another goal for DSM–V is to have at least a subset of the recommended severity assessments usable in primary care. The accumulated research with the PHQ–9 and the ongoing development of the PROMIS measures by the NIH suggest that this goal is feasible for depressive disorders.

References

Andrews, G. & Peters, L. (1998) The psychometric properties of the Composite International Diagnostic Interview. *Social Psychiatry and Psychiatric Epidemiology*, **33**, 80–88.

Bagby, R. M., Rector, N. A., Bindseil, K., *et al* (1998) Self-report ratings and informants' ratings of personalities of depressed outpatients. *American Journal of Psychiatry*, **155**, 437–438.

Bagby, R. M., Levitan, R. D., Kennedy, S. H., *et al* (1999) Selective alteration of personality in response to noradrenergic and serotonergic antidepressant medication in depressed sample: evidence of non-specificity. *Psychiatry Research*, **86**, 211–216.

Bailey, J. & Coppen, A. (1976) A comparison between the Hamilton Rating Scale and the Beck Inventory in the measurement of depression. *British Journal of Psychiatry*, **128**, 486–489.

Beck, A. T. & Steer, R. A. (1984) Internal consistencies of the original and revised Beck Depression Inventory. *Journal of Clinical Psychology*, **40**, 1365–1367.

Beck, A. T., Ward, C. H., Mendelson, M., *et al* (1961) An inventory for measuring depression. *Archives of General Psychiatry*, **4**, 561–571.

Beck, A. T., Rush, A. J., Shaw, B. F., *et al* (1979) *Cognitive Therapy of Depression*. Guilford Press.

Cella, D., Yount, S., Rothrock, N., *et al* (2007) The Patient Reported Outcomes Measurement Information System (PROMIS): progress of an NIH Roadmap Cooperative Group during its first two years. *Medical Care*, **45**, S3–S11.

Cicchetti, D. V. & Prusoff, B. A. (1983) Reliability of depression and associated clinical symptoms. *Archives of General Psychiatry*, **40**, 987–990.

Conwell, Y., Forbes, N. T., Cox, C., *et al* (1993) Validation of a measure of physical illness burden at autopsy: the Cumulative Illness Rating Scale. *Journal of American Geriatric Society*, **41**, 38–41.

Costa, P. T. & McCrae, R. R. (1988) Personality in adulthood: a six-year longitudinal study of self-reports and spouse ratings on the NEO Personality Inventory. *Journal of Personality and Social Psychology*, **54**, 853–863.

Costa, P. T. & McCrae, R. R. (1992) *Revised NEO Personality Inventory (NEO–PI–R) and NEO Five-Factor Inventory (NEO–FFI) Professional Manual*. Psychological Assessment Resources.

Coulehan, J. L., Schulberg, H. C., Block, M. R., *et al* (1997) Treating depressed primary care patients improves their physical, mental, and social functioning. *Archives of Internal Medicine*, **157**, 1113–1120.

Cox, B. J., Swinson, R. P., Kuch, K., *et al* (1993) Self-report differentiation of anxiety and depression in an anxiety disorders sample. *Psychological Assessment*, **5**, 484–486.

Derogatis, L. R. (1983) *SCL–90–R Administration, Scoring, and Procedures Manual – II*. Clinical Psychometric Research.

Derogatis, L. R. & Cleary, P. A. (1977) Factorial invariance across gender for the primary symptom dimensions of the SCL–90. *British Journal of Social and Clinical Psychology*, **16**, 347–356.

Derogatis, L. R., Lipman, R. S., Rickels, K., *et al* (1974) The Hopkins Symptom Checklist (HSCL): a self-report symptom inventory. *Behavioral Science*, **19**, 1–15.

Derogatis, L. R., Rickels, K. & Rock, A. F. (1976) The SCL–90 and the MMPI: a step in the validation of a new self-report scale. *British Journal of Psychiatry*, **128**, 280–289.

Dietrich, A. J., Oxman, T. E., Williams, J. W., *et al* (2004) Re-engineering systems for the treatment of depression in primary care: cluster randomised controlled trial. *BMJ*, **329**, 602.

Digman, J. M. (1990) Personality structure: emergence of the five-factor model. *Annual Review of Psychology*, **41**, 417–440.

Duffy, F. F., Chung, H., Trivedi, M., *et al* (2008) Systematic use of patient-rated depression severity monitoring: is it helpful and feasible in clinical psychiatry? *Psychiatric Services*, **59**, 1148–1154.

Edwards, B. C., Lambert, M. J., Moran, P. W., *et al* (1984) A meta-analytic comparison of the Beck Depression Inventory and the Hamilton Rating Scale for Depression as measures of treatment outcome. *British Journal of Clinical Psychology*, **23**, 93–99.

Endicott, J., Spitzer, R. L., Fleiss, J. L., *et al* (1976) The Global Assessment Scale: a procedure for measuring overall severity of psychiatric disturbance. *Archives of General Psychiatry*, **33**, 766–771.

Fava, M., Rush, A. J., Trivedi, M. H., *et al* (2003) Background and rationale for the sequenced treatment alternatives to relieve depression (STAR*D) study. *Psychiatric Clinics of North America*, **26**, 457–494.

Gilbody, S., Bower, P., Fletcher, J., *et al* (2006) Collaborative care for depression: a cumulative meta-analysis and review of longer-term outcomes. *Archives of Internal Medicine*, **166**, 2314–2321.

Greenberg, P. E., Kessler, R. C., Birnbaum, H. G., *et al* (2003) The economic burden of depression in the United States: how did it change between 1990 and 2000? *Journal of Clinical Psychiatry*, **64**, 1465–1475.

Guy, W. (ed.) (1976) *ECDEU Assessment Manual for Psychopharmacology*. DHHS pub. No. ADM 76–336. US Department of Health, Education, and Welfare.

Hamilton, M. (1960) A rating scale for depression. *Journal of Neurology, Neurosurgery, and Psychiatry*, **12**, 56–62.

Hamilton, M. (1967) Development of a rating scale for primary depressive illness. *British Journal of Social and Clinical Psychology*, **6**, 278–296.

Hays, R. D., Wells, K. B., Sherbourne, C. D., *et al* (1995) Functioning and well-being outcomes of patients with depression compared with chronic general medical illnesses. *Archives of General Psychiatry*, **52**, 11–19.

Jackson, J. L., Passamonti, M. & Kroenke, K. (2007) Outcome and impact of mental disorders in primary care at 5 years. *Psychosomatic Medicine*, **69**, 270–276.

Katon, W. (1996) The impact of major depression on chronic medical illness. *General Hospital Psychiatry*, **18**, 215–219.

Katon, W., Von Korff, M., Lin, E., *et al* (1990) Distressed high utilizers of medical care: DSM–III–R diagnoses and treatment needs. *General Hospital Psychiatry*, **12**, 355–362.

Katon, W., Von Korff, M., Lin, E., *et al* (1992) Adequacy and duration of antidepressant treatment in primary care. *Medical Care*, **30**, 67–76.

Katon, W., Von Korff, M., Lin, E., *et al* (1995) Collaborative management to achieve treatment guidelines: impact on depression in primary care. *JAMA*, **273**, 1026–1031.

Katon, W., Robinson, P., Von Korff, M., *et al* (1996) A multifacted intervention to improve treatment of depression in primary care. *Archives of General Psychiatry*, **53**, 924–932.

Kessler, L. G., Burns, B. J., Shapiro, S., *et al* (1987) Psychiatric diagnoses of medical service users: evidence from the Epidemiologic Catchment Area program. *American Journal of Public Health*, **77**, 18–24.

Kessler, R. C., Zhao, S., Katz, S. J., *et al* (1999) Past-year use of outpatient services for psychiatric problems in the National Comorbidity Survey. *American Journal of Psychiatry*, **156**, 115–123.

Kessler, R. C., Berglund, P., Demler, O., *et al* (2003) The epidemiology of major depressive disorder: results from the National Comorbidity Survey Replication (NCS–R). *JAMA*, **289**, 3095–3105.

Kroenke, K. & Spitzer, R. L. (2002) The PHQ–9: a new depression and diagnostic severity measure. *Psychiatric Annals*, **32**, 509–521.

Kroenke, K., Spitzer, R. L. & Williams, J. B. (2001) The PHQ–9: validity of a brief depression severity measure. *Journal of General Internal Medicine*, **16**, 606–613.

Lambert, M. J., Hatch, D. R., Kingston, M. D., *et al* (1986) Zung, Beck, and Hamilton rating scales as measures of treatment outcome: a meta-analytic comparison. *Journal of Consulting and Clinical Psychology*, **54**, 54–59.

Lefevre, F., Reifler, D., Lee, P., *et al* (1999) Screening for undetected mental disorders in high utilizers of primary care services. *Journal of General Internal Medicine*, **14**, 425–431.

Leon, A. C., Shear, M. K., Portera, L., *et al* (1992) Assessing impairment in patients with panic disorder: the Sheehan Disability Scale. *Social Psychiatry and Psychiatric Epidemiology*, **27**, 78–82.

Leon, A. C., Olfson, M., Porter, L., *et al* (1997) Assessing psychiatric impairment in primary care with the Sheehan Disability Scale. *International Journal of Psychiatry in Medicine*, **27**, 93–105.

Lin, E. H., Von Korff, M., Katon, W., *et al* (1995) The role of the primary care physician in patients' adherence to antidepressant therapy. *Medical Care*, **33**, 67–74.

Lin, E. H. B., Katon, W. J., Simon, G. E., *et al* (1997) Achieving guidelines for the treatment of depression in primary care: is physician education enough? *Medical Care*, **35**, 831–842.

Löwe, B., Unutzer, J., Callahan, C. M., *et al* (2004a) Monitoring depression treatment outcomes with the PHQ–9. *Medical Care*, **42**, 1194–1201.

Löwe, B., Grafe, K., Zipfel, S., *et al* (2004b) Diagnosing ICD–10 depressive episodes: superior criterion validity of the PHQ. *Psychotherapy and Psychosomatics*, **73**, 386–390.

Löwe, B., Kroenke, K., Herzog, W., *et al* (2004c) Measuring depression outcomes with a brief self-report instrument: sensitivity to change of the PHQ–9. *Journal of Affective Disorders*, **81**, 61–66.

Löwe, B., Spitzer, R. L., Grafe, K., *et al* (2004d) Comparative validity of three screening questionnaires for DSM–IV depressive disorders and physicians' diagnoses. *Journal of Affective Disorders*, **78**, 131–140.

Löwe, B., Schenkel, I., Carney-Doebbeling, C., *et al* (2006) Responsiveness of the PHQ–9 to psychopharmacological depression treatment. *Psychosomatics,* **47**, 62–67.

Luborsky, L. (1962) Clinicians' judgements of mental health. *Archives of General Psychiatry*, **31**, 407–417.

McHorney, C. A., Ware, J. E., Lu, J. F. R., *et al* (1994) The MOS 36-item short form health survey (SF–36): III. Tests of data quality, scaling assumptions, and reliability across diverse patient groups. *Medical Care*, **32**, 40–66.

Miller, A. L., Crimson, M. L., Rush, A. J., *et al* (2004) The Texas medication algorithm project: clinical results for schizophrenia. *Schizophrenia Bulletin*, **30**, 627–647.

Moran, P. W. & Lambert, M. J. (1983) A review of current assessment tools for monitoring changes in depression. In *The Measurement of Psychotherapy Outcome in Research and Evaluation* (eds M. J. Lambert, E. R. Christensen & S. S. DeJulio), pp. 263–303. Wiley.

Morgan, C. D., Wiederman, M. W. & Magnus, R. D. (1998) Discriminant validity of the SCL–90 dimensions of anxiety and depression. *Assessment*, **5**, 197–201.

Mossey, J. M. & Roos, L. L. (1987) Using insurance claims data to measure health status: the Illness Scale. *Journal of Chronic Diseases*, **40** (suppl. 1), 41S–50S.

Murray, C. J. L. & Lopez, A. D. (1996a) The global burden of disease in 1990: final results and their sensitivity to alternative epidemiological perspectives, discount rates, age-weights and disability weights. In *The Global Burden of Disease: A Comprehensive Assessment of Mortality and Disability from Diseases, Injuries, and Risk Factors in 1990 and Projected to 2020* (eds C. J. L. Murray & A. D. Lopez), pp. 247–293. Harvard School of Public Health.

Murray, C. J. L. & Lopez, A. D. (1996b) Alternative visions of the future: projecting mortality and disability, 1990–2020. In *The Global Burden of Disease: A Comprehensive Assessment of Mortality and Disability from Diseases, Injuries, and Risk Factors in 1990 and Projected to 2020* (eds C. J. L. Murray & A. D. Lopez), pp. 325–395. Harvard School of Public Health.

Narrow, W. E., Regier, D. A., Rae, D. S., *et al* (1993) Use of services by persons with mental and addictive disorders: findings from the NIMH ECA Program. *Archives of General Psychiatry*, **50**, 95–107.

Narrow, W. E., Rae, D. S., Robins, L. N., *et al* (2002) Revised prevalence estimates of mental disorders in the United States: using a clinical significance criterion to reconcile 2 surveys' estimates. *Archives of General Psychiatry*, **59**, 115–123.

Nease, D. E., Nutting, P. A., Dickinson, W. P., *et al* (2008) Inducing sustainable improvement in depression care in primary care practices. *Joint Commission Journal on Quality and Patient Safety*, **34**, 247–255.

Nordgren, J. C. (1995) Instruments for assessing depression in adults. In *Handbook of Depression* (ed. E. E. Beckham & W. R. Leber), pp. 591–599. Guilford Press.

Oxman, T. E., Dietrich, A. J., Williams, J. W., *et al* (2002) A three-component model for reengineering systems for the treatment of depression in primary care. *Psychosomatics*, **43**, 441–450.

Parkerson, G. R., Broadhead, W. E. & Chiu-kit, J. T. (1993) The Duke Severity of Illness Checklist (DUSOI) for measurement of severity and comorbidity. *Journal of Clinical Epidemiology*, **46**, 379–393.

Parkerson, G. R., Hammond, W. E. & Yarnall, K. S. H. (1994) Feasibility and potential clinical usefulness of a computerised severity of illness measure. *Archives of Family Medicine*, **3**, 968–973.

Pearson, S. D., Katznelick, D. J., Simon, G. E., *et al* (1999) Depression among high utilizers of medical care. *Journal of General Internal Medicine*, **14**, 461–468.

Potts, M. K., Daniels, M., Burnam, M. A., *et al* (1990) A structured interview version of the Hamilton Depression Rating Scale: evidence of reliability and versatility of administration. *Journal of Psychiatric Research*, **24**, 335–350.

Radloff, L. S. (1977) The CES–D Scale: a self-report depression scale for research in the general population. *Applied Psychological Measurement*, **3**, 385–401.

Radloff, L. S. & Locke, B. Z. (1986) The Community Mental Health Assessment Survey and the CES–D scale. In *Community Surveys of Psychiatric Disorders* (eds M. M. Weissman, J. D. Myers & C. E. Ross), pp. 177–189. Rutgers University Press.

Regier, D. A., Narrow, W. E., Manderscheid, R. W., *et al* (1993) The DeFacto U.S. Mental and Addictive Disorders Service System: ECA prospective one-year rates of disorders and services. *Archives of General Psychiatry*, **50**, 85–94.

Rehm, L. P. & O'Hara, M. W. (1985) Item characteristics of the Hamilton Rating Scale for Depression. *Journal of Psychiatric Research*, **19**, 31–41.

Richter, P., Werner, J., Bastine, R., *et al* (1997) Measuring treatment outcome by the Beck Depression Inventory. *Psychopathology*, **30**, 234–240.

Robins, L. N., Wing, J., Wittchen, H.-U., *et al* (1988) The Composite International Diagnostic Interview: an epidemiologic instrument suitable for use in conjunction with different diagnostic systems and in different cultures. *Archives of General Psychiatry*, **45**, 1069–1077.

Rost, K., Zhang, M., Fortney, J., *et al* (1998) Persistently poor outcomes of undetected major depression in primary care. *General Hospital Psychiatry*, **20**, 12–20.

Rush, A. J., Giles, D. E., Schlesser, M. A., *et al* (1986) The Inventory for Depressive Symptomatology (IDS): preliminary findings. *Psychiatry Research*, **18**, 65–87.

Rush, A. J., Gullion, C. M., Basco, M. R., *et al* (1996) The Inventory of Depressive Symptomatology (IDS): psychometric properties. *Psychological Medicine*, **26**, 477–486.

Rush, A. J., Crismon, M. L., Kashner, T. M., *et al* (2003a) Texas Medication Algorithm Project, phase 3 (TMAP-3): rationale and study design. *Journal of Clinical Psychiatry*, **64**, 357–369.

Rush, A. J., Trivedi, M. H., Ibrahim, H. M., *et al* (2003b) The 16-item Quick Inventory of Depressive Symptomatology (QIDS), Clinician Rating (QIDS–C), and Self-Report (QIDS–SR): a psychometric evaluation in patients with chronic major depression. *Biological Psychiatry*, **54**, 573–583.

Rush, A. J., Trivedi, M. H., Carmody, T. J., *et al* (2004*a*) One-year clinical outcomes of depressed public sector outpatients: a benchmark for subsequent studies. *Biological Psychiatry*, **56**, 46–53.

Rush, A. J., Fava, M., Wisniewski, S. R., *et al* (2004*b*) Sequenced Treatment Alternatives to Relieve Depression (STAR*D): rationale and design. *Controlled Clinical Trials*, **25**, 119–142.

Rush, A. J., Bernstein, I. H., Trivedi, M. H., *et al* (2006) An evaluation of the Quick Inventory of Depressive Symptomatology and the Hamilton Rating Scale for Depression: a STAR*D report. *Biological Psychiatry*, **59**, 493–501.

Salvi, F., Miller, M. D., Grilli, A., *et al* (2008) A manual of guidelines to score the modified Cumulative Illness Rating Scale and its validation in acute hospitalized elderly patients. *Journal of the American Geriatric Society*, **56**, 1926–1931.

Schulberg, H. C., Block, M. R., Madonia, M. J., *et al* (1996) Treating major depression in primary care practice: eight-month clinical outcomes. *Archives of General Psychiatry*, **53**, 913–919.

Schulberg, H. C., Katon, W., Simon, G. E., *et al* (1998) Treating major depression in primary care practice: an update of the Agency for Health Care Policy and Research practice guidelines. *Archives of General Psychiatry*, **55**, 1121–1127.

Sheehan, D. V., Harnett-Sheehan, K. & Raj, B. A. (1996) The measurement of disability. *International Clinical Psychopharmacology*, **11** (suppl. 3), 89–95.

Shiels, C., Eccles, M., Hutchinson, A., *et al* (1997) The inter-rater reliability of a generic measure of severity of illness. *Family Practice*, **14**, 466–471.

Simon, G. E. & Katzelnick, D. J. (1997) Depression, use of medical services and cost-offset effects. *Journal of Psychosomatic Research*, **42**, 333–344.

Simon, G. E. & Von Korff, M. (1995) Recognition, management, and outcomes of depression in primary care. *Archives of Family Medicine*, **4**, 99–105.

Simon, G. E., Von Korff, M., Wagner, E. H., *et al* (1993) Patterns of antidepressant use in community practice. *General Hospital Psychiatry*, **15**, 399–408.

Simon, G. E., Lin, E. H., Katon, W., *et al* (1995*a*) Outcomes of 'inadequate' antidepressant treatment. *Journal of General Internal Medicine*, **10**, 663–670.

Simon, G. E., Von Korff, M. & Barlow, W. (1995*b*) Health care costs of primary care patients with recognized depression. *Archives of General Psychiatry*, **52**, 850–856.

Spitzer, R. L., Williams, J. B. W., Kroneke, K., *et al* (1994) Utility of a new procedure for diagnosing mental disorders in primary care: the PRIME–MD 1000 Study. *JAMA*, **272**, 1749–1756.

Stewart, A. L., Hays, R. D. & Ware, J. E. (1988) The MOS short-form general health survey. Reliability and validity in a patient population. *Medical Care*, **26**, 724–735.

Suppes, T., Rush, A. J., Dennehy, E. B., *et al* (2003) Texas Medication Algorithm project, phase 3 (TMAP–3): clinical results for patients with a history of mania. *Journal of Clinical Psychiatry*, **64**, 370–382.

Trivedi, M. H., Rush, A. J., Crismon, M. L., *et al* (2004*a*) Clinical results for patients with major depressive disorder in the Texas Medication Algorithm Project. *Archives of General Psychiatry*, **61**, 669–680.

Trivedi, M. H., Rush, A. J., Ibrahim, H. M., *et al* (2004*b*) The Inventory of Depressive Symptomatology, Clinician Rating (IDS–C) and the Quick Inventory of Depressive Symptomatology, Clinician Rating (QIDS–C) and Self Report (QIDS–SR) in public sector patients with mood disorders: a psychometric evaluation. *Psychological Medicine*, **34**, 73–82.

Trivedi, M. H., Rush, A. J., Wisniewski, S. R., *et al* (2006) Evaluation of outcomes with citalopram for depression using measurement-based care in STAR*D: implication for clinical practice. *American Journal of Psychiatry*, **163**, 28–40.

Unützer, J., Patrick, D. L., Simon, G., *et al* (1997) Depressive symptoms and the cost of health services in HMO patients aged 65 years and older. *JAMA*, **277**, 1618–1623.

Unützer, L., Katon, W., Williams, J. W., *et al* (2001) Improving primary care for depression in late life: the design of a multicenter randomized trial. *Medical Care*, **39**, 785–799.

Unützer, L., Katon, W., Callahan, C. M., *et al* (2002) Collaborative care management of late-life depression in the primary care setting: a randomized controlled trial. *JAMA*, **288**, 2836–2845.

van der Feltz-Cornelis, C. M., Lyons, J. S., Huyse, F. J., *et al* (1997) Health services research on mental health in primary care. *International Journal of Psychiatry in Medicine*, **27**, 1–21.

Von Korff, M., Wagner, E. H. & Saunders, K. (1992). A chronic disease score from automated pharmacy data. *Journal of Clinical Epidemiology*, **45**, 197–203.

Ware, J. E. & Sherbourne, C. D. (1992) The MOS 36-item short form health survey (SF–36): I. Conceptual framework and item selection. *Medical Care*, **30**, 473–483.

Ware, J. E., Kosinski, M. & Keller, S. D. (1996) A 12-item short-form health survey: construction of scales and preliminary tests of reliability and validity. *Medical Care*, **34**, 220–233.

Wells, K. B., Hays, R. D., Burnam, M. A., *et al* (1989) Detection of depressive disorder for patients receiving prepaid or fee-for-service care. *JAMA*, **262**, 3298–3302.

Wells, K. B., Sherbourne, C. D., Schoenbaum, M., *et al* (1999) *One-year Impact of Disseminating Quality Improvement for Depression to Managed, Primary Care Practices: Results from a Randomized, Controlled Trial.* Working paper no. P-143. RAND.

Williams, J. B. W. (1988) A structured interview guide for the Hamilton Depression Rating Scale. *Archives of General Psychiatry*, **45**, 742–747.

Williams, J. W., Rost, K., Dietrich, A. J., *et al* (1999) Primary care physicians' approach to depressive disorders: effects of physician specialty and practice structure. *Archives of Family Medicine*, **8**, 58–67.

Wisniewski, S. R., Rush, A. J., Balasubramani, G. K., *et al* (2006) Self-rated global measure of the frequency, intensity, and burden of side-effects. *Journal of Psychiatric Practice*, **12**, 71–79.

World Health Organization (1997) *Composite International Diagnostic Interview, version 2.1.* WHO.

World Health Organization (2000) WHO *Disability Assessment Schedule II (WHODAS II).* WHO.

Zanarini, M. C., Skodol, A. E., Bender, D., *et al* (2000) The Collaborative Longitudinal Personality Disorders Study: reliability of axis I and II diagnoses. *Journal of Personality Disorders*, **14**, 291–299.

Zitman, F. G., Mennen, M. F. G., Griez, E., *et al* (1990) The different version of the Hamilton Depression Rating Scale. *Psychopharmacology Series*, **9**, 28–34.

Index

Compiled by Linda English

Quality of Life Questionnaire in
    Schizophrenia (S–QOL) 154
Quality of Life Scale (QLS) 150–152, 160
Quality of Life Self-Assessment Inventory
    (QLS–100) 148–149
quality-of-life measures 8, 39–40
    and affective disorders 155–158
    and anxiety disorders 155–158
    and content validity 47
    counterintuitive results 160
    and depression 157, 245–246
    developed by World Health
        Organization 294–295
    interpretation 159–160
    research needs 160–162
    and schizophrenia 150–155, 159, 317
    selection 158–159
    and severe mental disorders 135–168,
        317
    and social disability 179
    state or trait 161
    subjective, and satisfaction with
        services 101
quantitative assessment 30
quasi-experiments 18
questionnaires, descriptive 30–31
Quick Inventory of Depressive
    Symptomatology (QIDS) 243,
    330–331

random effects model 23, 25
randomisation 17, 24
    allocation of patients to treatments 17
    cluster 16, 17, 21–22, 25, 26
    of experimental units 19
    randomised controlled trials 16, 17
rating scales 30, 31
    analogue 37–39
    based on 'wide' or 'restrictive'
        concept of mental disorder 32
    central tendency error 35, 38
    consistency 41–42
    cost–utility evaluation 51
    detection 33
    diagnostic 32
    dichotomous categorical scale 37
    external redundancy 50
    follow-up 33
    general and specific 32
    graphic 38
    interviewer-administered 33, 34, 35
    meta-analysis of 50
    multidimensional 34

multi-item 33
purpose 32–33
self-administered 33
sensitivity to change 50–51
state 32–33
symptom 32, 35–36
target content areas and population
    groups 32
trait 32
transferability 42
unidimensional 34
unitary (global) 33, 39
receiver operating characteristics (ROC)
    analysis 48, 49, 50
recovery 6
    clinical 63, 64, 67
    collaborative recovery model (CRM)
        and AIMhi study 69–71
    definitions 64, 66–67
    in depression 238, 240
    -focused mental health services 67–68
    FOCUS study 74–75
    NODPAM study 72–74
    personal 63, 65–66, 67, 69
    use of outcomes to support recovery
        63–79
Re-engineering Systems for Treatment of
    Depression in Primary Care
    (RESPECT) 325
REHAB scale 91
Rejection Experiences Scale (RES) 209
reliability 5, 23–24
    coefficients for measuring 43–44
    in context of GT 44–45
    and cultures 53
    external 42–45
    inter-informant 43
    internal 41–42
    inter-observer 43
    inter-rater 23, 33
    intra-observer 43
    and validity 45–46
Role Activity Performance Scale (RAPS)
    174

Satisfaction with Life Domains Scale
    (SLDS) 137–140
satisfaction with services 6, 8, 99–115
    and adherence behaviour 102
    and care-seeking behaviour 102
    and clinical routine 103–104
    methodological issues in measurement
        104–105